D....
Masquerading
As Foods

DELICIOUSLY Killing American-AFRIKANS and All Peoples

Volume 1 of 3

SUZAR

Dr. S. Epps, N.D., D.M.

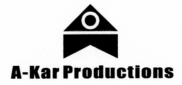

A-Kar Productions

Published by
A-Kar Productions
P.O. Box 386
Oak View, CA 93022
Website: www.a-kar.com

Also by Suzar:

• *Unfood By The UnPeople*
(vol. 2 of Drugs Masquerading as Foods) © 1999

• *Don't Worry, Be Healthy!*
(vol. 3 of Drugs Masquerading as Foods) © 1999

• *Blacked Out Through Whitewash* (vol.1) © 1999

• *The numerous book releases from the 7-volume series of B.O.T.W.*

Available Soon:
• *Creation's Great Blak Mother & the Blak Woman*
(vol. 2 of Blacked Out Through Whitewash) © 1999

• *Resurrecting Bab-El, The Book of Books of Books*
(vol. 3 of Blacked Out Through Whitewash) © 1999

Dedicated to the Loving
Great Blak Mother
Of Creation

May, '05
Lindsey,
    This Cook is being shared
with you so that you can expand
your knowledge.
    You are such an accomplished
young woman. I know there is
more to come. This family is
very proud of you. You're
quite impressive.
    Always stay prayerful,
focused and informed.
    Hugs & Kisses, and I
love you!
                    Aunt
                    Doris

My Gratitude to
Myra & Joseph Burch
Sonia Patton Williams
Jamaal Goree
Connie Kelly
Irasha Pearl
Tarik ibn Freeman
Willie Southall
Arvel & Bobbie Chappell
Linda & Walter Shrider
Doctah B
Clayton Silver

Contents

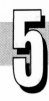

The Top Drugfood-Weapons Killing Us Slowly & Deliciously 71

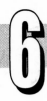

Supermarkets are disguised killer *Drugstores*

...and 99% of the "foods" in supermarkets and grocery stores are not foods but toxic *Drugs Masquerading As Foods*. Drugs *laced* with food. Healthfood stores are hardly better. And the American populace is deliciously deceived as they slowly kill themselves with each meal. If someone comes at you with a *dagger*, you know you're in danger and need to defend yourself, else get hurt or even killed. But if someone comes at you with a *donut*, the average person will take the donut and *eat* it, – and essentially get "cut up" inside as that deadly donut– which is 100% composed of *hard* drugfood– does its damage to the body in concert with all the other toxic killer drugfoods eaten by the same unsuspecting hungry victim. So if you are not eating TRUE *Health*-foods, then you are eating *Death*-foods by default! *Drugs Masquerading As Foods*. And you *are* a drugfood addict, whether or not you eat so-called "health foods." If you care about your precious health, there are actions you can take to defend your health from the constant *attacks* upon it. Attacks not only from Drugfood but from other *Disguised Weapons* softly assaulting us 24 hours a day. For yes, Drugfoods are also *disguised weapons of war* –and even *mind control*, –and the whole American populace is under attack ...in a "Quiet War" fought with "Silent Weapons." AFRIKANS are the most targeted in this Quiet War and consequently suffer the highest mortality rate than any other ethnic group in America.

This book and its other volumes (*Unfood By The UnPeople* and *Don't Worry, Be Healthy!*) show you how to defend, protect, and empower yourself, and survive –even achieve Fabulous Health. For such is possible in a *toxic* world if you know how and are willing to put forth the effort to achieve and maintain it. When Earth has finally been detoxed and healed, the task of maintaining our health will almost be as easy as breathing. Our disconnection from wholefoods is linked to our disconnection from our common mother, *Mother Nature*. In fact, our *Great Gap* from this *Divine Feminine Principle of Life* is resulting in accelerating Planetcide. It naturally follows that getting back in Harmony and Alignment with our Mother: *Nature* –is the real and true key to our real and true Health ...and survival. Are you ready? You are? OK, finish your hormoned, nitrated, dyed, irradiated, pesticide-enriched, antibiotic-ladden hamburger, –or your carcinogenic-mushroomed, calcium-leaching, digestion-proof, isolated-soy-protein veggie burger and let's begin.

Suzar

And You Thought You Were Eating Food

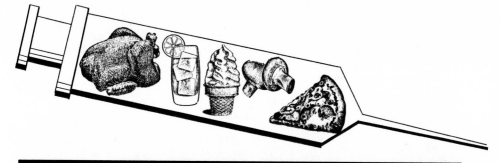

Yes <u>YOU</u> too, are an addict! —*a Drugfood Addict!*

You, yes *YOU*, dear American-*AFRIKAN* people and any people who eat in
America, including "healthfood" eaters, are ALL *drug addicts* unknowingly,
–slowly and pleasurably killing ourselves with the *meals of drugs* we eat daily,
deceived into thinking these drugs are *food*. They are not food; they are *Drugs
Masquerading As Foods.* If the disastrous effects of such drugfoods were to
occur shortly after we ate them, we would see them for what they are –killer
drugs. Then it might be easy to cut them out of our diet. But since they kill us
slowly, we fail to suspect the true nature of these insidious culprits (*kill*-prits).
As a result, we suffer their cumulative damaging effects over time and reap a
harvest of pain, low energy, fatigue, depression, mental problems, sickness,
dis-ease and ultimately, death. Ignorance may be bliss, but only until the effects
of this debilitating *die*-t catch up with us.

So you think you're *not* a drugfood addict?

What specific foods do you crave ("love") the most? Can you go one day
without it? OK, now can you go one week without eating it? three months? The
drugfoods that are the *most poisonous* to your body are the very ones you *crave
the most!* And *consume* the most. Americans are addicted to their drugfoods
and find the thought of change overwhelming. Further, the American diet is
permeated with outright chemical drugs. So even if you don't *take drugs*, if you
are eating any commercial, supermarket food, including most so-called "health
food," you are unknowingly eating –and are addicted to– many hidden drugs.
Any wonder we feel hopelessly attached, addicted to our drugfood? This is true
of the majority of coffee / chocolate /sugar /alcohol /cigarette "junkies."
Addiction to drugfood (like addiction to outright drugs) can be so great that
people are quite literally willing to die for them, and they often do just that! In
spite of this dilemma, changing our habits is as simple as this: you *can* change –
if you *want* to. Working as a team, family members can assist each other in the
disciplinary actions required for changing from drugfood to wholefood. Yes,
temptations will sometimes overcome discipline. Just brush those drug-crumbs
from your grinning face and get back on track. Happy is the person who knows
the art of starting again after each defeat. The rewards from eating right are
worth the endeavor.

In reality, Drugfoods are disguised *weapons* killing over 240,000 Americans every two months!

The diet of our colonizers is killing us and killing them also. This diet is so deadly, it kills at least 240,000* Americans prematurely every two months through degenerative diseases! **This amounts to a major war upon Americans. This war is happening right now in America and has been going on for many years. In fact, Americans are being killed at the rate of 3 to 4 atomic bombs every two months from just heart disease and cancer alone.** (The A-bomb dropped on Hiroshima killed 70,000 to 118,000 People of Color [Japanese]) The primary war zones include the supermarkets, grocery stores, drugstores, hospitals, and even healthstores to an extent. The battlefields are our stomachs, intestines, livers, kidneys and ultimately our whole bodies. In *The Golden Seven Plus One*, Dr. Samuel West wrote:

"One of the main purposes of this government document [*The Dietary Goals for the United States*] is to alert the people in the United States that there are interests, of **conspiring men** with evil designs in their hearts that are helping to create the present problems that are **destroying two hundred and forty thousand men, women, and children every two months.** It is calling for a national health education program to make people aware that medical practice cannot help because of the foods we are being encouraged to eat which act on the body as a deadly poison. **These foods are destroying more people than any war we have ever been engaged in.**"[1] "The wickedness of these men is now being revealed unto us *in a manner* that is truly *shaking the earth*. The 'foods' they are now promoting, which are actually physically and mentally addicting drugs, are playing a major role in destroying us in the form of heart disease, cancer, obesity, stroke, high blood pressure, hypoglycemia, diabetes, arthritis and the other killer and crippling diseases. Just think about it: from heart disease and cancer alone, there are over two hundred and forty thousand men, women, and children being slain every two months in the United States alone. This does not count the millions of others who are suffering from other killer and crippling diseases. We have never had such destruction of human life since the beginning of this nation."[2]

* The count is now much higher than this figure, released in 1977.   1) West, GS, 108.   2) Ibid., 97.

Degenerative diseases cause more than 2/3 of U.S. deaths!

The 1988 Surgeon General's Report on Nutrition and Health admitted that degenerative diseases *"now account for more than two-thirds of all deaths in the United States."* **The top five killers are heart disease, cancer, diabetes, lung disease, and liver disease.** These are all degenerative diseases with long incubation periods. For decades they grow silently inside you, usually emerging in a time of stress, fullblown and allegedly incurable (no such thing, really). All of these killer *dis-eases* are primarily the results of a killer drugfood diet.

America, in fact, is the sickest nation in the world

The facts and statistics bust the myth of health in America: [1]
- The U.S. Public Health Service recognizes a mere 3.5 million of us as healthy. That's only 1.5% of the population.
- **About *one billion* visits are made to physicians each year.**
- **250,000 people in the U.S. suffer from incurable disease.**
- 54% of all Americans die of heart disease. In 1990, 43% of U.S. deaths were results of cardiovascular disease. 50 million Americans suffer from severe heart disease. Risk of death from heart attack for the average American man is 50%.
- 58 million Americans have high blood pressure.
- 49% of Americans suffer from at least one chronic disease or disability.
- One of every 5 children under age 17 already has some chronic disorder.
- Nearly 90% of America's children cannot pass a minimum physical fitness test.
- Arthritis and rheumatic disorders affect 77% of adults. 40 million have arthritis.
- Over 50% in this country suffer chronic digestive disorders.
- 40 million Americans suffer mental illness. Over 8 million children are retarded.
- 50 million have headaches. 20 million are migraine sufferers.
- 98.5% of Americans have bad teeth; 31 million have no teeth.
- 60% of Americans have defective vision; 27.9 million have visual impairments.
- 20 million have hearing impairments. 16 million Americans suffer ulcers.
- 70-80% are overweight; 80 million are obese. 80 million suffer allergies
- Nearly 7 million have urinary infections. 11.4 million have hemorrhoids.

Disease & Drugs are BIG business.
$ickness, not health, is a TRILLION dollar-a-year *industry.*

America's deadly drugdiet keeps most American-Afrikans and basically the whole American population in a state of chronic sub-health and diminished energy, making it easier for us to be exploited and manipulated by the "conspiring men" who appear to control everything and, in fact are responsible for the promotion and profusion of drugfoods *and drugs.* Their vast wealth is uncountable. Apparently, the main way they keep their bank accounts flooded is by keeping us sick and *buying drugs* (55 billion aspirin tablets are consumed yearly in the US, to say nothing of other drugs). They control the FDA (Food & Drug Administration) and AMA (American Medical Association), own the major drug, chemical, and oil corporations, industrial farming corporations and much more. $ickness, not health, is a mega *industry* in America and they intend to keep it that way! **America spends over a trillion dollars a year[2] for "health care" –which is "disease maintenance,"** really. Each year $136

1) Statistical Abstract of the United States 1992, by US Dept. of Commerce /Bureau of the Census. 2) Quillin, 8.

billion is spent for heart disease; $70 billion is spent for cancer. Nearly a fifth (18%) of the Gross National Product is used to treat illness when lost economic productivity and premature death are accounted for. **Most of our health problems come from the so-called food we eat.** Drugfood. Drugs laced with food. *Drugs Masquerading As Foods*....which contain large amounts of drug-chemical-additives, which are non-nutritive, toxic "trash" that 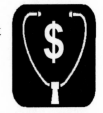 contaminate our cells. Over 100 million Americans suffer a chronic illness –caused from manmade toxins in their environment and especially in the (drug)food they eat. And no wonder, because nearly a billion pounds of toxic *white*man-made chemicals (poisons, drugs, "additives") are annually put in America's food. Over 25,000 new synthetic poisons are created and added each year. Very few are ever tested for toxicity. Yet the FDA and AMA suppress and even ban safe, harmless, natural substances (herbs, nutrients, vitamins, etc.) that are proven to heal so-called incurable dis-eases. **The FDA has approved hundreds of cancer-causing drugs & synthetic hormones** (that are still on the market, killing people), **while closing down healthfood stores (at gunpoint!) and holistic clinics, and forcing holistic professionals out of business.**

"FDA has become an extension of the drug industry."
Richard Burroughs, Ph.D.

"Doctors Kill More People Than Guns and Traffic Accidents Combined"

[By Don Harkins / The Idaho Observer - April, 1999 / 5-29-99 /
www.sightings.com/politics2/doctors.htm]

"Last year, commented Dr. Welch, the pharmaceutical industry did $182 billion in drug sales world wide. In contrast to that figure, it cost approximately $183 billion to treat **adverse reactions** from all of those drugs. ..According to JAMA [Journal of the American Medical Association], **doctors kill more people than auto accidents and guns**. With that in mind, one has to wonder why gun control is such a hot legislative issue when, perhaps, we should be more concerned about doctor control. ..The number of people that doctors kill per day from medical malpractice is roughly equal to the amount of people that would die if every day, three jumbo jets crashed and killed everybody on board, commented Dr. Welch who added, in defense of his own profession, just imagine what headlines would result if a chiropractor or a naturopath accidentally killed just one patient? .. Another JAMA statistic stated that 1/5 (20 percent) of all people who see an allopath will suffer an iatrogenic (doctor-induced) injury. ..Again, according to JAMA, 16 percent of all people who die in the hospital are determined by autopsy to have died of something other than their admission diagnosis. In other words, the doctor had no idea what was really wrong with the patient and, therefore, the patient may have died for want of appropriate care that would have been subsequent to an accurate diagnosis. ... Another trade publication, American Medical News, stated that **28 percent of people admitted to hospitals are there because they have suffered an adverse reaction to prescribed drugs.**"

America has no medical freedom

Although the medical profession did not begin to grow into the powerful monopoly it is today until around 1900, as far back as 1789, Dr. Benjamin Rush, a signer of the Declaration of Independence and physician to George Washington, urged that the first Amendment to the Constitution be expanded to protect us from such monopolies. The first Amendment states: *"Congress shall make no law prohibiting the free exercise of religion, or abridging the freedom of speech, or the press."* Apparently knowing the nature of his people and how they can be, even with themselves, Dr. Rush wanted to include these words, *"or abridging the rights of citizens to secure medical treatment from doctors of their own choice."* [1] Dr. Rush prophetically warned: *"Unless we put medical freedom into the Constitution, the time will come when medicine will organize into an undercover dictatorship...To restrict the art of healing to one class of men and deny equal privileges to others will constitute the Bastille of medical science. ...The Constitution of this republic should make special privilege for medical freedom as well as religious freedom."* [2] His prophecy is reality today, unfortunately.

This is why Americans are denied access to many natural methods proven so successful in ending some of the most agonizing dis-eases of today. This is why drug-pushing medical schools are "accredited" while holistic schools teaching natural (i.e., "alternative") medicine are not accredited. Americans, especially American-Afrikans, have become the victims of the Drug & Medical Monopoly. The money is in treating sick people with drugs, not in making them healthy with a wholesome diet. In the last two decades there has been a mounting concerted effort on the part of government regulatory agencies to punish and harass medical professionals who recommend or practice nutritional and herbal medicine, and other natural therapies for health and preventing illness. Healthfood stores and manufacturers of herbs and nutritional supplements have been the target of FDA seizures in an attempt to block the manufacture and sale of many natural substances (like primrose oil, laetrile, citrus seed extract, certain herbs) which have been proven to heal or prevent diseases. The FDA's suppression of natural medicine and nutritional supplements is a war for power with billions of dollars and America's health at stake.

"You may lose your right to important information about vitamins, minerals and herbs."

Recall that in the early 1990's, the FDA, AMA tried to make it so that you needed a prescription from a medical doctor just to buy vitamins and other common nutrients (so you would have to pay super high prices for them). Well they haven't stopped. They will keep on trying to get their way utterly. It's up to the American people to reverse this, if they can at all. The majority seem unmindful, unaware, and apparently don't care. Americans still have power if they ACT and continue to act/counteract. Because the Controllers never stop.

1) Preston, H, 56.   2) Preston, 56; Burton, AM, 17.

When the FDA reared up again only a few years later, one group that acted was *Citizens For Health.* Excerpts from their flyer (urging people to *act*) is very revealing and summarizes the Controllers' intent:

"Dear Friend, ...FDA has proposed new rules which will deny your access to essential information about your health choices. But if you act now...you can make a difference and protect those rights. ...FDA wants to define aging, pregnancy and menopause as diseases! ...What does that mean for you? Producers of dietary supplements will not be able to tell you how new scientific research has been linked to supplements that address these and other conditions... FDA could reclassify many natural health products as drugs. Your access to many vitamins, minerals and herbs could be greatly restricted based on how your "intend" to used those products...

- Government agencies have proposed barriers to many products and services that emphasize alternative options and preventive care...
- The legal climate is restrictive in many states where nonconventional practitioners have literally been run out of town.
- Many physicians are being prohibited from offering alternative medicines to their patients.
- Government intervention is preventing parents from using alternative health practices for their children.
- Alternative therapies are being used in child custody cases as a basis for an unfit parenting claim."

One medical doctor with a conscience, J. Hodge, wrote:

"The medical monopoly or medical trust, euphemistically called the American Medical Association, is not merely the meanest monopoly ever organized, but the most arrogant, dangerous and despotic organization which ever menaced a free people in this or any other age. Any and all other methods of healing the sick by means of safe, simple and natural remedies is sure to be assailed and denounced by the arrogant leaders of the AMA doctor's trust as 'fakes, frauds and humbugs'. Every practitioner of the healing art who does not ally himself with the medical trust is denounced as a 'dangerous quack' and imposter by the predatory trust doctors. Every sanitarian who attempts to restore the sick to a state of health by natural means without resort to the knife or vaccines, is at once pounced upon by these medical tyrants and fanatics, bitterly denounced, vilified and persecuted to the fullest extent." [1]

Another (holistic) doctor, R. Preston wrote:

"So thoroughly does the AMA...control health in the United States that it does not merely stifle medical doctors from taking a nutritional approach to health, but it also, through the Food and Drug Administration, the Post Office, the IRS and any one else they can find, destroys anyone who dares to speak out. ..It hounds and harasses health writers and lecturers. They are arrested and frequently convicted of such ridiculous charges... Undercover agents are used with tape recording devices to attempt to trick them into

1) Preston, H, 54-55.

saying something that will be convicting. The news media [which the Controllers own] loves to publish public interest articles about so-called health frauds, warning the public not to trust anyone who is not an AMA drug-pushing doctor." [1]

It's bad for Caucasians, worse for Afrikans.

The AMA and FDA (who work/conspire together, –being branches of the Controllers) want to keep all of us sick and dependent in order to ensure their copious, continuous cash flow at the expense of our health. **If the Controllers are doing this to their own kind, what do they care about People of Color? In fact, whites (the killer khemical korporations) still manufacture lethal, banned chemicals and sell them to "thirdworld" nations (code term for Blacks, People of Color).** This is disguised *genocide* which People of Color pay for with their money, their health and their lives. **If Blacks do not look out for their own health who will?** And while it is true that Albinos are also suffering and getting poisoned by the very same toxic food they abundantly manufacture and consume, the effect is worse for Afrikans. The toxic western diet is more harmful to Blacks than to Caucasians. As detailed by Carol Barnes in *"MELANIN, The Chemical Key to Black Greatness,"* many toxic additives bind chemically with our Melanin, producing even more adverse effects.

Why do we cling to killer drugfood (dietary slavery)?

One could argue that this colonized diet is yet another form of disguised slavery for Afrikans, for our ancestors in Afrika ate no such fraudulent food and nor could even conceive of it. But the truth is that almost all Americans, Afrikan or otherwise, immensely enjoy and willingly participate in and cling to this dietary slavery. Reasons for this include:

● **Fatal ignorance.** We are kept ignorant of the life-saving simple truth. We do not know how to live wholistically like our Afrikan ancestors and have not taken the time and effort to learn the basic principles of purifying /regenerating our body.

● **We are constantly encouraged** to eat these killer drugfoods. They are abundantly available, gloriously advertised everywhere, and considered "normal."

● *Addiction* **to these drugfoods** and resistance to change because we love this deadly diet. Catering to our appetites, we eat ourselves into the grave.

● *Addiction* **to a seriously unbalanced pathological, fear-based culture** that is killing us, everybody else, and the planet. Dick Gregory stated, *"The rat race has made us ignore our nutritional needs while we remain preoccupied with tailoring our lives to European standards."*[2]

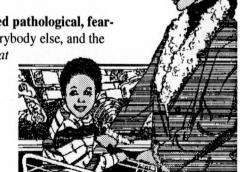

1) Preston, H, 55.   2) Afrika, AH, Intro.

SOUL-food is killer slave-food sending Afrikans to early graves.

"Soul-food" is a misnomer. Any way you prepare it, it is still perverted drugfood. The fondness (*addiction*) which many American-Afrikans have for "soul-food" is directly inherited from slavery –like their *lastnames* (= the names of their former slavemasters) and *child-whipping* (slavemasters or the "crackers" constantly "cracked" the whip upon Blacks, thus Blacks whip their children). Slaves were fed the most inferior, unwanted food, including the rejected parts of the pig. "Modern" soul-foods include ham, pig hoofs, pig intestines (*shit*-terlings), fried chicken, fried okra, fried rice, greasy overcooked green vegetables, shortening, grits, potato salad, etc.

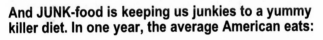

And JUNK-food is keeping us junkies to a yummy killer diet. In one year, the average American eats:

- 180 pounds of refined sugar
- 60 pounds of cakes & cookies
- 24 gallons of ice cream
- 756 donuts
- 22 pounds of candy
- 200 sticks of gum
- 365 cans of soda pop
- 90 pounds of fats & oils
- 50 pounds of salt
- 7 pounds of potato chips
- 7 pounds of corn chips, popcorn, pretzels
- 190 pounds of meat

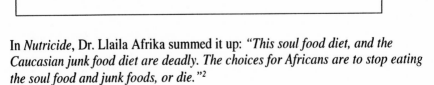

In *Nutricide*, Dr. Llaila Afrika summed it up: *"This soul food diet, and the Caucasian junk food diet are deadly. The choices for Africans are to stop eating the soul food and junk foods, or die."*[2]

1) Afrika, N, 240

Do Blacks *really* lead the nation in mortality rates from drugfood diseases?!

Blacks apparently have a higher risk for disease and premature death than any other group in America. Dr. Barbara Dixon stated it succinctly, *"If you are black and live in the United States, you are more likely to die sooner, and of a major disease, than members of any group ... African Americans lead in the mortality rates from the nation's six biggest killers: heart disease, cancer, stroke, liver disease, infant mortality, accidental death, and homicide."* [1]

- **Blacks have the highest rates** of hypertension and death from stroke /heart attack in the world.
- **Death from diabetes** and respiratory diseases are much higher among Blacks.
- **Lupus** is highest among Afrikan women.
- **Asthma** is 3 times higher in Blacks than Whites.
- **Uterine fibroid tumors** is an epidemic striking 75% of Black women vs. 33% of whites. [2]
- **Infertility is higher** among Afrikans, along with breast and lung cancer.
- **The rise in the reported death rate from prostate cancer** in Black men was nearly double that of whites, from 1980-1988. [3] (Blacks: 5.7%; whites: 2.5%)

These statistics might be exaggerated –hence a form of *psychological warfare* to make Blacks think they are dying off in droves (for whites do not always tell the truth about Blacks). But if they *are* the truth, then Blacks –along with the rest of the population– definitely need to change their eating habits, else keep slowly killing themselves...deliciously.

1) Dixon, xiii. 2) Afrika, N, 214. 3) Colburn, OSF, 180.

In addition to eating drugfood, People of Color around the world are growing and "refining" (debasing) their foods just as their *masters* taught them.
These nations are slowly destroying their people and their land, especially their precious topsoil, the foundation of life since it feeds the plants that sustains humanity.

Afrikans around the globe are infected, enamored with, and fatally addicted to toxic, anti-Nature white Caucasian culture. Ignorant of their true suppressed incredible history /herstory, and divorced from their wholistic roots by their colonizers, Afrikans seek to be like their colonizers. As long as People of Color around the world continue eating the drugfoods of their colonizers and "refining" their food like their colonizers, they will continue to suffer the chronic poor health and epidemic killer-diseases of the same. Knowledge of truth will heal this... hopefully.

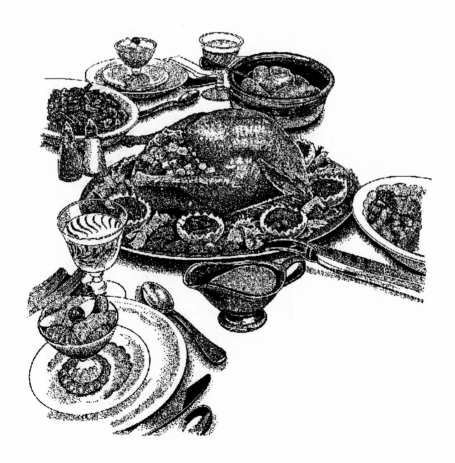

To eat wholistically is a return to our Afrikan roots

Albino scientists have proven, to the chagrin of many Albinos, that Afrikan people were the ancestors of all so-called races. (White people /*Caucasians* are *albinos*; white skin is a form of albinism.) Our Afrikan ancestors "ate right." They lived on a diet of whole foods while living close to Nature. Accordingly, they enjoyed superb lasting health, free of diabetes, cancer, heart disease and the other epidemic diseases of European culture. For us to do likewise is a return to our Afrikan roots, at least at the physical nutritional level. This is the way to lifelong health for any people. This will make and keep us sound. Sickly diseased people, Black or otherwise, do not have the energy to liberate themselves from oppressive systems which promote their exploitation, manipulation, sub-health, and eventual demise.

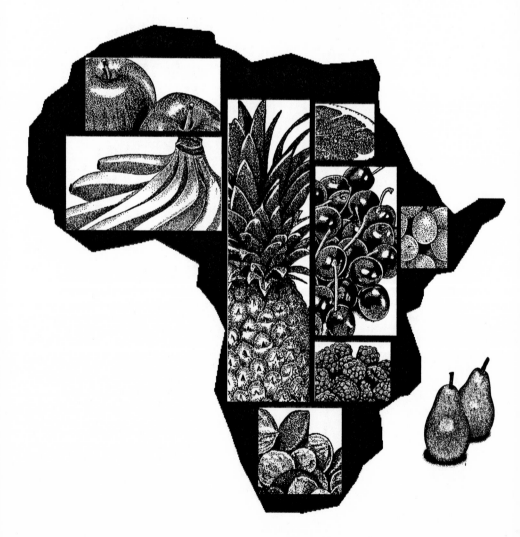

What is your most precious material possession?

Your car? house? wedding ring? computer? business? Let me tell you what it really is: your Physical Body! For without it, your other material possessions become useless to you. Your Physical Body is more precious than money, gold, real estate, stocks, and diamonds. But people often take better care of their other possessions while taking their Body for granted. This is a serious error, for our health and sense of well being is in direct relationship to how well we take care of our Body. As you get your Physical Body together, the rest of you will follow (emotional body, mental body, spiritual body) and also be easier to get together. In fact, don't be surprised if problems on other levels (depression, low self-esteem, lethargy, etc.) diminish or even disappear as you build your physical health. For all the parts of ourselves are inseparably connected. What we do to one affects the others. We realize just how *precious* our health is when we lose it.

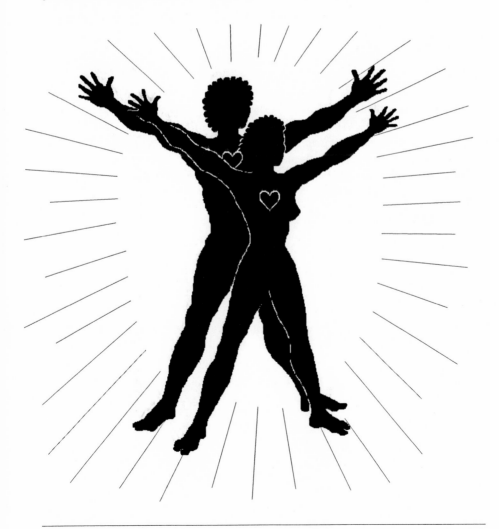

Incredible facts about your awesome precious Body

Heart & Blood

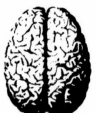

- The heart will beat, even if removed from the body (*automaticity*), as long as it has food. Only the heart-muscle can do this.
- Your heart beats over 100,000 times in a day.
- Your heart pumps 1,440 gallons of blood each day.
- Your heart pumps all your blood through your circulatory system and kidneys every 7 minutes. It pumps blood all the way around your body in just 30 seconds.
- Your blood travels over 170,000 miles in a day.
- There are 62,000 miles of blood vessels in your body –a distance twice around the world! In each eye alone are about 80 miles of blood vessels if stretched out from end to end.
- Your blood contains 25-30 trillion red blood cells. Their combined surface would cover about 200 square feet.

Brain & Nerves

- You are born with all the brain cells you will ever have.
- The brain is composed of about 15 billion (15,000,000,000) powerful brain cells that are about 90% water.
- Humans use only a fraction (less than 1/10th) of their brain capacity.
- Each half of the brain controls the opposite side of the body.
- Your nervous system sends messages as fast as 185 miles per hour.
- Your brain & nerves cannot function without (neuro) Melanin.

Lungs & Breathing

- There are over 300 million air sacs in the lungs.
- You breathe about 23,000 times in a day, inhaling about 438 cubic feet of air, weighing more than your food and drink combined (about 34 pounds).
- A pair of lungs have about a *billion* air cells. Their combined surface, if laid out 1 cell high, would cover 40-50 feet squared or the area of a tennis court.

Skin

- Over 600,000 skin cells would fit into an area the size of a postage stamp. The entire surface of the skin has about 7 million pores (perspiratory tubes), each about a 1/4 inch long. Laid out end to end, they'd extend 28 miles.
- The skin breathes like the lungs, absorbing oxygen and exhaling carbonic acid gas and watery vapor.
- The skin excretes organic matter, toxins, and saline matter in solution, like the kidneys. The average amount of fluid waste discharged through the skin every 24 hours is about 2 pounds.
- In one square inch of skin are 625 sweat glands, 90 oils glands, 19 million cells, 19 feet of blood vessels, 19,000 sensory cells, 65 hairs... and millions of microscopic animals.

Organs
- Your organs are duplicated in each cell of your body.
- Your liver is a chemical factory and detoxifier which filters toxins at a rate of a quart of blood per minute. It regenerates its own tissue, even if 80% of its cells are damaged.
- As much as 500 gallons of blood pass through the kidneys each day to be filtered of waste. Your kidneys filter the body's entire volume of blood 60 times each day.
- Your ears enable you to keep your balance, plus hear.

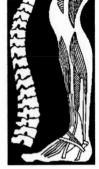

Bones & Muscles
- Bones are blood factories, besides being a flesh-hanger. Bone marrow can produce 5 billion red blood cells a day.
- The human skeleton has 206 bones; over 50 in the hands.
- The skull appears to be one bone but is really 29 separate bones fused together.
- 650 muscles cover the body. Over 200 are used when you walk. Smiling uses only 17 muscles but a frown uses 43.

Cells & Growth
- From the time of conception to adulthood, your body grows from one cell to one quadrillion cells (1,000,000,000,000,000).
- Blood is renewed at the rate of millions of cells per second.
- The stomach lining completely regenerates in a week, a healthy liver regenerates in 6 weeks, and the skin surface in a month.
- No cell in your body is over 2 years old! (except for your irreplaceable brain cells, and even with these – the *atoms* are continually being replaced).
- Every year over 96% of your body is completely replaced, even the structure of the DNA of your genes, reconstructed from the food you eat (or rather, the nutrients you *assimilate*).
- Each cell is a storehouse for some 5000 enzymes needed to implement chemical reactions.
- Each of your cells is responsible for supervising 1000 to 10,000 different chemical reactions.
- In the human body, some 6 trillion reactions occur every second and each of them is correlated with every other reaction.

See how superb your *Physical* Body is?
(To say nothing about your *other* bodies –emotional, mental, and spiritual bodies existing within your physical body at higher vibratory rates). Your Body is a self-cleaning, self-healing, irreplaceable mechanism which deserves Nature's best. All you have to do is feed it properly, give it sunshine, avoid poisoning it, and stay out of its way. What is your Body worth? ...Priceless! So treat it like it's priceless. In the **"body-parts market," organs literally cost $everal hundred thousand dollars!** Take good care of your priceless body and it will take good care of you!

Incredible facts about Black Melanin

As Dr. Richard King observed, the central role Melanin plays in the body has been *"suppressed to maintain the mythological inferiority of blacks as part and parcel of racism, and the defensive clinging to whiteness as some token of superiority."*

● **Your brain and nerves cannot function without Black Melanin!** Melanin is necessary in order for your eyes to see, your ears to hear, and your brain and nervous system to operate! Melanin in the brain increases from the lower primates and reaches its peak in the BLACK HUMAN.

● **Your body cannot function without Black Melanin.** It is found throughout your body,[1] in almost every organ, even in the blood (of Blacks). It is centrally involved in the control of almost all physio /psychological activities. It is essentially linked to the DNA of the genes, serving as the organizing principle for DNA. It is the major organizing molecule for living systems.

● **Melanin is necessary for humans to reproduce.** It is present at the inception of life: a Melanin sheath covers both the sperm and the egg.

● **Black Melanin is the super absorber and transmuter of all forms of energy.** It stores, transforms and conducts energy. Like the rods and cones of the eye, Melanin can absorb radiant sunlight energy and convert it to sound or electromagnetic energy and back again.[2]

● **Exposing your skin to sunlight** recharges the *battery* of your Melanin.

● **Melanin is an anti-oxidant which destroys free-radicals.** Free-radicals accelerate aging. Melanin slows aging and protects you from damaging effects of sunlight. The darker your skin (genetically) the less it ages. Thus whites often have wrinkled skin in their 30s while Blacks often have smooth, unwrinkled skin even in "old" age.

● **Melanin is found** *everywhere* ...in animals, insects, plants, fruits, soil, streams, lakes, oceans, clouds and even in meterorites and comets.

Melanin gives Black people advanced mental and physical ability.

Carol Barnes wrote: *"...your mental processes (brain power) are controlled by the same chemical that gives Black humans their superior physical (athletics, rhythmic dancing) abilities. This chemical...is Melanin!"* Melanin in the brain increases from the lower primates and reaches its peak in the Black Hue-man. The abundance of Melanin in Afrikans produces a superior organism mentally and physically. Black infants sit, stand, crawl, walk sooner, and demonstrate more advanced cognitive skills than whites because of their abundance of Melanin. Melanin is the neuro-chemical basis for what is called "SOUL" in Black people. Melanin refines the nervous system in such a way that messages from the brain reach other areas of the body more rapidly in Afrikans than in other. In the same way Blacks excel in athletics, Blacks can excel in all other areas as well (like they did in the past) once the road blocks are removed.

For more information

Melanin: The Chemical Key to Black Greatness	Carol Barnes
Handbook for a Melinated, Melatonin-Friendly Lifestyle	Dr. Patricia Newton
African Origin of Biological Psychiatry	Dr. Richard King

1) Cousens, SN, 31. 2) Ibid, 62, 94.

The Five Fatal Foremost Traits of Killer Drugfoods

The commercial foods of the "Western Diet" are legal disguised drugs...food-laced drugs

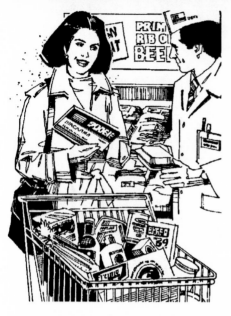

"Refining" is a deceptive term for the modern-western-Albino practice of debasing, bastardizing, fractionating, and perverting food into poison. In their health books, Albinos refer to their diet as "the western diet" ; "foods of commerce" and the "Standard American Diet" (S.A.D.). Yes indeed, the Western Diet is truly *SAD*. And *B.A.D. B*reaking *A*merica *D*own. And *M.A.D. M*ultiplying America's *D*iseases, and *M*aking *A*merica *D*ammed (clogged, constipated). As described by one westerner, the Western Diet consists of a *"high intake of refined carbohydrates, saturated fats, processed foods and cholesterol, and an extremely low intake of dietary fiber."*

Western commercial food is counterfeit killer drugfood.

Foodless food. **Food-laced drugs.** It is so processed, pesticided, preserved, chemicalized, cosmeticized, carbonated, bleached, dyed, hormoned, hydrogenated, hybrid, acidified, alkalized, buffered, irradiated, denatured, and devitalized that it is no longer food. **It has been turned into poisonous drugs. Drugfood affects our bodies just like drugs, and like drugs, it is highly addictive.** These drugfoods degenerate our bodies, corrupt our health, diminish our minds, dim our souls, and kill us slowly, insidiously. We eat these drugfoods every day, week after week, month after month, year after year, and ultimately pay for it with our most precious assets; our *health* and eventually our lives –over 240,000 lives every two months.

Overview Summary

The five, fatal foremost traits of America's killer drugfoods:
1. Perverted *before* birth.
2. Grown in poison.
3. Sprayed with death.
4. DEAD –especially from cooking and irradiation.
5. Processed and embalmed with chemical poisons.

Let's look more closely at these anti-life practices...

Drugfoods are killers because they are made with Produce that is...

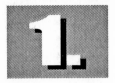

Perverted *before* birth.

They start off wrong and *wronged*. Deliberately perverted from Nature. Hybrid. Seedless. Sterile. Biologically castrated. Genetically altered from their natural pattern to grow in unnatural ways, unnaturally fast, unnaturally large, in unnatural debased soil. Nutrient-poor hybrid strains of grains and vegetables were developed just to grow better in soil degraded from using unnatural artificial NPK fertilizers.[1] **Even worse and unthinkable; some vegetables, genetically altered to contain their own insect-killing toxin, are now registered as a pesticide and not a vegetable at all!** (*Weed Technology*, June 1994) The unnatural specially bred strains of grain that produced the "green revolution" are very vulnerable to pests and adverse weather conditions. Much produce has even been genetically altered with DNA segments from animal genes to affect their natural character (vegetarians beware), thus your peach may think it's a pig. Biotech companies and food manufacturers use genetic meddling techniques to manipulate genes in produce to "enhance shelf life, size, taste, and resistance to pests." Examples are tomatoes with flounder genes, potatoes with silkworm genes, and corn with firefly genes.[2] What's this doing to the cells in your precious body when you eat such unnatural **"Frankenfood"**?

Dr. Afrika wrote:

"...tobacco plus tomato gene splicing has created frost-resistant tomato plants. The same cancer causing potential exist in the combination of 'tobacco tomato' plant as the toxic cooked oil from the tobacco plant. Some other freaks available to consumers are 'chicken/potato' animal which increases potato immunity. 'Insect (Wax Moth)/Potato' plant resists bruises in processing. Human/Pig (swine) cell animals."[3]

Another author wrote:

"The United Nations Food and Agriculture Organization (FAO) predicts that by the year 2000, 67% of the seeds used in underdeveloped countries will be 'improved.' This means they will be altered to yield more production, but will also be more vulnerable to pests. Therefore, they will require more pesticides. Weir and Shapiro indicate that pesticide companies are ...starting to corner the market on global seed businesses; the creation of seeds which require fertilizers and pesticides is the work of these parent companies."[4]

1) Colgan, NN, 15.   2) Pappas, 233.   3) Afrika, N, 191-192.   4) Rappoport, 52.

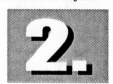

Grown in poison.

Commercial produce is grown in abused, bastardized, mineral-poor, depleted soil which is saturated with poisonous synthetic chemical fertilizers. The chemical poisons from the fertilizers are absorbed into the plants we eat.

> "American farmers now apply more than 20 million tons of chemical fertilizers to our farmlands every year, more than the combined weight of the entire human population of the country."[1]

Nutrition begins with the soil, the foundation of life on the planet. The health of humanity (and the plants and animals) depends upon the health of the soil. The Albino practice of commercial mass production plants thousands of acres in monoculture. This is not Nature's way. It causes serious deficiency, thus the farmers add more and more chemical fertilizers. These highly concentrated artificial fertilizers kill the bacterial life of the soil, which is as important for fruits and vegetables as bacillus acidophilus is for the human intestinal tract.

Chemical fertilizers also kill or chase away the earthworms in the soil. Earthworms are invaluable in helping the formation of humus that is the plant's nourishment. They also aerate the top-soil so that plant roots can spread out in search of nutrition. Artificial fertilizers poison the soil and upset the economy of nature, over-stimulating the plants and hurrying up their growth. The plants are big and oversize, but their aroma and flavor is lacking because they are deficient in minerals and vitamins. And though big, they have failed to mature. They fill the stomach but give little nourishment.

This is one reason why so many Americans are overweight –*overweight* yes, but undernourished, *mal*nourished (mal=bad). *Ever* eating because they are *ever* hungry because their bodies are *ever* craving the nourishment it can *never* get on a diet of toxic, foodless drugfoods. Over 79 million Americans are fat; far more than half are overweight.

1) Robbins, DNA, 357.

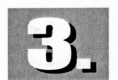

Sprayed with death.

Would you eat a salad that's been sprayed with Raid® insecticide? I wouldn't either. The commercial produce which looks so pretty all neatly stacked in the supermarkets is heavily sprayed with pesticides, herbicides and other "cides" (killers) which not only kill bugs and weeds, but kill you also –little by little with each mouthful. 35% of the food consumed in the U.S. has detectable pesticide residues. Over 400 pesticides are licensed for use on our foods.

- In 1951, the quantity of pesticides produced in the U.S. was sufficient to kill 15 billion human beings – about six times the world's population.[1]
- "Today 2.6 billion pounds of pesticides are spread on America every year. That's...10 pounds for every breathing one of us."[2]
- In his eye-opening book, *Diet for a New America*, John Robbins wrote: *"We [Albinos] produce pesticides today at a rate more than 13,000 times faster than we did only 35 years ago. Our environment and food chains are being inundated by a virtual avalanche of pesticides. What three decades ago took us six years to produce, we now produce every couple of hours."*[3]
- More than 50,000 pesticide products are used in America today.[4]
- All children born in the United States today have traces of pesticides in their tissues.[5] In fact, likely everyone on earth, including the animals, have toxic pesticide residues in their flesh!

This is the food we are eating today. Its cellulose fibers contain residues of the poison sprays, dusts, powders placed on the plant and filtering into the soil where it is absorbed by the plant roots. Hence, washing, though it may remove a little, is generally ineffective. Even minute amounts are very contaminating and irritating to our cells.

Bred to hold more poison without dying

The big pesticide corporations (which are also deadly chemical/drug corps, plus they own large shares of seed companies) are now inserting special genes in their seeds. Why? To allow these seeds to grow into food crops which will absorb more pesticides than ever without curling up and dying.[7] This means you will be eating more poison (unless you buy organically grown food). The soil will be drenched with more poison. And those heartless corporations will be making more money selling pesticides to farmers.

Insects don't attack healthy plants!

When plants are forced into quick development, they are not able to draw the normal amount of minerals from the soil, thus are mineral-deficient. The vitality of such plants is not sufficient to withstand the attacks of insect pests and fungus –Nature's way of purging them– so chemical poisons are sprayed on commer-

1) Wickenden, OD. 2) Colgan, 25. 3) Robbins, DN 313. 4) Colgan, 26. 5) Winter, PYF 5

cial crops to kill insects. Few people know that <u>insects only attack inferior and unhealthy plants, not good healthy ones</u>.[1] This is Nature's way of protecting us from unfit harmful food. In the name of profit, commercial establishments overstep this protection by killing the insects with pesticides, thereby allowing inferior, nutritionally deficient, health-damaging produce to grow anyway.

Nazi pesticides

Pesticides are vastly concentrated, potent chemicals intentionally developed to kill living creatures. In fact, many of them were originally developed in Nazi Germany (an Albino nation) to kill humans and have actually been used to kill millions of humans. Many of them are lethal nerve gasses, such as malathion and parathion. **A chemist who had swallowed an infinitesimal dose (0.00424 of an ounce) of parathion was instantly paralyzed and died before he could take an antidote he had prepared in advance and had at hand.**[2] Malathion is allegedly being sprayed on fruit trees, but "it's people that are being sprayed."[3] This spraying often happens in communities having large Black populations.

Black Genocide through White Pesticides

White American chemical corporations not only *still make deadly banned chemicals* –but sell them to so-called *Thirdworld* or *"developing"* nations (code terms for People of Color) by the millions of pounds each year. Yes this is genocide; pesticides are a major weapon against Colored People more than against the bugs. Pesticide contamination of food is much higher in "developing" countries. <u>About 3 million cases of pesticide-poisoning occur annually, with over 200,000 deaths. And 99% of these deaths occur in "developing" countries even though 80% of pesticides are used in "developed" (i.e., white, Western) countries</u>.[4] In 1990 over 120 million pounds of pesticides were exported overseas from America. Over 18 million pounds were classified as extremely toxic, including banned cancer-causing chlordane, mirex, and heptachlor, plus other lethal chemicals that cause birth-defects, infertility, nerve-damage, etc. To some degree, whites suffer from this practice as well, since much food imported to America is contaminated with pesticides banned in America (the same ones manufactured in America). In the book, *Our Stolen Future*, we read: ***"In 1991, the United States exported at least 4.1 million pounds of pesticides that had been banned, canceled, or voluntarily suspended for use in the United States, including 96 tons of DDT. These exports included 40 million pounds of compounds known to be <u>endocrine disruptors</u>."***[5] (*Endocrine disruptors* impair the reproductive organs and cause infertility, reduced sperm-count, tiny penises, cancer of the uterus, prostate, breast, etc.)

In addition, Melanin is made toxic from pesticides & herbicides.

Herbicides (paraquats, dioxin) and other manmade toxins bind irreversibly with Melanin and remain in the Black human throughout life causing many disorders. This may be a significant overlooked, unsuspected factor contributing to the super high mortality rate of American Afrikans with degenerative diseases.

---

1) Kulvinskas, LTC, 144. 2) Robbins, DF, 314. 3) Valerian. 4) Steinman, LH, 155. 5) Colburn, OSF, 138.

A glimpse of chemical horrors haunting your drugfoods

While a few lethal pesticides /chemicals have been banned in America, *most* of the remaining *thousands* are still being used. These killers include:

● **Dioxin:**

The DI of DIoxin is DIE. Dioxin is called the most toxic chemical ever made. A single drop can kill 1000 people; an ounce can kill a million.[1] Even at lowest levels possible for testing (1 part per trillion), dioxin causes cancer, birth defects, miscarriages and death in lab animals.[2] The EPA reports that levels in the population are high enough to cause infertility, cancer and damage to the immune system. Dioxin traces are found in virtually all the bleached-white stuff you come into contact with: white paper, napkins, paper towels, coffee filters, toilet paper, tampons, disposable diapers, and even white underwear. All deceptively snow white yet filthy with the worse of toxins. Traces may also be in the meat (especially beef), dairy and eggs in your supermarket. It contributes to the extreme cancer-causing nature of commercial meats. Millions of pounds of this herbicide have been sprayed on American soil. Dioxin is also one of the breakdown by-products formed when chlorine (regular bleach) is used to bleach paper, fabrics or home surfaces. (A less toxic replacement is hydrogen peroxide)

● **Dieldrin:**

Also appropriately begins with *DIE*. Dieldrin is 5 times more poisonous than DDT when swallowed, and 40 times more so when absorbed by the skin. Is one of the most potent carcinogens ever known. Causes cancer in lab animals at every dosage tested, down to the tiniest concentrations measurable by scientific equipment. Though banned, it's permanently with us. A test in 1974 by the FDA revealed that it exists in the flesh of 99.5% of the American people.[3]

● **DDT:**

A most toxic banned pesticide, now exist in some degree in nearly every person on Earth, even in babies, before and after birth.[4]

● **PCBs:**

Likely, every person and living creature on Earth carry PCBs in their flesh. PCBs (polychlorinated biphenyls) apparently contaminate the whole planet and are found everywhere: in soil, air, water, oceans. Introduced in 1929, PCBs were widely used for decades before its toxicity was realized. PCBs are considered to be the chief reason for the drastically increased sterility rate and the declining sperm count of men around the globe. The average sperm count of the American male is today **only 70% of what it was only 30 years ago.** A recent government study found PCBs present in 100% of the human sperm samples tested. A few parts *per billion* can cause birth defects and cancer. High PCB levels correlate to low sperm count.[5] As detailed in *Our Stolen Future*, PCBs are also linked to neurological damage (especially in the womb), brain damage, lowered intelligence, learning disabilities, hyper-activity/reactiveness, thyroid disruption, and abnormal sexual development in males, including very small penises.

1) Robbins, DNA, 321.   2) Ibid.   3) Ibid., 319.   4) Clark, SHB, 33.   5) Robbins, DNA, 330.

These killers are extremely stable.

Ominously, they do not break down for decades or centuries! As a result, they stay in our food chain. They accumulate in the tissues of animals, and as one animal eats another, they build up in ever higher concentrations at each higher rung on the food chain. Humans sit at the top of the chain whenever they eat fish, chicken, meat, eggs or dairy products. From these foods come 95% to 99% of the toxic chemical residues in the American diet.[1] Eat these if you want to include pesticides in your diet.

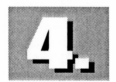

DEAD –especially from cooking & irradiation.

Food irradiation exposes food to the equivalent of 30 million chest X-rays.

Commercial supermarket food is often irradiated (exposed to massive doses of nuclear radiation to kill insects and germs). Originated and developed by white people, food irradiation is a technology designed to use radioactive **waste products from weapons manufacture** to extend the shelf life of meats, grains, and produce. This practice continues, despite many tests (by other whites) proving the dangers of irradiated foods and linking it with numerous diseases. Though the FDA states that irradiated food is safe, tests show that food irradiation destroys food nutrients, disrupts the normal bio-energy field of the food, and creates dangerous new free radicals. Food irradiation is done with the radioactive materials, **cobalt-60** which is produced in **nuclear reactors**, and **cesium-137** which is produced from **nuclear wastes** (that's right!) and, according to the U.S. Department of State, **will minimize U.S.** *nuclear waste disposal.* (!!!)

Cecium-137 is the most radioactive of waste materials and the one promoted by the Department of Energy for food irradiation. The food does not become radioactive, unless there is equipment or human error, but electrons are knocked out of orbit and <u>massive molecular rearrangement takes place</u>. New chemicals called Unique Radiolytic Products (URPS) are formed in the foods. Most URPS are unknown and untested. There is <u>no way to determine</u> if a food has been irradiated, or at what dosage, or how many times. The first commercial instance of food irradiation took place in 1957 in the Albino country of Germany, where it was used to sterilize spices. *"The results were so disturbing the government banned the procedure the following year."*[2]

1) Robbins, DNA, 315.   2) Valerian, 0140.

Why is nuclear irradiation & irradiated food harmful?

- **"Consumption of irradiated rice** has been linked with the development of pituitary, thyroid, heart and lung disturbances, and development of tumors."[1]
- **Has dangerous results.** Animals fed irradiated food developed damage to their testicles, kidneys, and chromosomes. Mice fed a diet high in irradiated chicken died sooner and had a higher rate of tumors.
- **When children and animals were fed irradiated wheat,** they developed increased abnormality of their chromosomes (called polyphoidy).[2]
- **Irradiation creates new toxins /chemicals in foods** called radiolytic products. These toxins include formaldehyde and cancer-causing substances like benzene (in irradiated beef). Others are unique to the irradiation process and no one knows what effects these have on human health.
- **Radiation-deranged food transfers its derangement directly to your cells.** Studies at Cornell University showed that eating irradiated sugar can produce the same results as irradiation directly applied to the cell.

  "Scientists experimented with carrot tissue and coconut milk... both high in natural sugars. They bombarded them with cobalt 60, causing radiation-induced cell mutations in both foods. Moreover, the chemicals produced by sugar breakdown in the [irradiated] foods were seen [to] transfer radiation effects into the cells of fruit flies, resulting in stunted growth and chromosome damage. All living cells contain sugar, the report emphasized, and human beings may suffer similar consequences from long-term consumption of irradiated food."[3]
- **Irradiation destroys essential vitamins and nutrients** that are naturally present in food.
- **Irradiated seeds and plants do not grow.** Irradiation stunts growth and prevents sprouting, depending on the level of irradiation.
- **Aflatoxin** (a cancer-causing mold poison), may grow more readily on irradiated foods.
- **Irradiation plants pose environmental threats to workers and surrounding communities.** The transportation of nuclear materials to irradiation facilities also poses severe public health risks.

Cooking & Microwaving are other forms of irradiating food.

All drugfood is cooked food. Cooking turns food into drugs. Note that high temperatures are used in manufacturing drugs and processed drugfood. Any wonder that most addicting substances are cooked: tobacco, coffee, alcohol, cocaine, sugar, etc. Microwaving vibrates food molecules up to over 2 billion times per second, deranging the structure of the molecules and making the food even more toxic than if it were cooked conventionally. A German study found that the body responds to microwaved food as if it were an infectious agent (see page 61). It causes pathological changes in the blood /body cells. In 1992, Dr. Hans Hertel did a study of the blood chemistry of persons eating microwaved food. Major changes occurred, similar to those with cancer.

1) Valerian, 0141.   2) Ibid.   3) Winter, PYF, 241.

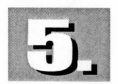

Processed and embalmed with chemical poisons.

If the "food" has any virtues left after going through the previously described abominable practices, this is effectively demolished in food processing, the final phase of the **War Against Wholistic Food.** Commercial drugfood is excessively, massively, ridiculously over-processed. It is fractionated, bleached, dyed, gassed, hormoned, homogenized, hydrolyzed, hydrogenated, carbonated, acetylated, bromated, flavored, deflavored, acidified, alkalinized, buffered, sulfated, nitrated, scented, deodorized, texturized, creamed, emulsified, thickened, thinned, defoamed, stabilized, preserved, waxed...

The use of chemicals in foods has soared from 419 million pounds in 1955 to more than <u>800 million today</u>. Each of us eats more than 50 pounds of additives a year.[1]

Read the labels before you buy *any* food!

When additives combine, new, mutant, worse chemicals are created.
The poisonous chemicals we ingest when we eat commercial drugfoods interact with those that are already in our body, forming mutant, second generation chemicals far more harmful that the originals. *"Another great problem with testing additives is how they interact with each other and with the **sixty-three thousand other chemicals [!!!]** in common use today. In 1976, the Journal of Food Sciences carried a report on a small-scale attempt to determine the extent of the problem. When three additives were tested one at a time on rats, the animals stayed well. Two at a time, the rates became ill, and with a three-additive combination, all the animals died within fourteen days."[2]*

Have a frothy, delicious, chilled glass of Ethyl Methylphenylglycidate
It tastes just like strawberries. This clear, liquid chemical artificially imparts a very berry taste to ice cream, beverages, candy, gum, and other delights when not being used in perfumes. It's even listed as GRAS (Generally Recognized As Safe), even though it retards the growth of rats and atrophies their testicles, and paralyzes the muscles of female rats.[3] Still want some? Jes help yourself! In the next section, let's sample some more delectable "additives" until we pass out.

1) Winter, PIYF, 5. 2) Ibid., 259. 3) Winter, FA, 173.

Khemical Kuisine: Food In Your Poison?

Virtually no food items in American supermarkets are free of *chemical additives*, including table salt. Over a billion pounds of chemicals are used each year! These chemicals are drugs. They have absolutely no nutritive or beneficial effect upon the body. Many of them are known to be dangerous and even lethal when ingested outright, even in minute amounts. Following are a few of over 3000 chemicals added to the beautifully packaged, enticing, innocent-looking but killer kounterfeit foods enjoyed by the typical, unsuspecting hungry American:

● **Piperonal**, a vanilla-flavor substitute is also used to kill lice.[1]

● **Butyraldehyde** provides a delicious nut like flavor, but is also an important ingredient in rubber cement and synthetic resins.[2]

● **Aldehyde C-17** imparts a delectable cherry flavor when it is not serving as an important constituent in synthetic rubber and certain plastics.[3]
8-hydroxyquinoline helps preserve cottage cheese when it is not being used in contraceptives and rectal suppositories.[4]

● **Alginic acid** gives your cheese spread a uniform flavor and color when it is not making celluloid and synthetic ivory.[5]

● **Ethyl acetate** makes a great pineapple taste when it is not being used as a solvent for cleaning leather and plastics.[6]

● **Polyvinylpyrrolidone** gives clarity and storage life to beer, ale, jellies, cider, wines, and fruit juices when it is not helping out with aerosol hair sprays.[7]

● **BVO** (bromated vegetable oil) is used as an emulsifier in some foods and as a clouding agent in many popular soft drinks. The main ingredient of BVO is **bromate**, a poison. Just 2-4 ounces of a 2% solution of BVO can severely poison a child. Bromates are also used in bromated flours, bromated wholewheat flour and hair products such as permanent-wave neutralizers. It harms the central nervous system and causes skin eruptions when topically applied.

● The **food colors: bordeaux, amaranth, orange**, and **procean** are all derived from compounding nitrogen and benzene, which is also a commonly used motor fuel. Some of the same **dyes** coloring your clothes may be used to dye your food. Ice cream, sherbert, maraschino cherries, drinks...all beautifully deadly colored. **Coal tar dyes** produce cancer, reduced fertility, and malformed fetuses.[8]

● Ice cream is treated with **formaldehyde**, a chemical used to embalm corpses. Commercial ice cream also contains curcumin, carmoisine, sodium alginate, carrageenan, sodium carboxymethyl cellulose (made by treating cellulose with alkali & monochloroacetic acid), mono/di-glycerides of fatty acids derived from slaughterhouse by-products, and gelatin made from beef bones, calf or pork skin.

● The dictionary informs us that **potassium nitrate** (saltpeter) is *"used to pickle meat and in the manufacture of pyrotechnics, explosives, matches, rocket propellants, and fertilizers."*

● **Cochineal**, used to produce a bright red color in food, is made from the bodies of dried cochineal bugs.

1) Preston, HYM, 69. 2-7) Ibid. 8) Hunter, FD, 57-61.

- **Nitrates** used to preserve meats and camouflage its rotten smell were key ingredients for manufacturing bombs and shells.
- Vegetable oils are processed with **gasoline solvent** and **sodium hydroxide** (known as **Draino** and caustic soda).
- Caramel is prepared from **ammonia**; it is suspected in the manifestation of some mental disorders in children.[1]
- The **package itself** is a major unlisted ingredient! **BHT** and **BHA** (bishydroxytoluene & bishydroxyanisole) are food preservatives and seizure triggers. *"They are often put on the boxes of cereals, rather than the cereals themselves, so the cereals can be pronounced preservative-free. Imagine how much the box must be drenched with to prevent oxygen leakage into the interior?"*[2] And many foods are wrapped in **aluminum**, a harmful metal.
- **HVP** is used to create a beefy taste in hot dogs, barbecue sauce, and soups, plus add a creamy texture to processed foods, frozen dinners and nondairy creamers. They make HVP by boiling vegetables in sulfuric acid, neutralizing the soup with caustic soda, and then drying it to a brown sludge.
- **Calcium sulfate** is a fancy name for **gypsum** or **plaster of Paris**, a chalklike concrete used for patching holes in walls and making plaster casts of sculptures, furniture and ornaments. A large number of dairies use plaster of Paris in their cottage cheese to thicken it up and cause it stick together![3] It is also an ingredient in some veggie burgers in healthfood stores.
- Once ingested, **sulfites** are converted to deadly **sulfur dioxide gas**, responsible for acid rain. Reactions include suppression of immunity, allergic reactions, and severe asthma attacks which sometimes lead to death. Sulfites are sprayed on fresh foods like shrimp and fruit /salad bars in restaurants to keep them looking fresh and prevent browning with exposure to air. Sulfites are also lurking in maraschino cherries (they're bleached white, then dyed bright red), canned soups, frozen vegetables, fruit juices, dried fruit, hard candy, potato salad, white and brown sugar, molasses, vinegar, cole slaw, sauerkraut, gravies, sauces, french fries, hard liquor, wine, wine coolers, drugs and more.[4]
- The same **talc** (chalk) of talcum/baby/makeup powder is put in powdery foods to make them "free-flowing." Talc and other **silicates** are often contaminated with **asbestos**,[5] for talc mineral beds may contain several forms of asbestos. Also, talc and some forms of asbestos are both forms of *hydrous magnesium silicate*. The only difference is in structure: talc is flaky or granular, while asbestos is fibrous. Once these tiny, razor-sharp, needle-like, asbestos particles are breathed in or ingested, they move through your body like a swordfish, impaling cells until your body routes it into a cyst or forms a cyst around it. There it remains, providing lifelong potential for cancer development. Talc silicates are found in dry soup mixes, salt, garlic powder, vanilla powder, baking powder, vitamins, dried egg yolk, powder on chewing gum, flavor fixative on polished rice, etc. Other names for silicates include anti-caking agents, sodium aluminosilicate, calcium aluminosilicate, & tricalcium silicate.

1) Valerian, 0140. 2) Clark, CA, 232-233. 3) Robbins, UP, 187. 4) Igram, ST, 225-226. 5) Hunter, FA, 85.

- **Olestra** is a sucrose polyester. A fat-substitute developed by Procter & Gamble that cannot be digested. It has no calories. It can supposedly replace regular fats in french fries and baked desserts. It causes tumors and liver changes in animals. It is one big greasy deception; a Drug Masquerading as *FAT*.

- **Can't pronounce it? Don't eat it!** —even if you can pronounce it. Here are a "few" more drug-chemicals added to our supermarket-foods:

Acetophenone	**Allyl anthranilate**	**Allyl isothiocyanate**
Aluminum ammonium sulfate	Aluminum oleate	Aluminum sodium silicate
Ammonium alginate	Ammonium carrageenan	Ammonium isovalerate
Arabingalactan	Aspergillus oryzae	Azodicarbonamide
Benzaldehyde	**Benzyl butyl acetate**	**Bisabolene**
Bovine somatotropin	Butylene glycol	Butylparaben
Calciferol	**Calcium acetate**	**Calcium acid phosphate**
Calcium iodate	Calcium pantothenate	Calcium propionate
Calcium stearoyl lactate	Caseinate	Chloropentafluorethane
Cinnamaldehyde	Cyanocobalamin	Cyclamate
Daminozide	**Dextrans**	**Diethylene glycol distearate**
Diethylenetriamine	Dilauryl thiodipropionate	Dimethyl polysiloxane
Disodium guanylate	Dioctyl sodium sulfosuccinate	Dodecyl gallate
Ergocalciferol	**Erythrobic acid**	**Ethylenediamine**
Ethyl methylphenylglycidate	Ethyl methylphenylglycidate	Eugenyl methyl ether
Ferric ammonium citrate	**Ferric sodium pyrophosphate**	**Ferric orthophosphate**
Furcelleran	Furfuryl acetate	Furyl acrolein
Glucono delta-lactone	**Glutamic acid**	**Glycerine**
Glycerol	Glyceryl triacetate	Glycyrrhizin
Heptylparaben	**Hydrogen peroxide**	**Hydroxypropyl cellulose**
Imidazolidinyl	**Indigotine**	**Isovaleric acid**
Magnesium sulfate	**Mannitol**	**Methane dichloride**
Methylparaben	Monosodium glutamate	Myristaldehyde
Octahydrocoumarin	**Ormetoprim**	**Oxystearin**
Phenylalanine	**Phenylmethyl cyclosiloxane**	**Polysorbates**
Potassium chloride	Potassium hydroxide	Potassium nitrate
Potassium phosphate	Propyl gallate	Propylene glycol
Quinine hydrochloride	**Quinine sulfate**	**Quizalofopethyl**
Rapeseed oil unsaponifiables	**Rhizopus oryzae**	**Rhodinyl Isovalerate**
Salicylaldehyde	**Silicon dioxide**	**Sodium bisulfite**
Sodium carbonate	Sodium carboxymethylcellulose	Sodium nitrite
Sorbitan monostearate	Sorbitol	Sulfur dioxide
Tallamphopropionate	**Tarragon**	**Tartaric acid**
Tertiary butylhydroquinone	Tetramethylthiuram	Titanium dioxide
Undecalactone	**Undecylenic acid**	**Undecylenyl alcohol**
Valeraldehyde	**Viburnum prunifolium**	**Vinegar naphtha**
Xanthophyll	**Xylenol**	**Xylitol**
Zedoary	**Zearalanol**	**Zinc ricinoleate**

This list of additives doesn't even include the (outright intentionally lethal) **pesticide-residues** in the same food. Sure, it's only a "leetle bit" of toxins in each food but each food has scores of different toxins. By their very nature, all it takes is a "leetle bit" of a toxin to cause problems; that's what makes it a toxin. And eaters usually eat more than one food in a single meal. In addition, toxins

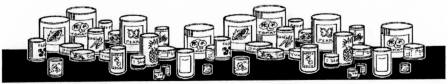

interact with each other to create new, mutant, worse toxins. Often, toxins are cumulative because most people do not periodically DE-toxify their bodies through fasting or cleansing diets (raw fruits & vegetables). Combine all the toxins we ingest with the toxins we encounter from our environment (plastics, styrofoam, house cleansers, nail polish, body-care products, polluted air, etc.). All the toxins in your food, body-care products and environment add to a continuous assault upon your health –keeping your body in continuous defense-mode. A *leetle* here and a *leetle* there equals a whole *lot* when the total is added! Multiply this 365 days a year and you get an idea of the fighting which your body (your overwhelmed organs of elimination: liver, kidneys, lungs, skin) must continuously do just to keep you alive. "Additives" in our food contribute to the waste which our body attempts to eliminate. If our bodies are spending most or all its time and energy getting rid of wastes, then how can it take the time and energy to REPAIR itself? It can't! That's why we break down...and eventually succumb to degenerative diseases and painful, premature demise. When the load of toxins in your body becomes too great, your body produces an emergency state of *rapid toxic discharge*. This state is called "dis-ease"! This is why 4 outta 10 Americans get cancer. Or why over 100,000 Americans die each month from degenerative disease. Thanks to the Standard American Diet. It's so S.A.D. All degenerative diseases are reactions to living on toxic drugfood.

Albinos have accomplished the impossible with their chemicals

Never before in known history have humans had available to them such a vast variety and quantity of food, all year round, all in a single place appropriately called the "super" market. An eater's paradise. This incredible feat is a major accomplishment of the Albinos, linked with their equally incredible industrial-ized factory-farms, –both complete with major destruction and disruption to Nature. Those same additives we sampled earlier and barely survived, are the chemicals making this feat possible:

- These chemicals preserve the food, making it last beyond its natural time, for weeks, months, and even lifetimes, without spoiling.
- These chemicals keep food appearing, smelling & tasting fresh, indefinitely.
- These chemicals keep food consistent in color, taste and texture; Hershey chocolate bars still taste exactly the way they did when you were a child; maraschino cherries all have the same uniform bright red color and taste; some breakfast cereals defy moisture and stay crunchy "even in milk."
- These chemicals give food an artificial cosmetic boost, lab-produced color brighter than flower petals; cucumbers with a shine you can see yourself in.
- They keep the food cheap. Why should producers pay $100 dollars for an ounce of real flavor extract when they can pay 10 cents for a chemical tasting like the real thang? Or use real blueberries in their muffins when they can use a chemical that artificially creates the same delightful effects?
- They make it possible to have inexpensive gourmet meals several times a day if you want. Buy them frozen, nuke 'em, and in moments you gotta gourmet dinner that shoulda taken hours to prepare.

The billion pounds of toxic chemicals enriching our foods explain why:

All Drugfoods are "DELICIOUS"! ...

only after "preparation," that is. Deliciousness is the 6th top trait of Drugfoods. They taste so *good* (to our *perverted* sense of taste). And that's really too *bad*. That's what makes them so irresistible. We *love* 'em. Is the *short-term* pleasure we get from eating Drugfoods worth the *long-term* health-stealing, happiness-stealing results? You bet! **Never in history has the route to disease and death been so pleasurable!** *Drugs Masquerading As Foods.* Delicious slow death. There are worse ways to exit. This unprecedented khemical kuisine perfectly aligns with the mechanistic artificial society that produced it, which is utterly gapped from Mother Nature and even in a *War Against Nature* and all things Natur-Real. Thus, the final trait: **(Hard) Drugfoods Are *All* Deadly!**

Thus, drugfood mucks you. Effects of a drugfood diet include:

- addiction
- foul polluted body
- foul body odors
- chronic constipation
- much mucus
- waking w/ encrusted eyes
- aches and pains
- negative outlook
- depression, irritability
- hyperactivity
- uncontrolled temper
- meaness

- apathy, zombie-ness
- moral degeneration
- criminal behavior
- chronic fatigue
- needing much sleep
- lethargy
- excessive or no appetite
- obesity
- dull or bloodshot eyes
- mental degeneration
- mental dullness, slow
- mental retardation

- impotency
- menstrual cramps
- reduced fertility
- decreased birthrate
- miscarriages, birth defects
- sterility
- accelerated aging
- physical degeneration
- chronic sickness
- degenerative diseases
- acute diseases
- premature death

- **creates toxins/filth; poison the bloodstream and cells**
- **clogs the lymph and elimination system**
- **robs, depletes the body of enzymes, vitamins, nutrients**
- **drains the body's lifeforce and enzyme reserve**
- **produces the ideal environment for parasites, flukes, germs**
- **throws off pH balance, making the body too acidic**
- **overworks, stresses, strains, enslaves digestive system, glands & organs**
- **makes your brain smaller and organs bigger (hence promotes stupidity?):**
  Harvard Medical School researchers found that on the American diet of processed, denatured foods, the kidneys, liver, pancreas, heart, endocrine glands, pituitary and thyroid gets BIGGER while the brain gets SMALLER. This is probably because the organs have to work overtime just to keep the body functioning, while using much of their energy to keep drugfood-toxins at bay. Scientists have verified that the brains of domesticated (i.e., *enslaved*) animals are smaller than that of wild animals.[1] And the fossil skulls of the Neanderthal man indicated they had larger, heavier brains than that of "modern" man.[2]
- **assaults and insults every cell and organ in your body**
- **makes you ugly; disfigures body, skin, face, smile; erodes natural beauty**
- **heaven in the mouth, hell in the stomach, colon, liver, heart**
- **the final "effect" is a big STOP SIGN called DEATH**

1) Afrika, AHH, 83.   2) Ibid.

No time for building health?
–then plenty of time for sickness & disease!

We realize how valuable our health is when we lose it. How much is your health worth to you? If you cannot find time for health –to practice healthful living, and learn how to eat /live wholistically, you will have plenty of time for illness, suffering, depression, dullness of spirit, unhappiness and dis-ease. Most people seem oblivious to the ominous dangers these drugfoods represent, and of the crucial importance of their food choices. Hospitals are full of people who were too busy to be concerned about healthful living. Graveyards are full of people who did not have time to properly take care of themselves and so they died as the karma of their harmful eating and lifestyle caught up with them.

Elderly people show us the end result of our daily drugdiet

Visit any home for the elderly and you will witness firsthand the insidious, cumulative degeneration which the American supermarket diet awards its faithful longterm eaters. This is why the vast majority of elderly people in America suffer from chronic degenerative diseases, constant health problems, senility, and chronic pain. The elderly people of the Hunzas in northern India live to be from 125 to 175 years or longer and maintain robust health, youthfulness and vitality throughout. Many even have children *after* the age of 100! [1]

Return to whole organic "real food" and save yourself!

The only REAL FOODS are pure fruits, vegetables and nuts –not chemically embalmed or destroyed with fire and microwaves, but organically grown and alive, and ideally, non-hybrid. A diet of such food will keep us healthy at any age. Compared to commercial drugfoods, organic whole food tastes better, is nontoxic and highly nutritious as Nature intended. Organic produce may not look as pretty because it is not cosmetically treated. Yes, it may be more expensive but isn't your health worth it? Since organic foods are far more nutritious (having twice as much nutrients), you will feel satisfied on *less* food, especially *after* you *purify* your inwardly foul, toxic body. Our bodies have evolved over eons on raw, natural organic food. It's truly unfortunate that we have been conditioned into killer eating habits by the culture. It may sometimes be hard to break these killer habits and addictions that give us much short-term pleasure. But if we love our health more than our addictions and have patience with ourselves, we can gradually replace health-busting eating habits with health-building ones. The short-term pleasure of living on drugfoods is not worth the longterm suffering and eventual premature death. The longterm rewards of living primarily on *real* foods will outweigh the temporary discomforts.

1) Flanagan, EA, 1.

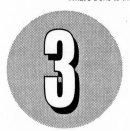

What's Done to
the Produce
is Done to
the Farm Animals

Farm Animals suffer the same treatment as the Produce

What's being done to the produce is also being done to the farm animals that people eat! These animals suffer the same process, treatment, and fate as the commercial drugfoods.

Overview Summary

The 5 fatal foremost traits of killer drugfoods apply to farm animals (as fleshfood) because they too are:
1. Perverted, bastardized *before* birth.
2. Grown in, and fed poisons.
3. Sprayed, doused with death.
4. DEAD(ER), especially from cooking /irradiation.
5. Processed and embalmed with chemical poisons.
   Again, let's look at these anti-life practices...

Commercial fleshfood is killer drugfood because it's made with animals that are...

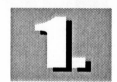

Perverted, bastardized *before* birth.

The farm animals are unnatural (crossbred, hybrid). As with commercial produce, their genes are artificially altered by Albino scientists. The new, "improved" animals that result are as grossly out of balance with Nature as their heartless re-creators. Robbins wrote: "...the genetic manipulators are continuing their efforts to 'improve' the pig, and convert this good-natured and robust creature into a more efficient piece of factory equipment. ...' *Breeding experts are trying to create pigs that have flat rumps, level backs, even toes, and other features that hold up better under factory conditions."*[1] Not just pigs, but *all* the farm animals have been /are being genetically mucked with and altered from their natural blueprint.

Your Unknowing Cannibalism May Eventually Drive You Insane

It's horrible enough that "most livestock are being fed genetically altered feed...and often diseased and discarded animal carcasses."[2] But even worse,

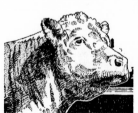

human genes are being added to the equation! **"Commercial pork has been genetically altered with DNA from human beings. Great time to decide to be vegetarian."**[3] This spells another way to get "prions." See pages 36 and 108 for the gory details.

1) Robbins, DNA, 86.
2) www.afrocentricnews.com/html/food.htm. 3) Ibid.

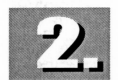

Grown in, and fed, poisons (and feces) just to keep their diseased bodies alive.

They are fed poisons because their appalling *living* conditions ("deathing" conditions, really) in modern factory farms are abominably unhealthy / unsanitary /filthy /feces-ful, and grossly unnatural. They are all fed drugs (poisons) and **they are all drug addicts! Factory-farm animals are subjected to many horrible toxic chemicals.** They are intentionally fed many toxic compounds never encountered by animals raised in a more natural way.

- Animal feed contains DDT, pesticides, hormones, stilbesterol, antibiotics, and tranquilizers. Animal feed is also often grown on land that is heavily sprayed with the most dangerous pesticides.
- Cancerous pesticides are fed to animals to keep their manure free of flies.
- The diet of commercial chickens include sulfa drugs, hormones, antibiotics, nitrofurans, arsenicals, and feces.
- Over 90% of today's chickens are fed arsenic compounds.[1]
- Livestock is also fed huge quantities of often contaminated *fish.* Yes, *fish!* – which is NOT a natural food of cows. And this is "trash fish" that can't be fixed up to sell to humans. It is fed to factory-farm animals solely to enrich the owners of the "factory trawlers" wiping out fish stocks in our oceans.

Pigs are routinely fed recycled raw feces [2] **(pig/chicken manure) /waste** which contains drug residues and high levels of toxic, heavy metals such as arsenic, lead and copper. In some farm-factories, the diet of cattle may include sawdust laced with ammonia and feathers, shredded newspaper (with toxic ink from the print), "plastic hay," processed sewage, inedible tallow and grease, poultry litter, cement dust, and cardboard scraps, plus insecticides, antibiotics and hormones. This mess is artificially flavored and scented to trick the animals into eating it.[3] Sounds familiar? It should, for essentially this is the delicious and deadly American *die*-t; chemical junk flavored and "done up" as real food, then deceptively presented to us as such.

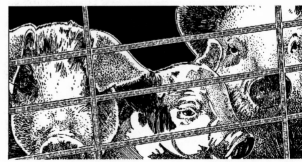

1) Robbins, DNA, 65.   2) Ibid., 93; Inglis, 48.   3) Robbins, DNA, 110.

Brain-Dissolving Cannibal-Flesh: Cows are being fed cows! Chickens are being fed chickens!

This is diabolical! The flesh of such *cannibal-ed* animals contains a new class of freak-poison with its own special name: "PRION," or outta-control protein requiring the heat of 3500 degrees to be destroyed! Humans can't digest such unnatural stuff; we can't even properly digest "normal" toxic flesh. Eating such drugflesh can result in brain-dissolving, dementia-insanity diseases (such as *Mad Cow Disease*) in both animals and humans who eat them. (see page 108)

Animal flesh has the highest concentration of pesticides.

Foods of animal origin are the major source of pesticide residues in the diet. *"Recent studies indicate that of all the toxic chemical residues in the American diet, almost all, 95% to 99%, comes from meat, fish, dairy products and eggs. If you want to include pesticides in your diet, these are the foods to eat."*[1]

Only 10% of the meat adulterated with pesticides and chemicals, or contaminated with filth and diseased organs is condemned by food inspectors. The other 90 percent gets through to the unsuspecting consumer.[2] **America would become a nation of vegetarians if there were strict enforcement of pesticide residues in red meat, dairy produce eggs, fowl and fish.**

Even fish and seafood are now deadly.

Normally, fish would be the most wholesome animal flesh to consume, but now, fish is just as bad or worse than eating red meat. The lakes, rivers and oceans they live in are polluted. Fish have a remarkable ability to absorb and concentrate toxic chemicals from their watery environments. They literally breathe the water they swim in, so they are also continually accumulating more and more contaminants in this manner. The net effect is almost as if they were underwater magnets for toxic chemicals. The EPA estimates **fish can accumulate up to 9 million times the level of PCBs in the waters in which they live!** By the food chain effect, fish may thus become loaded with enormous concentrations of these toxic chemicals. Shell fish that filter water (oysters, clams, mussels, scallops, etc.) are especially saturated with pesticides. DDT levels in the oceans have damaged a major source of the world's oxygen supply – the microscopic phytoplankton.[3] Fish and seafood get contaminated with additional poisons from the **chemicalized ice** they are packed in for shipment.

1) Robbins, DNA, 315.   2) Kulvinskas, STC, 14.   3) Robbins, DNA, 331.

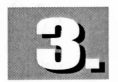

Sprayed, injected with death.

Shot up with drugs, hormones and antibiotics because their environment is full of feces and filth. Because they are usually diseased, they are injected with antibiotics. A government report found that over 90% of chickens from most of the country's flocks are infected with chicken cancer (leukosis).[1] Literally hundreds of drugs are used on livestock. Factory-farm-animals are dipped in, and sprayed with many toxic compounds. They are injected with dyes so that their meat and yolks will appear to be a 'healthy-looking' yellow.[2] Pesticides are also injected to kill worms in their stomachs.[2] Cattle, pigs, sheep and other livestock are often routinely doused with *toxaphen* to kill the parasites they breed in the crowded, filthy conditions of modern factory farms. Toxaphen is in the same family with DDT, dieldrin and PCBs. In the most microscopic doses, it produces cancer, birth defects, and causes bones to dissolve in lab animals. It is used every day in America on animals whose flesh Americans eat.

Nearly HALF of America's antibiotics are used on meat animals!

In 1991, the Centers for Disease Control in Atlanta released figures showing that approximately half of the 15 million pounds of antibiotics produced yearly in America, are used on livestock and poultry. *"We [Albinos] have bred such sickly food animals, that in order to keep them from becoming infected, over 90% of pigs and veal calves, 60% of cattle, and 95% of all poultry have antibiotics routinely added to their feed. Residues of these drugs are in much of meat that you eat."* [3] Antibiotics and chemicals cannot protect meats. The U.S. Meat Inspection Services recognizes over 42 diseases which make flesh-eating dangerous and antibiotics useless.[4] The continued eating of antibiotics in animal corpses causes human resistance to medicines and immunity to penicillin.

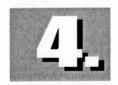

DEAD(ER), especially from cooking /irradiation.

Animals fed irradiated food develop damage to their testicles, kidneys and chromosomes. After the animals are slaughtered and neatly packaged, their flesh is irradiated with nuclear radiation. (Effects of irradiated food on pages 25, 61) Once purchased, animal flesh is further debased by cooking and microwaving. Much fleshfood is already conveniently pre-cooked. Microwaved and radiation-deranged food is even more harmful than cooked food.

1) Robbins, DNA, 67   2) Ibid., 68.   3) Colgan, 16.   4) Afrika, AHH, 96.

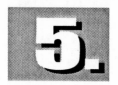

Processed and embalmed with chemical poisons.

This is done to keep bad meat deceptively looking and smelling fresh, thus salable. Meat, the most perishable and expensive of all foods, is also one of the most tampered with. *"After an animal is slaughtered, or dies from disease, it is shipped off to the processing house. The meat is doctored up, for the benefit of the gullible public, with aesthetic beautifiers, stink reducers, taste accentuators, color additives, drug camouflagers, nutritive enhancers, bleaching agents and death certificate. No corpse gets such a face lift by the embalmers and with good reason, for the corpse is soon buried, whereas salami, hotdogs, bologna, and chicken may sit on the shelves for months."* [1]

Meat is dyed red with sodium nicotinate otherwise it would turn yellow-grey.[2] Nitrites are also used to give meat a bright red color. Sometimes it is put in older meat to make it look fresh, red. It is a cheap preservative. Potassium or sodium nitrate/nitrite is used to fix color in cured meats. It reacts chemically with the myoglobin molecule to impart blood-redness to processed meats, convey tanginess to the palate, and to resist the growth of *Clostridium botulinum* spores, which can cause botulism. Sodium nitrite /nitrate (saltpeter) is present in very high levels in **hot dogs, bacon, ham and canned fish. It is in all processed meat: cured meats, bacon, bologna, frankfurters, deviled ham, meat spread, potted meats, spiced ham, Vienna sausages, smoke-cured tuna fish products, smoke-cured shad /salmon.**

The problem is that nitrates/nitrites combine with natural stomach and food chemicals (secondary amines) to create nitrosamines, among the most powerful cancer-causing agents known.[3] Studies from two separate institutes found that very small doses of nitrite or nitrosamines caused cancer in animals.[4] Animals feeding on high levels of this chemical develop cancerous tumors. **At levels higher than 10 parts per *billion*, sodium nitrite is a potential cancer hazard.**[5] The FDA nevertheless allows 200 parts per million (ppm) in processed meats. Nitrates are used in matches and to improve the burning properties of tobacco. **And nitrates were key ingredients for manufacturing bombs and shells during World War I.**[7] Such toxins are still quietly bombing people.

---

1)Kulvinskas STC 14. 2)Ibid. 3) Winter PYF 74. 4)Ibid. 75. 5)Whittlesey 106. 6)Valerian 0159. 7)Ibid. 0136.

What's Done to the Produce & Animals is Being Done to Us!

We are suffering the same fate as the supermarket-produce & factory-farm animals we eat!

And at the end (and along the way), like them, we too are being "eaten"! –that is, *exploited* for our lifeforce, power, emotional energy, money, time, health, happiness, and ultimately our lives:

Overview Summary

The five, fatal foremost traits of killer drugfoods apply to us:
1. Perverted (cheated, mutated, damaged) *before* birth.
2. Grown in, and fed, poisons.
3. Sprayed, dosed, injected with death (poisons).
4. Half DEAD and DYING faster, from being slowly cooked / irradiated with harmful radiations.
5. Processed & embalmed with chemical poisons.

Again, let's look at these evil (anti-life) practices...

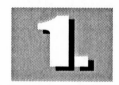

Perverted (cheated, mutated) *before* birth.

You were damaged and shortchanged before you were born, actually before you were *conceived*, because your parents were biologically damaged from being born into and harmed by ever-growing toxicity, both internal (their bodies) and external (the environment).

- **Though Afrikan babies** are born with the most advanced neurological system, by the time they are two years of age, this has reversed! Further, Afrikans in America have the highest infant mortality rate.
- Millions of women are *x-rayed* while pregnant.
- Millions of women are sonagramed while pregnant. **Sonagrams** cause leukemia (blood cancer), the chief cause of death amongst babies /children.
- **Nearly 100% of American women** of child-bearing-age suffer debilitating *leukorrhea* and its consequent monthly hemorrhaging. This disease is regarded as normal. This disease, called *menstruation*, is not to be confused with *ovulation*, a normal healthy process.[1] Women that live on a natural, organic, rawfood plant diet do not have bloody menstruation. Only a "civilized" diet produces this disease (in humans and domesticated animals).

1) Fry, BS, 57.

- **Almost every baby** born in America has already been drugged, exposed to toxins before birth, by doctors or their mother's drug /cigarette /alcohol / drugfood habits. Because of widespread drug-use and conceiving children under the influence of drugs, middleclass white American moms (especially) are finding that their children often die with their first infection.
- **Your parent's flesh was polluted:**
  - All children born in the U.S. have traces of pesticides in their tissues.[1]
  - Your parents' childhood vaccines (and *yours* for that matter) may have altered their DNA /RNA (hence influencing your own), turning them/ you into biological mutants.
  - A Minnesota study found strong links between birth defects and pesticide-exposure in that state's farming regions.[2]
- **Everyone is suffering damage** from half a century of exposure to endocrine-disrupting chemicals called hormone-impostors (described later).
- **Imitating whites, we Afrikans** continue poisoning our **babies** after birth. Feeding them *cows' milk* in *plastic* bottles; they suck from plastic/rubber nipples; we give them pacifiers and teething toys made of *plastic* or *PVC* (polyvinyl chloride or vinyl). Toxins leach from this plastic, especially when pressured...as in sucking, nibbling. The softeners of the plastic *(phthalates)* are toxic. Effects on lab animals include damage to the liver, kidneys and reproductive tract.[3] Some European countries have banned PVC toys.

Therefore, we all were biologically cheated before we were born.

Just because you *seem* to have what you're supposed to have (two eyes, two legs, a belly button, ability to see, etc.) does not mean that you got everything you were supposed to. Many biological defects are not outwardly visible. None of us are biologically where we should be, had conditions been "right." Evidence is everywhere you look. Huge numbers of sick, diseased, deformed, demented, psychotic, "off", imbecilic, "slow", retarded, "handicapped," eyeglass-wearing, or otherwise impaired humans fill this country. America is a nation of biological degenerates getting worse with each generation. America is the sickest country in the world. One of five Americans under age 17 already has some chronic disabling disease. Over 7 million children are "mentally retarded," disturbed or otherwise seriously handicapped because of brain problems. This would hardly exist if folks were mainly eating organic, raw, wholefoods. Everyone should be geniuses, especially the *Original People*.

People do not know how to make babies right!

To make the most perfect baby your body is capable of, it is imperative that both the mother and father FIRST detoxify their bodies through fasting, etc. Then rebuild for at least nine months by eating primarily raw organic fruits, nuts, veggies. During pregnancy and nursing years, again it is imperative the mother primarily eat these foods. Geniuses will be born to such parents –or at least brilliant children. A child conceived in a foul, impure, degenerating body fed on drugfoods and dead animals will not be born at its highest biological potential.

1) Winter, PYF, 5.   2) Colborn, OSF, 257.   3) Whole Life Times, 9/98, p7.

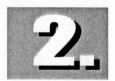

Grown in, and fed poisons.
We live in a toxic environment and eat toxic food.

We are inundated in a sea of synthetic poisons continuously being created by Albinos /their technology. More than 2 million are known, thousands are added each year, and over 100,000 are now on the market. The vast volume of health-mucking poisonous chemicals manufactured each year is staggering –*billions* of pounds. Very *few* are ever tested for toxicity.

- An article in the *Washington Post* stated that at least 60,000 chemicals are in use in the environment, and less than 2% have been tested for toxicity.[1]
- Five billion pounds of pesticides alone are spread far and wide not only on agricultural fields but in schools, parks, restaurants, supermarkets, homes and gardens.
- Pesticides in the air /water /earth travel hundreds of thousands of miles from the place they are first used. They may also persist for years in the soil, in their original form or in broken-down products.
- We fill the sky with 130 million tons of noxious chemicals, carbon monoxides, hydrocarbons, nitrogen oxides, sulfur oxides, etc. People living in New York City may inhale the equivalents of 730 pounds of chemicals a year.[2]
- "Some 600,000 young children living in slums [Melanated neighborhoods – no doubt] are threatened with lead poisoning, and 50,000 to 100,000 are likely to required immediate treatment. Slum houses are old, and interior walls have been covered with lead paint –some of it half lead– which peels from the wall. The lead tastes sweetish and the children eat it....airborne lead settles in the dust of the city streets... Playing children swallow or inhale this leaded dust... The result at the least is mental retardation [or cerebral palsy]; at the most, death. Damage to the brain is permanent."[3]
- Millions of children sit in classrooms for six hours a day breathing residues of the chemicals used to construct the schools, especially schools built between 1950 and 1968.
- All children born in the U.S. have traces of pesticide in their tissues.
- Most people carry *several hundred* "persistent" (non-biodegradable) chemicals in their bodies, including synthetic xeno-hormones.[4]
- The water from our faucets are toxic chemical soups.
- We daily wear clothes of permanent-press fabrics, outgassing formaldehyde.

> The use of chemicals in foods has soared from 419 million pounds in 1955 to more than 800 million today. **Each of us eats more than 50 pounds of food additives a year**, according to Roper Scheuplein, Ph.D. Office of Toxicological Sciences.[5] A third of all our food is contaminated with DDT and other lethal chemicals.[6]

1)Valerian, 0141.   2) Winter, PYF, 8.   3) Shroeder, 43.   4) Colborn, 140.   5) Winter, PYF, 5.   6) Davidson, 114.

Babies are endangered through breast milk.

Because America's diet is so toxic, the majority of nursing, drugfood-nourished moms have contaminated breast milk unfit for any living creature, especially their babes. Most mothers' milk is so high in DDT, PCB's, dieldrin, heptachlor, that it would be subject to confiscation and destruction by the FDA were it to be sold across state lines. Why are poisons concentrated in her milk? A nursing woman's body draws on its body fat reservoirs to make milk. Stored in her fat reservoirs are virtually all the toxic chemicals she has ever ingested, inhaled, or absorbed through her skin. Breast-fed babies thereby may consume large amounts of the most toxic substances known to man. In spite of this, nursing moms should still nurse their babies for numerous reasons. They can greatly reduce risk to their young: the amount of animal fat she eats and amount of toxins in her milk are connected. The less flesh, butter, eggs, cheese, milk in her diet, the less toxins in her breast milk. If she is a vegetarian, the amount of pesticides in her milk will be only 1 or 2% of that of the national average.[1]

Brain damage from pesticides.

A study of the long term effect of common organophosphates (such as neurotoxic **malathion /parathion**) upon human electro-encephalograms shows that a single exposure can alter the electrical activity of an infant's brain for years and possibly cause abnormal behavior and learning patterns. Harvard Medical school studies concluded that *"there is a dangerous possibility that organophosphate pesticides have the potential for causing long-term brain damage."* Organophosphates also decrease sex drive, impair concentration, and cause memory loss, schizophrenia, depression, irritability and more.

Melanin is made toxic from herbicides.

Herbicides bind irreversibly with Melanin and remain in Blacks throughout life causing many disorders. This may be a key unsuspected factor contributing to the super high mortality rate of Afrikan Americans with degenerative diseases.

Metal poisoning is pervasive in Albino society.

Your flesh is already polluted or even degenerating from metal-poisoning from metal cookware/utensils (aluminum /stainless steel), metal worn against your skin (jewelry, eyeglasses), metal in your mouth (dental fillings), in drugfoods, bodycare products, and the poisoned environment. In the U.S. alone, lead from industrial sources and leaded petrol contribute more than 600,000 tons of lead to the air [2] to be inhaled or ingested after depositing on crops, soil or fresh water.

1) Robbins, DNA, 345, 346 . 2) Murray, EN, 32.

ANGER-provoking agents and Genocide is put in the beer /wine /alcohol sold in Black neighborhoods

In one of his lectures, Malcom X said that an agent is deliberately put in the alcoholic beverages (especially cheap ones) sold in Afrikan neighborhoods, which triggers anger; it makes its drinkers mad. You likely won't find *malt liquor* in white neighborhoods. The alcoholic drinks available in Black communities are not the same as those sold in white communities. Blacks, especially males, drink this stuff and it makes them angry. They act out this induced anger on each other. This contributes to the high rate of Black-on-Black crimes. Black people themselves have noticed other Blacks becoming angry after drinking these brews. One brand, called MD 20 20 has even been nicknamed "Mad Dog" by Afrikans. A high percentage of Black-on-Black crimes is in fact, alcohol-related. This is a slick, hidden form of genocide, making the victims responsible and making them pay for it with money, jail time, and often their lives.

Other deadly poisons in malt liquor and beer include: petroleum, isobutenol (natural gas), sugar, alcohol, wood and starch alcohol.[1] These poisons deteriorate the brain, sex organs, liver, pancreas and lungs. They are highest in deadly malt liquor, which is consumed heaviest by Black men.

"My scientists have come up with a drug that can be smuggled into their [Black South Afrikans] brews to effect slow poisoning results and fertility destruction." So wrote P. W. Botha, former President of South Africa, in the August 18, 1985 edition of the South African *Sunday Times*.

Malt liquor has been shown to cause sperm-related fertility problems and genetic birth defects.[2] Thus, many Afrikans believe it is being used as a weapon of **genocide on Blacks**, for well-deliberated marketing strategies target Blacks and other minorities. The "**40 oz. malt**" is the worse culprit. In his book, *Message 'n a Bottle - The 40oz. Scandal*, Alfred "Coach" Powell provides uncommon insights and decodes secret messages contained in the ads and labels of malt liquor products, designed to manipulate and control people (especially Afrikans) through symbols.

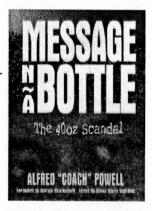

1) Lecture, Dr. L. Afrika.   2) Awadu, PW, 26.

Nitrates messing with us

You met Nitrates in Chapter 3. You thought you only got them in meats. Recall
that nitrates were key ingredients for manufacturing bombs. Sound delicious?
Nitrates change to *nitrites* on exposure to air. Nitrates /nitrites combine with
natural stomach and food chemicals to create **nitrosamines**, among the most
powerful cancer-causing agents known. **Besides causing cancers, nitrates are
linked to heart diseases, diabetes, and strokes.**[1] Nitrates have also caused
death from methemo-globinemia (cuts off oxygen to the brain). Too much
nitrate in the water is the cause of "**blue baby syndrome.**" The infant's lips,
nails and body becomes a marked blue hue. The cause is that bacteria (in an
unsterilized feeding bottle or child's gut) convert nitrate into nitrite. The
haemoglobin in the baby's blood takes up the nitrite instead of oxygen, resulting
in respiratory failure.[2] **Main sources of nitrates /nitrites:**
- **Cigarette smoke** is the #1 source of nitrosamines according to K. Prasad,
  author of *Vitamins Against Cancer*. Nitrates largely account for the
  powerful cancer-causing effect of tobacco smoke.
- **Cosmetics** is the 2nd leading source! Many brands contain DEA & TEA
  (diethanolamine & triethanolamine), which reacts with other chemicals to
  form nitrosamines.
- **Shampoo**: Both, *Sodium Lauryl Sulfate* and *Sodium Laureth Sulfate,* cause
  carcinogenic nitrates and dioxins to form in shampoos and cleansers by
  reacting with other product ingredients.
- **Meat /fleshfood** from regular supermarkets (especially processed meats).
- **Tap water** from water tables in areas of heavy agriculture /farming.
- **Certain vegetables** (see chapter 6) which become high in nitrate when
  synthetic fertilizers are used.

Some good news: fresh fruit (especially), also raw vegetables /herbs are rich in
bioflavonoids and other nutrients which block the transformation of nitrates into
carcinogenic nitrosamines.[3] Eat them a lot! (eat fruit on an empty stomach).
Citrus fruit have over 50 anti-cancer compounds.

And Hormone-Impostors ...here, there, everywhere, bringing chemical castration to animals and humans

Hormone-impostors, estrogen-impostors, estrogen-mimics, xeno-hormones,
xeno-estrogens, hormone-disrupters all mean the same and point to certain
petrochemical, non-biodegradable, fat-soluble toxic chemicals which "exert
harmful estrogenic effects." In other words they mess up the hormone system of
humans and animals. By so doing, they reduce or annihilate our ability to
reproduce. These chemicals have become prevalent everywhere –since western
chemical corporations invented and unleashed petrochemicals 50 years ago.
Once in our bodies, hormone-impostors behave like hormones, binding to
estrogen receptors in our cells and causing reproductive /genital disorders to
humans and animals. These hormone-disrupting chemicals cause uterine, breast,

1) Igram, ST, 228.   2) Valerian 0159.   3) Igram, ST, 228-229.

testicular, and prostate cancers. They cause endocrine disruption, sperm count reduction, infertility, endometriosis, and other genital abnormalities such as undescended testicles, extremely small penises, etc. They can also alter the nervous system and brain, and impair the immune system. **They are the main reason wildlife (on land and in water) is dying and disappearing. They are the reason for the plummet of human sperm counts over last 50 years.** The average male sperm count has dropped 45% in the period from 1940 to 1990. And the volume of sperm ejaculated has dropped 25%. Whose sperm? Mostly white men. The initial study by Danish researchers –61 studies– involved about 15,000 men from 20 countries –mostly white of course, but they also had men (tokens?) from Afrika, Asia, and South America.[1]

These hormone-disrupters are in our environment and diet, –more present in processed synthesized foods, fastfoods, animal fats and meats. Common in plastics, paints, textiles, detergents, paper products, pesticides, herbicides. **These chemicals can act** *together*; and small, seemingly insignificant amounts of individual chemicals can have a major cumulative effect –as demonstrated by cancer cells in culture. When estrogen-sensitive breast-cancer cells were exposed individually to 10 types of estrogen-mimics, it hardly made a difference in their growth. But when they were exposed to all 10 chemicals at the same time, the cancer cells grew like crazy, rapidly proliferating.[2]

Xeno-hormones and <u>DES</u> have similar effects (DES is the synthetic female hormone given to cattle to speed their growth). This was determined in an experiment by Albinos (British researchers), who fed low doses of xeno-hormones and DES to pregnant rats and charted the outcome with the rats' offspring. *"Octylphenol and butyl benzyl phthalate* [Ugly awkward words for ugly xeno-hormones, giving a clue to their real nature] *produced effects similar to DES, and the males exposed to these estrogenic chemicals in early life had smaller testicles and reduced sperm production of as much as 21 percent when they reached adulthood."* [3] As previously noted (chapter 2, page 22), **white America deliberately sells tens of millions of pounds of known endocrine-disrupting chemicals to Thirdworld nations (i.e., Afrikans, People of Color); this is disguised** *Black Genocide Through White Pesticides.* Created and brought to you by white people (the chemical-drug corporations), all these synthetic estrogenic chemicals are chemically castrating humans and animals, including their creators. **They are threatening the survival of Humanity and Wildlife. They are putting all lifeforms on the endangered-species list.**

Got Plastic? Got Xeno-hormones!

Hormone-disrupting chemicals also migrate into your food and drink directly from the plastic in which food is packaged, bottled or stored. Throughout your life you been eating food outta plastic packaging, containers, bottles, plus styrofoam. And a large percentage of the stuff you daily come into contact with is plastic, including synthetic fabrics. Plastic, plastic everywhere. You grasp the implication of this? Then you see the accelerating threat to our future.

1) Colborn, OSF, 172-173.   2) Ibid, 140.   3) Ibid., 255.

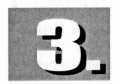

Dosed, doused, injected with death (poisons).

We take poisons (drugs) to keep us "well" and functioning.

Like the weakened produce and weakened farm animals, the humans are weakened also, from eating them. As with the produce and animals, because of our weakened state we are most vulnerable to disease. So like the dosed produce and animals, we heavily dose ourselves with poisons (drugs) to suppress symptoms of disease and keep our selves remaining functional, obedient, productive sheep, *sheeple*. In addition to being drugfood addicts, Americans have clusters of other addictions to tobacco, alcohol, crack, cocaine, sleeping pills, amphetamines. But that ain't enough. We go to *commercial* doctors (MDs who are legal drug pushers and servants of the deadly pharmaceutical [*drug*] companies) and get *shot* ...shot up with more drugs.

> Dosage and intent are the only differences between drugs and poisons.

Adverse Drug-Reactions is the 4th top cause of death in the U.S.

(–after heart disease, cancer & stroke).[1] And another 2.2 million people have serious, non-fatal reactions. Prescribed hospital drugs are so toxic they kill over 137,000 Americans every year. Outside the hospitals, the death toll from the same drugs is undoubtedly much higher, but is frequently unreported or listed simply as heart failure.[2] In hearings before Rep. Elton Gallegly on 18 February 1994, Mitchell Zeller of the FDA coolly announced that the number of deaths in America from "normal" uses of prescription drugs is an estimated 150,000 per year. That's an obscene 900,000 deaths between 1985 and 1990. Publicly, the FDA keeps very quiet about these figures, because they approved the prescription drug use in the first place.[3]

The American Death Game

It starts with a single simple aspirin for a simple headache. When one aspirin no longer masks the headache, pop two. Next use a stronger drug. By now you need to take something for the ulcers caused by the aspirin. This medication will disrupt your liver. If an infection develops, take penicillin. That will stop infections just starting, while damaging the spleen and red blood cells so that anemia develops. Hide the symptoms with sulfa drugs, unaware that your kidneys are breaking down. You can go a long time this way. By now the medications will be so confused, they won't know what they're supposed to be doing. It matters not. If you follow every step as outlined, you can make an appointment with your undertaker. This is the game most Americans play, except for the few ignorant ones who go back to Nature.

1) New Life Magazine, July/Aug 89.   2) Colgan, NN, 51.   3) Ibid., 108 .

America, home of the drugged (self-poisoned)

● Besides *tap water*, another way Americans are unknowingly being kept drugged is by all the *"enriched"* bread /commercial foods they eat, "enriched" with synthetic, lab-made substances deceptively labled *vitamins*. In reality, they are not foods but *chemicals* that are harmful drugs. Outright drugs are made from the same coal-tar as the "vitamins."

● Americans are the most medicated people in the world; each year swallowing billions of doses of therapeutic pills, powders, capsules, and elixirs. An estimated 13 billion barbiturate and amphetamine pills ("speed") are taken annually by Americans.

● Over 50 million aspirins are taken *daily* in America. This amounts to 40 million pounds (20,000 tons) yearly.

● Nearly every American has been subjected to narcotic drugs by their physicians or commonly sold nostrums they've been induced to buy, notably the analgesics, opium based drugs (cough medicines) and amphetamines, barbiturates, etc.

● Over 200 million Americans are hooked on one or more drug habits. The drugs of most frequent use are sugar, salt, caffeine (in coffee, soft drinks), nicotine, alcohol, aspirin, theine (in tea), theobromine (in cocoa and chocolate) and distilled vinegar. Over 100 million Americans drink alcohol, a narcotic drug, with over 13 million being alcoholics. Over 100 million narcotize themselves with cigarettes or other narcotic products.

Brain & MELANIN-damage from neuroleptic drugs

A million Americans have brain damage from neuroleptic drugs such as Thorazine and Moban. All neuroleptics can and do cause brain damage. Neuroleptics (for treatment of psychosis) bind to and chemically react with Melanin due to structural similarities.[1] Carol Barnes documents the harmful effects of drugs on Melanin centers within the Black Human in his book: *Melanin: The Chemical Key to Black Greatness*.

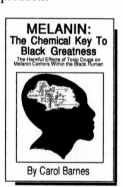

MELANIN:
The Chemical Key To
Black Greatness
The Harmful Effects of Toxic Drugs on
Melanin Centers Within the Black Human

By Carol Barnes

"Study Says Hospitals Give Blacks More Drugs, Less Time Than Whites"

That was the title of an article in the San Francisco Chronicle (5/20/96), where we read: *"Citing results of a five-year study, a Berkeley professor is charging that mentally ill black patients are being overmedicated with anti-psychotic drugs at county hospital emergency rooms. ...Inattention by mostly white hospital staffers, he contends, and the race of the individual patients played a role in determining why black patients were prescribed more drugs than whites, Latinos or Asian Americans in the same study. ....Segal and his team concluded that white psychiatric clinicians spent significantly less time with African American patients than with patients of other races* [and] *were more likely to prescribe anti-psychotic drugs to blacks and were giving blacks significantly higher dosages of anti-psychotic drugs."*

1) Barnes, MCK, 86.

Our helpless children are being legally drugged

School children are legally forced to take drugs

Ritalin, a cheap form of speed (methylphenidate), is the main means used to control "hyperactive" children in schools. To justify the use of this drug, the term ADD (Attention Deficit Disorder, a bogus syndrome) was coined. Ritalin has increased 97% in use since 1985. In 1996 it was prescribed to over 3 million schoolchildren. Students are forced to take the drug or face expulsion.[1] Ritalin makes drug addicts. Ritalin can cause depression, tremors, hyperactivity, withdrawal symptoms, cancer, cysts, and liver tumors. It is wrongly prescribed when environmental toxins are the actual cause of behavioral problems. Health-wise parents have discovered that cutting out "refined" sugar /starches /foods from their children's diet, and feeding them organically grown wholefoods usually solves the hyperactivity problem.

Foster children as young as 3 are being routinely drugged

Following are excerpts from an article entitled *"Caretakers Routinely Drug Foster Children,"* in the Los Angeles Times (5/17/98, A1, A30):

Children under state protection in California group and foster homes are being drugged with potent, dangerous psychiatric medications, at times just to keep them obedient and docile for their overburdened caretakers. ...A review of hundreds of confidential court files and prescription records, observations at group homes as well as interviews with judges, attorneys, child welfare workers and doctors across the state, revealed that youngsters are being drugged in combinations and dosages that experts in psychiatric medication say are risky — and can cause irreversible harm. ...Many child psychiatrists, attorneys and children's advocates say the apparently widespread practice of drugging amounts to a form of medical experimentation on some of the state's most vulnerable kids—those taken from parents who abused them. ..In many instances, the doctors who prescribe what their colleagues call "chemical straitjackets" aren't psychiatrists and have little training in the highly specialized field of psychiatric medications. ...An estimated 800,000 children and adolescents nationwide last year were prescribed antidepressants such as Prozac, Paxil and Zoloft, according to IMS America, an industry research firm that surveys physicians. Another half a million children, aged 6 to 12, were prescribed Tegretol and Depakote, two adult anti-manic, antiseizure drugs... And in 1996 some 3.25 million in that age group were prescribed drugs such as Ritalin to control hyperactivity... A lot of these kids suffer from *a deficit in attention*, not attention deficit disorder... If we were to get more one-on-one with these kids over a longer period of time... they wouldn't need all those meds." ...Under the influence of such drugs, children have suffered from drug-induced psychoses, hallucinations, abnormal heart activity, uncontrollable tremors, liver problems and loss of bowel control, according to health professionals, attorneys and court records...These drugs can result in a toxic reaction, either something that makes the child really sick or ...makes the kid dead," said Dr. Chadwick from the Center for Child Protection in San Diego.

1) Valerian 0280.

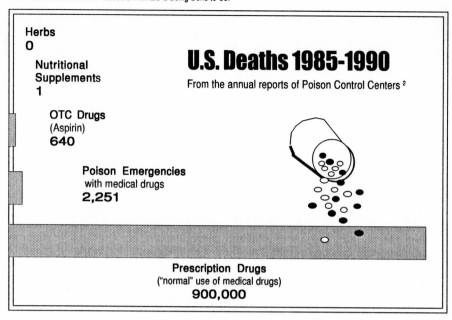

U.S. Deaths 1985-1990

From the annual reports of Poison Control Centers [2]

Herbs
0

Nutritional
Supplements
1

OTC Drugs
(Aspirin)
640

Poison Emergencies
with medical drugs
2,251

Prescription Drugs
("normal" use of medical drugs)
900,000

Drugs don't heal; they only suppress symptoms, lower your vitality, and destroy vitamins & nutrients

Drugs form chemical unions that paralyze nerves, destroy cells, suspend vital action, thus causing symptoms of disease to disappear. The person so treated is sicker than before, though appearing and perhaps feeling better. **Every action performed by the body in defense against drugs weakens it!** Drugs which have a stimulant rather than narcotic action goad the body into extraordinary eliminative activity; but this exhausts an already exhausted body, resulting in the person being worse off than before. <u>**Our body cannot be poisoned into health!**</u> All healing that takes place after the administration of drugs does so in spite of the drugs, not because of them. Medical doctors are legal drug pushers; servants of the Controllers via the AMA, drug companies, etc. **When such doctors go on strike, the death rate drops about 50%!** Over a million people are annually killed by doctors.

Most drugs also interfere with normal enzyme and vitamin action in the body, causing derangement in metabolism and vital body processes.[2] Many drugs damage the liver, kidneys and can cause serious diseases, including impotence, infertility, birth defects and cancer.[3] Results of the liberal use of antibiotics and cortisone includes widespread yeast disorders and immunity, resistance to medicines, and immunity to penicillin. **AZT, the central drug prescribed for AIDS,** terminates DNA synthesis in the body. It also attacks the bone marrow, where immune-system cells are manufactured, and so creates the symptoms of AIDS.

1) Colgan, NN, 107-108.   2) Airola, HGW, 175-6.   3) Ibid.

Of course, there are situations in which drugs are necessary and can be life-saving. But drugs should be used only in absolute emergencies, and only if ordered by a competent doctor.

Drugs aggressively destroy vital vitamins and minerals and/or prevent their absorption. Examples:

- **Medical literature itself admits that** *aspirin* causes a greater amount of disease than it cures and is even responsible for its own unique and potentially fatal disease: *Reye's Syndrome.* Thousands die of aspirin each year. Strokes (cerebral hemorrhage) can even result from taking aspirin, since it weakens the blood vessel walls of the brain. For every aspirin tablet consumed, the body loses several million molecules of beta carotene, selenium, essential fatty acids, and vitamins C, E, K.[1]

- *High-blood-pressure medications* promote potassium deficiency because it causes large quantities of precious potassium to leak into the urine. Physicians attempt to minimize this by prescribing potassium-sparing diuretics. But the diuretics themselves (thiazide diuretics, Diazide, chlorothiazide, etc.) aggressively deplete tissue stores of potassium,[2] hence are linked with "sudden death syndrome."

- **The drug of** *cigarette smoke* **consumes /destroys vitamin C in the body at a more rapid rate than it can be consumed.**[3] A pack wipes out some 700 mg: three packs, 2000 mg. Thus, smokers suffer from "totally negative Vitamin C status," a very dangerous condition which leaves one vulnerable to lung infections, liver diseases, cancer, blood vessel fragility, emphysema and many other disorders.

- **In commercial foods,** *additives* **and** *pesticides*, which are poisons /toxins / drugs themselves, also destroy nutrients. The preservatives BHT and BHA destroy vitamins A, E, C. Sulfites oxidize /destroy vitamins A, E, C, B12, molybdenum, riboflavin, and folic acid. Food dyes inactivate vitamins C, B6, and folic acid. Pesticide residues destroy vitamins C, E, B6, digestive enzymes, selenium, etc. Chlorine inactivates thiamine, destroys vitamins.

Drugs cannot act on the body; the body acts on drugs.

As noted by one doctor: *"Drugs and serums do not and cannot act on the body. They are dead matter, and dead matter is powerless to act. ..It is the body that acts, and not the drug, serum, or body waste. It is the danger inherent in the poisonous nature of these things that prompts the body to act. The action is in self-defense, and is produced by a calling out of the body's reserve forces; just as the danger of the enemy prompted the man to act in self-defense, and struggle until his strength was exhausted. The effects of the abnormal action is beating heart, throbbing brain, rapid respiration, profuse perspiration, vomiting, diarrhoea, skin eruptions, fevers, etc. The nature and locality of the symptoms is what determine the name the physicians give them, and that*

1) Igram, STN, 131.   2) Ibid.   3) Ibid., 5.

is incidental and immaterial. The more poisonous any substance is, the more dangerous it is, and the quicker and harder the body acts– sending a large dose of salts or castor oil through the alimentary canal with a rush. Such treatment, instead of its being curative, is destructive; for it is a terrible shock to the nervous system, and may be continued until the body will utterly collapse from the exhaustion induced by its own violent efforts of self-protection." [1]

Vaccines, inoculations, immunizations = getting poisoned

I knew vaccines were bad for people but I was appalled to find out just how bad. In *Epidemic*, Keidi Obi Awadu –*The Conscious Rasta*, summarizes information about the horrors of vaccination and how they are causing epidemics of diseases upon our children. Vaccination /Inoculation / Immunization (three words for the same thing) is part of the war against us, keeping us unhealthy and diminished. **Vaccines are time-release poisons** which often cause crippling, if not fatal disease later in life. **Childhood vaccination is mandatory in many states.** If American parents knew the truth about vaccination, they would unite to remove this deadly, anti-life practice from America's school system. **Vaccines actually <u>cause us to become genetic mutants</u> because they are made with genetic material from animals –plus outright toxins and decaying matter– injected into our blood!**[2]

Ghastly lethal poisons in vaccines

Carcinogenic and toxic chemicals used as deactivators and carriers of vaccine material are: **aluminum** (a neuro-toxin associated with Alzheimer's disease, dementia & seizures), **thimerosal** (a sodium salt derived from deadly mercury; thimerosal has been linked to brain and kidney damage, immune and neurological disorders; it is a component of vaccines for DPT, tetanus, hepatitis B and Hib), **methylene glycol** (antifreeze), **formaldehyde** (embalming fluid, a cancer-causing chemical shown to be injurious to the liver and to trigger gene mutations), **carbolic acid** (a deadly poison used as a disinfectant), **antibiotics** (Neomycin, Streptomycin and other drugs), **acetone** (a solvent used in fingernail polish remover), and traces of other **toxic chemicals** (sodium hydroxide, sorbitol, benzethonium chloride, methylparaben...).[3] The Hepatitis-A vaccine is made from human feces.

Overview of vaccine wickedness

In *Matrix III*, Valerian informs us:[4] "The term 'immunization' was derived from the [Albino] belief that the injection of a foreign body of infection into the human system (which already possesses a natural immune system) will confer life-long immunity from a specific disease. The word immunization is synonymous with the word inoculation. Despite this belief, there has always existed the observation that immunizations cause disease, and it is considered heresy in the medical community to make mention of this fact.

1) Clements, LLH, 42.   2 Awadu, E, 10.   3) Ibid., 9, 10.   4) Valerian, 0165-0166.

"Immunizations also are responsible, according to some medical experts, for many health problems. Dr. Herbert Snow, senior surgeon at the Cancer Hospital of London, once stated that immunization or inoculation causes permanent disease to the heart ... In the March 4, 1977 issue [of Science], researchers ... warned that, 'Live virus vaccines against influenza or poliomyelitis may in each instance produce the disease it intended to prevent... the live virus against measles and mumps may produce such side effects as encephalitic (brain damage). ...In the magazine Health Freedom News, July /August 1986, an article noted that 'Vaccine is linked to brain damage....At the annual AMA Convention in 1955, the Surgeon General of the United States, Leonard Scheele, said that 'no batch of vaccine can be proven safe before it is given to children.' James R. Shannon of the National Institute of Health declared that the only safe vaccine is a vaccine that is never used.'

"In the United States and many other countries, there are compulsory immunization programs for children. Because of the financial prospects, physicians are asking that children be vaccinated earlier in their lives. It is no small coincidence that the agencies responsible for the promotion of immunizations, such as the CDC, FDA, AMA and the WHO are also involved with the large drug firms who make it their business to treat the diseases the vaccines cause. It is also these same agencies that have drafted the procedures which forced the states to enact compulsory immunization legislation."

Horrid "side effects" of vaccines

As documented in *Immunizations: The People Speak!*, by Neil Z. Miller:
"The following conditions have each been investigated as a consequence of, or have been scientifically confirmed as resulting from, one or more of the vaccines: fever, rashes, itching, bruises, headache, pain, soreness, sore throat, inflamed sinuses, swelling, diarrhea, projectile vomiting, excessive sleepiness, inconsolable crying, high-pitched screaming, tics, tremors, seizures, collapse, convulsions, anaphylactic shock, loss of consciousness, breathing problems, cranial nerve palsies, encephalitis, grand mal epilepsy, neurological disorders, weak muscles, paralysis, polio, aseptic meningitis, epiglottitis, multiple sclerosis, Reye's syndrome, Guillain-Barre syndrome, chronic fatigue syndrome, sudden infant death syndrome (SIDS), blood-clotting disorders, urinary and abdominal complications, juvenile-onset diabetes, pneumonia, liver abnormalities, arthralgia, rheumatoid arthritis, unilateral nerve deafness, polyneuritis, measles, atypical measles, pertussis, mumps, meningitis, inner-ear nerve damage, recurrent abscess formation, demyelinating neuropathy, EEG abnormalities, dyslexia, visual defects, hearing loss, speech impediments, T-lymphocyte blood count reductions, haemophilus influenza, influenza, smallpox, AIDS, cancer, leukemia, lupus erythematosus, genetic mutations, autoimmune disorders, autism, childhood schizophrenia, brain tumors, developmental disabilities, learning disorders, hyperactivity disorder, juvenile delinquency, drug abuse, alcoholism, violent crime, mental retardation, brain damage, and death."   [!!!]

And tobacco is the safest, healthiest ingredient in cigarettes.

It's mainly the other stuff in cigarettes that is killing people. **Nicotine** is but one of some 18 or more poisons taken into the system when smoking is indulged. Ingredients in cigarettes, as disclosed by Canadian /British suppliers, include: [1]

- **shellac**   • **acetone**   • **turpentine**
- **acetaldehyde** and **glyocal** (animal carcinogens)
- **methyl aslicylate** (causes birth defects in hamsters)
- **licorice root** containing **glycyrrhizic acid** (produces cancer-causing polycyclic aromatic hydrocarbons when burned)
- **catechol** (carcinogenic by-product of heated sugars used for flavoring)
- **other additives** that strengthen the effect of cancer-causing compounds when heated

The list of additives in American brands is filed in the Department of Health and Human Services and protected from public scrutiny by criminal penalties against anyone disclosing it.[2]

Other deadly ingredients in cigarettes:

- Large amounts of **benzene /hydrogen cyanide**. The latter is considered dangerous at levels of 10 ppm; the concentration in cigarette smoke is 1,600 ppm.[3]
- **Sugar**: the addition of sugar to tobacco creates a carcinogenic substance within the nicotine tar.[4]
- **Opium** (added to the cigarette paper): "Since a small amount of this substance can be highly addictive, it explains why hand rolled tobacco using other types of paper does not satisfy the craving that regular cigarettes do." [5]
- **Gunpowder**, added to the paper to make the it burn evenly.
- **Radiation** (see page 62). **Cadmium,** a very toxic heavy metal.
- Every puff starts a chain reaction leading to **nitrosamine** formation (potent carcinogen) within the lungs, liver, digestive tract, tissues. Heavy smoking also makes one crave toxic meat, another (indirect) source of nitrosamines.

Healthy ways to help stop unhealthy smoking

- *Doctah B's Incredible Herbal Stop-Smoking Formula.* Non addictive. You smoke it and drink a tea. Habit is gone within a month. (213) 427-8419.
- A homeopathic solution called *Nico-Stop* with a money-back guarantee. By Lehning Laboratories; distributed by Enzymatic Therapy. 1-800-783-2286.
- Take an **Epsom salt bath** with 1/2 pound of the salts. This pulls nicotine and tar from the skin. Shower afterward and dry off with a white towel. The brownish residue on the towel from nicotine excreted by the skin enforces desire to stop smoking.[6]
- **Aversion therapy:** Stop smoking except for 1 hour daily. Smoke constantly during that hour. Take 15 drops of **lobelia tincture** 1/2 hour before the 1st cigarette and again at 15 minutes before the last cigarette. Take the same quantity of lobelia every 15 minutes during remainder of the smoking hour. This produce nausea. Its association with smoking can eliminate desire for cigarettes in just 5-6 days.
- **Fasting**. Also, chewing on a piece of **licorice root** is helpful.

1) Valerian, 0151.   2) Ibid.   3) Anderson, YH, 91.   4) Valerian, 0150.   5) Ibid., 0153.   6) Burton, 823.

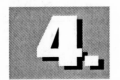

Half DEAD and DYING faster, from being cooked 24 hours a day in harmful EMF radiations.

You are being irradiated every single day, 24 hours a day, 7 days a week with harmful ELFs (EMFs). You literally live in a sea of harmful ELFs /EMFs! "Extremely Low Frequencies" are the same thing as Electromagnetic Frequencies" or electromagnetic radiation. ELFs/EMFs radiate from every single electrical item or appliance in your environment:

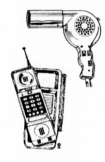

• watches	• TVs	• all electrical outlets
• radios	• computers	• washing machines
• stereos	• telephones	• electric heaters
• headsets	• beepers	• cellular phones
• vibrators	• power lines	• electric blankets, pads
• clocks	• electric lights	• wires/cables of any kinds
• hairdryers	• microwave ovens	• electric system in cars, etc.

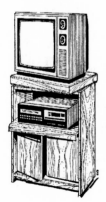

Thus, your biomagnetic field is constantly being irradiated / slowly cooked with ELFs /EMFs. Most of the electromagnetic spectrum is already known to be injurious to health (microwaves, X-rays, gamma rays, ultraviolet rays, etc.). From just X-rays alone, an estimated more than 45,000 fatal cancers are induced each year.[1] And cobalt therapy cooks the flesh, ensuring the cancer patient's death. All living creatures are sensitive to electrical, electromagnetic and magnetic influences. Just because most of us do not perceive these energies does not mean that they are not affecting our essential life functions. EMFs are continuously disrupting our body's own bio-magnetic field, within which millions of electrical impulses *regulate the activity of every single cell.* With electrical and magnetic energy reaching us from power lines and cabling, microwave radar and communications, TV and radio broadcasting, industrial and domestic electromagnetic devices, it is estimated that **we are getting 200 million times more radiation than our ancestors** took in from the sun and cosmic sources. **ELF fields exist wherever electricity flows and are thus virtually unavoidable.** At frequencies below 300 hertz, electrical and magnetic fields behave independently: *electrical fields show little penetration through body tissues, while magnetic fields penetrate the body readily.*[2]

1) Cousens, CE, 384.   2) Valerian, 0393.

Why is electromagnetic radiation (ELFs /EMFs) harmful?

- **Alters permeability of the blood brain barrier.** The blood brain barrier is the body's special defense mechanism that prevents foreign substances from entering the brain.
- **"Bodily functions most affected are those which are most active at night**: electrical meridians that regulate the liver, gallbladder, lungs and large intestine. During sleep, the normal detoxification process is blocked by electromagnetic (EM) stress on those meridians. In order to reduce EM effects it is necessary to consider eliminating current from appliances in the bedroom, including electric blankets, waterbed heaters and clock radios."[1]
- **Proliferates disease.** Disrupts motor functions.
- **Alters the behavior of cells**, tissues, organs, and organisms.[2]
- **Alters hormone levels**, cellular chemistry, and immune system processes.[3]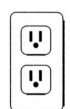
- **Alters time-perception** in animals and humans.[4]
- **Can rupture cellular structure.**[5]
- **Causes sterility.**[6] **Causes defects**, developmental abnormalities and alterations in embryos.[6, 11] Accelerates fetal mortality rates.[6]
- **Entrainment** of human and animal brainwaves, and the DNA transaction process.[6]
- **Cause cataracts** and eye problems.[7]
- **Create fatigue, depression**, fear, and disorientation.[8]
- **Alter moods**, cause memory loss.[9]
- **Impinges on the pineal gland**, suppressing its production of the hormone melatonin. This can cause the liver to be unable to achieve its proper nighttime detoxification mode.[10]
- **Increases rate of cancer-cell division**; increases incidences of certain cancers. [11]
- **Alterations in neurochemicals** resulting in behavioral abnormalities such as suicide. [11]
- **Alterations in biological cycles.** [11]
  Stress responses in exposed animals that, if prolonged, lead to declines in immune-system efficiency. [11]
- **Alterations in learning ability.** [11]
- **Can cause chromosomal damage.**[12]
- **Miscarriage is much higher** among pregnant women who use electric blankets than those who do not.[13]

---

1) Anderson, YH, 37.   2) Valerian, 0301.   3) Ibid., 0301.   4) Ibid., 0301.   5) Ibid.   6) Ibid.   7) Ibid., 0302.   8) Ibid.   9) Ibid.   10) Anderson, YH, 42, 43.   11) Ibid., 36.   12) Davidson, 113.   13) Becker, 269.

- **"Using an electric razor** regularly may boost a man's risk of developing leukemia because the razors are used on the facial skin near to the pineal gland in the brain. It is speculated that the magnetic field might suppress the pineal gland's production of a hormone believed to help the body protect itself against cancer."[1]
- **A pulsating low-intensity EMF** (one that's cycling on /off) will cause a release of noradrenaline in most people within 15 minutes. This may result in increased hospital admissions during times of magnetic disturbance.[2]
- **Adversely affects the energy-meridians of the body.** Example: a man who developed a chronic foot inflammation (which responded to no treatments) discovered his beeper to be the cause. He always wore his beeper on his left side, on the same acupuncture meridian of his foot. The inflammation disappeared only when he stopped wearing the beeper. "When a much stronger field is superimposed, it can block the flow of the meridian, resulting in energy imbalances, functional disturbances and toxicity buildup. Over longer periods of time, clinical disease is the result."[3]

And ELFs /EMFs from overhead power lines:

- **Causes leukemia:** Studies in America, England, and Sweden show that leukemia and other cancers increases greatly among people living near overhead power cables. After extensive studies showing the bad effects (leukemia, especially) of EMFs on over 500,000 people living near power lines for over 25 years, the government of Sweden now lists EMFs, along with tobacco, as a Class 2 Carcinogen. A study in Portland, Oregon discovered that neighborhoods with the highest levels of FM radiation also had the highest rates of leukemia.[4] Leukemia is higher among amateur radio operators than among the general population
- **A study in Sweden** involving half a million people concluded that living near power lines increased the leukemia rate in children by about four times over normal incidence. In adults, cancers were one and a half to three times more likely to occur. A study of 252 leukemia cases in Denver, Colorado also linked power lines to childhood cancers.[6]
- **A Boston University researcher** claims that people who say they live near transmission lines are twice as likely to show symptoms of depression as those who do not.[7]
- **A Syracuse hospital** reported that plant growth is stunted as far away as 1,000 feet from power lines.
- **As far away as 1,000 feet from power lines,** "behavioral effects, like decreases in human reaction time, are observed, and people living closer than that distances had changes in their blood chemistry and electrocardiograms."[8]

1) Anderson, YH, 41.   2) Ibid., 43.   3) Ibid., 41.
4) Becker, 28.   5) Ibid., 218.   6) Anderson, YH, 38, 39.   7) Ibid., 39.   8) Ibid.

Why is artificial light harmful?

- **Cause disorders** ranging from lack of vitality to lowered resistance to disease, and hyperactivity. Can lead to aggressive behavior, heart disease and even cancer.[1] The body cannot handle this intervention in a natural human relationship with the environment any more than it can handle albino drugfood, chemical additives, pesticides, etc. The body breaks down on the cellular level.
- **In a typical study, children in school** under the standard cool white fluorescent lighting demonstrated nervous fatigue, irritability, lapses of attention, and hyperactive behavior. Within a week after new fullspectrum lights were installed, the children's behavior greatly improved.[2]
- **Too much artificial fluorescent light** interferes with the natural development of the child and subjects the nervous system of the adult to inordinate stress.[3]

Why is artificial light /radiation from television harmful?

- **Television is fluorescent;** the mechanism by which it illuminates is almost identical with fluorescent lighting. Thus, the harmful effects of fluorescent light (as described by Ott in *Health and Light*) is directly applicable to television.[4]
- **Television /Microwave towers:** The Federal Communications Commission (FCC) emissions figures from TV towers show that the radiation level within a one-mile radius of a major TV broadcasting tower can be ten times higher than the limit the former Soviet Union considered safe for its citizens.[5]
- **TV set radiation** caused rat litters, which usually contained 8-12, to drop off to 1-2, and many simply did not survive.[6]
- **Hyperactivity in children** has been directly linked to radiation from TV (and fluorescent light), to which children are especially susceptible.[7]
- **The** *flicker* **from TV sets can cause epileptic seizures.**[8] You do not consciously perceive the *flickering* of your TV screen because the flicker rate is higher than the "flicker-fusion" rate of the human eye. Whether you perceive it or not, your body reacts to it and is affected by it.[9]
- When female rats were regularly exposed to TV radiation before and after pregnancy, their growth rates diminished and the weights of their fetuses were greatly reduced.[10]
- When male rats were exposed for 35-50 days to TV sets, it reduced the size of their testicles, slowed their growth, and affected the functions of their brains.[11]

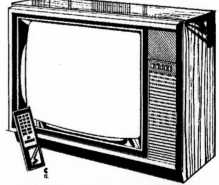

1) Mander, FA, 178. 2) Ott, HL, 203. 3) Ott, LR, 20. 4) Mander, FA, 172, 179 . 5) Anderson,YH, 43. 6) Ott, HL, 133. 7) Ibid., 135. 8) Ibid., 131. 9) Mander, FA, 192. 10) Becker, 273. 11) Ibid., 273

Why is artificial light /radiation from computers harmful?

- Health problems associated with computer use include **miscarriages, birth defects, cataracts and other vision problems, fatigue, skin rashes, headaches, nausea, and sleeplessness.**[1]
- The International Journal of Cancer, May 1992, published a study that found an almost **fivefold increase in brain tumors** among women who worked at VDT's (computer terminals /visual display terminals).[2]
  - **Causes miscarriages**: A huge proportion of miscarriages and embryonic deformities occur among pregnant women working on computers.[3] In a study done on a group of 1,583 pregnant women, the miscarriage rate of computer users was twice that of non-computer users.[4] A 1988 study found a double rate of miscarriage among women using computers more than 30 hours per week.[5]

Sunlight is a primal element of life. Artificial light is *druglight*.

All life originates and develops under the influence of *Sunlight*. Sunlight influences the vital processes of all plants, animals, and humans. There is a concrete relationship between light and our bodies. **Light is food.** And food, really, is condensed Sunlight. "Food" originally started out as light. We eat light for nourishment and growth. Humans eat light through their skin, eyes, and the antennae of their *hair*, a process made possible by *Melanin*, the receiver of all wavelengths of light and energy. Melanin is the chlorophyll of HUE-mans. Like plants, we soak up and transmute Sunlight nutrient into our energy system.

Natural Sunlight is composed of all the radiant wavelengths of energy (spectra) that we call "light." Artificial light from any source –whether incandescent or fluorescent– is fractionated light which leaves out many segments of the spectral range in natural light (Sunlight). For example, incandescent light emphasizes the spectrum portion near the infrared while minimizing or leaving out others. The body can be seriously affected by changes in light spectra. In his research, John Ott found that differences in cancer rates resulted from differences in light sources. Pink fluorescent light produced the highest rates of cancer in rats; natural daylight produced the lowest.[6] Other light changes cause aggressiveness, hyperactive behavior, aimlessness, disorientation, and changes in sexual patterns among animals.[7]

1) *Terminal Shock*, by R. DeMatteo.   2) Anderson, YH, 39.   3) Davidson, SE, 112.
4) Becker, 276.   5) Anderson, YH, 39.   6) Mander, FA, 174.   7) Ibid., 175.

There is a link between light and human health.

Your health is largely dependent upon your exposure to natural Sunlight kissing your skin and entering your eyes. If there is drugfood, then there is *druglight*. **Artificial light is *druglight*!** Like drugfood, *druglight* harms our health on all levels. Artificial light is inferior to natural light – like toxic drugfood is inferior to natural living wholefood. Like drugfood, some druglight is more harmful than others.

Since life evolved under the influence of Sunlight, humanity has developed many physiological responses to solar light. Our exposure to artificial light (*druglight*) has harmful effects of which we are not aware. **Spending most of our time indoors under *druglight* is very unhealthy,** for *druglight* is fractionated, thus unbalanced. Everyone needs daily exposure to full-spectrum Sunlight. Apparently, TV light (hard-druglight equivalent to hard drugfood) has been a surrogate light source, satisfying our need for light, but in the wrong way, a destructive way.

Ott explains the connection between eye-received light and our cell structure: Light passes via neurochemical channels into and through the pineal and pituitary glands and therefore into the animal and human endocrine systems. This interaction affects hormonal structures, sexuality, fertility, growth and many other aspects of cell structure. **The KIND of light passing through the eyes** determine the reactions of human cells. Experiments on plants and animals demonstrate that even minute changes in "color" (wavelength spectra), say, between one kind of artificial light and another, or between natural light and artificial light, cause important biochemical alterations.[1] Books about light written by white people (all whites are albinos) have an obvious prejudice; they OMIT discussing *Melanin*, especially in regards to Sunlight hitting the *SKIN*. Since white people have a serious obvious Melanin-deficiency, the importance of light in regards to the *skin* and *Melanin* is rarely or barely addressed by white authors. Instead, they emphasize the significance of light passing through the EYES.

Yes, light is food. Artificial light is adverse food.

We are eating the wrong kind of food (drugfood of varying degrees) and the wrong kind of light (druglight or artificial light). The type of light we are exposed to (hence, ingest) affects many aspects of our health and vitality. This is especially true for the Black Human and Melanated People. As you change the light, you change the spectra / light-nourishment that finds its way to the cells; as you alter cells you alter the human body.

1) Mander, FA, 175.

Why is Microwave Radiation harmful?

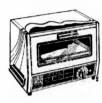

Microwave systems operate at _billions_ of cps!

...while electrical power systems operate at 50-60 cps (cycles per second), just above the highest naturally occurring frequency of 30 cps.

Microwaves are high frequency electromagnetic waves that alternate in positive and negative directions, causing vibration of food molecules up to 2.5 billion times per second! This creates friction which produces heat. This also alters the structure of the food molecules, making the food far more toxic than regularly cooked food.

- **Causes brain tumors, cancer, and immune-system decline.** Between 1940-1977, there was an unprecedented increase in the use of microwaves. During this period, the incidence of primary brain tumors among American-Afrikans rose from 2.15 to 3.85 per 100,000, and among European Americans from 3.80 to 5.80 per 100,000. A 1985 U.S. Navy study also showed that microwaves cause brain tumors; radar operators had a significantly higher rate of brain tumors than navy personnel who were not exposed.[1] Children of fathers employed in occupations with EMF-field exposure have a high risk of developing brain cancer before the age of two.[2]

- **Causes cancer in lab animals,** especially cancer of the pituitary, thyroid and adrenal glands. Because stress resistance is connected with these glands, we must conclude that microwave exposure produce an very high levels of stress.[3]

- **Microwave communications** systems are a vast health hazard threat, described in _Zapping America_, by Paul Brodeur.

- **"exposure to micro-waves** ...produces stress, a decline in immune-system competency, and changes in the genetic apparatus. Thus, the levels of exposure that the government says are 'safe' are in fact not safe at all."[4]

- **When located near microwave relay towers,** farm animal productivity diminishes: dairy herds located within two miles of microwave relay tower produced way less milk; chickens produce a fraction of their usual egg quota.[5]

- **Implicated as a cause of cataracts.**[6]

- **Connected with developing Alzheimer's disease.**[7]

Microwaved Food

- **Microwaving food alters the structure of the food molecules** and can cause chemical changes beyond those associated with being exposed to heat.[8]

- **Among findings of a German study** of blood samples of people fed microwaved food: 1) drop in lymphocytes and rise in leukocyte counts, hence **the body was responding to the food as if it were an infectious agent.** 2) pathological changes in the blood and body cells. 3) rise in lipoprotein levels (measures of cholesterol). 4) radiation levels of light-emitting bacteria were highest in those consuming microwaved food, suggesting that the energy had been transferred from food to subject.[9] **(also see page 25)**

- **In the blood chemistry of persons eating microwaved food,** major changes occur, similar to people with cancer.

1) Becker, 199.   2) Ibid., 200.   3) Valerian, 0290. 4) Becker, 200.   5) Ott, HL, 135.
6) Anderson, YH, 38. 7) Ibid./Valerian, 0142.   8) Burton, AM, 185.   9) Lifestyle News/Jan. 95.

Why is X-radiation harmful?

X-rays cause leukemia, cancer, birth defects, etc...

"**X-rays have been used and abused** indiscriminately by doctors, hospitals, dentists and chiropractors for decades, ignoring their great potential danger. X-rays are cumulative, so that even small amounts, such as those emitted from a color TV, a wristwatch or an alarm clock, can be dangerous as they add to the total amount received from all sources...Over exposure can cause leukemia, cancer, birth defects and a later development of leukemia in a child born of a mother who received abdominal x-rays during pregnancy."[1]

There is no "safe" dose of radiation since radiation is cumulative. Consider these facts:*

- **Radiation is far more toxic than chemicals or pesticides.** Radioactive isotopes which concentrate in specific organs are very damaging because each electron emitted by a radioactive nucleus has several million electron volts of energy which is enough energy to disrupt millions of molecules in the living cell.

- **Longterm exposure** to low levels of radiation causes the most radiation damage to cells. It greatly increases the production of free radicals. In fact, this effect is 1000 times greater than from a single large exposure. (Free radicals are destructive, unbalanced molecules which accelerate aging, deteriorates the body, and causes cancer and other degenerative diseases.)

- **Low level radiation is 1000 or more times more damaging** to our health than estimated. This helps explain why leukemia and other cancers are occurring 100 to 1000 times more than the initially predicted rate at Hiroshima.

- **An estimated more than 45,000 fatal cancers** are induced yearly by X-rays.

- **Pregnant women endanger their unborn child** whenever they expose themselves to radiation (diagnostic X-rays, dental X-rays, chest X-rays, etc.). Their children have an increased risk of developing leukemia.

- **Radioactive isotopes** emit radiation as they decay. These isotopes have a long lifetime; Cesium-137 (used to irradiate our food) has a radioactive lifetime of 600 years. Accumulation of radioactive isotopes in vital organs creates the worst damage because it results in longterm exposure to a particular tissue.

- **Nuclear radiation is making Earth a planet of *mutants*.**

1) Airola, HGW, 174. 2) Cousens, CE, 385.
* From Chapter 26 of *Conscious Eating* by Dr. Gabriel Cousens

- **Cigarettes are a major source of self-induced radiation.** The pack-a-day smoker exposes themselves to the equivalent of **300 chest X-rays per year.**[1] Radium-226 is found in the phosphate fertilizers used for tobacco farming. When tobacco smoke is inhaled, its radioactive elements create alpha radiation exposure that is hundreds of times greater than naturally occurring background radiation.

Radiation-deranged food transfers its derangement directly to your cells

Studies at Cornell University showed that eating irradiated sugar can produce the same results as irradiation directly applied to the cell! "Scientists experimented with carrot tissue and coconut milk, both high in natural sugars. They bombarded them with cobalt 60, causing radiation-induced cell mutations in both foods. Morever, the chemicals produced by sugar breakdown in the [irradiated] foods were seen [to] transfer radiation effects into the cells of fruit flies, resulting in stunted growth and chromosome damage. All living cells contain sugar, the report emphasized, and human beings may suffer similar consequences from long-term consumption of irradiated food."[3]

Albino technology produces the main sources of excessive radiation:

All the sources of excessive radiation (except radon gas) are from Albino technology. The data is overwhelming that these are major threats to our health and safety:

1. Radioactive fallout from nuclear testing.
2. Major nuclear power plant accidents (such as Chernobyl). There were 2,974 accidents reported in 1985 alone.[4]
3. Unreported minor radioactive leakage from smaller mishaps at other nuclear plants.
4. Military nuclear activity, such as nuclear weapons plant site accidents, storage difficulties, & nuclear submarine accidents.
5. Accidents at sterilization & food irradiation facilities.
6. Routine leaks and emissions from common devices and products that use nuclear technology.
7. Radiation from medical radiation techniques such as X-rays, fluoroscopy, mammography and C.A.T. scans.
8. Cigarette smoking.

1) Cousens, CE, 38.   2) Ibid., 382.   3)Winter, PYF, 241.   4) Cousens, CE, 381-85

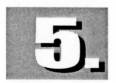

Processed, embalmed, treated with chemical poisons.

Would you spread your skin cream on a slice of bread and eat it? Or take a
hearty sip of your favorite perfume? A quick way to tell if a product is safe, ask:
"Is this safe to eat?" If the answer is NO, then it ain't safe. If you use it
anyway, you still *are* eating it *–through your skin,* toxins and all. Some of
everything you put *on* your skin or scalp goes *through* it into your bloodstream.

Personal-care products are *Poison*-care products

All the lotions, potions, creams, grease, soap, shampoo, bubble bath, shower gel,
toothpaste, mouthwash, deodorant, colognes, perfumes, cosmetics, sprays, and
water you bathe in –have outright chemical poisons brazenly composing them.
In just a single perfume scent alone, 600 chemicals may be used![1] Unknowingly
you use many harmful and even deadly products that you put on your face,
under your arms, between your legs, on your scalp, and in your mouth. The
majority of Afrikans and the rest of the unsuspecting American population
remain unwarned that **over 80% of products on the market today contain one
or more chemical ingredients that are documented to cause cancer or other
adverse reactions in humans and animals.** These beautifully packaged
products contain carcinogenic chemicals that are damaging your hair, teeth,
skin, scalp, brain, genitals, and making you age faster. Because of their higher
exposure to chemicals, hairdressers, manicurists and cosmetologists develop
multiple myeloma (cancer) at four times the rate of the general population.

Billions of pounds of chemicals are put in our foods & body products

Chemical behavior modifiers (drug formulas) were synthesized in Germany
under Hitler, and were part of the Nuremburg trial papers. Though not released
to the public, they were released /duplicated on the world trade market for
capital gain. In due course, they became known as preservatives and additives.[1]
A billion pounds of these drug toxins are added annually to commercial food
and all the other commercial products; soaps, toilet paper, toothpastes, mouth
washes, deodorants, disposable diapers, cosmetics, deodorized sanitary pads,
hair sprays, detergents, mineral oil, colognes, and all other synthetic products.
*"All drugs are addicting and alter the behavior and biochemical make-up of the
individual. The victim of the drug trade is the world population."*[2]

---

1) Steinman, LH, 129.   2) Afrika, AHH, 100.

Ten Common Toxic Chemicals in your Body-care Stuff

Read the ingredients of your body-care products, even "healthy" ones. You'll likely find several or all of the following chemicals. This is a list of just *ten* out of *tens-of-thousands* of toxic chemicals lurking in your body-care products:

Alcohol: As an ingredient in ingestible products, it causes body tissues to be more vulnerable to cancers. Mouthwashes with an alcohol content of 25% or more have been implicated in mouth, tongue, and throat cancers. Alcohol is a colorless, volatile, flammable liquid produced by fermenting yeast and starches. Is is also found in beverages and medicine.

Aluminum: A metallic element used in manufacturing aircraft components, prosthetic devices, and as an ingredient in deodorants (especially anti-perspirants), lipstick, face powder, vaginal douches, baking soda, antacids and antiseptics. Aluminum goes right to the brain, where it causes Alzheimer's Disease. It is cumulative in the brain tissues.

Collagen: An insoluble fibrous protein that is too large to penetrate the skin. The collagen found in most skin care products is derived from animal fat and ground up chicken feet. This ingredient forms a layer of film that suffocates the skin.

DEA: Readily absorbed through skin, DEA (diethanolamine) is a potentially cancer-causing chemical in shampoos, tooth-paste, bubble baths and many mainstream cosmetics. Reacts with nitrates in cosmetics to form other carcinogens.

Formaldehyde: A toxic, colorless, irritant, carcinogenic gas. When combined with water, formaldehyde is used as a disinfectant, fixative, or preservative of corpses in funeral homes. Found in many cosmetic products, nail care systems, and the clothes you wear. Formaldehyde is chemically bonded in fabrics to yield permanent press finishes added to clothing, sheets. Even when not stated on the label, all polyester /cotton-blend fabrics have formaldehyde finishes.

Lye: A highly concentrated watery solution of sodium hydroxide or potassium hydroxide. Lye is combined with animal fats to make bar soaps which corrode and dry out the skin. Lye is also the active ingredient in hair-relaxers, epidemically used by Afrikan women all over the world, victims of AANS (Acquired Anti-Nappy Syndrome). If only they knew that the same power that makes atoms spin and galaxies spiral is the same power causing their precious antennae ("hair") to SPIRAL out of their heads, giving them the super SPIRI-tual "hair of the gods."

Mineral Oil: A derivative of crude oil (petroleum) that is used industrially as a cutting fluid and lubricating oil. Forms an oily film over the skin to lock moisture, toxins and wastes, but hinders normal skin respiration by keeping oxygen out.

Petrolatum: A petroleum-based grease used industrially as a grease component. Petrolatum exhibits many of the same harmful properties as mineral oil. Around the world, Afrikans "grease" their "ashy" skin with toxic petroleum jelly (Vasoline, etc.) or "baby oil." A much healthier and non-toxic replacement is virgin olive oil.

Propylene Glycol: Called a humectant in cosmetics, it is really "industrial anti-freeze" and the major ingredient in brake and hydraulic fluid. It can be a strong skin irritant. Safety Sheets warn to avoid skin contact as it is systemic and can cause liver abnormalities and kidney damage.

Sodium Lauryl Sulfate (SLS) & Sodium Laureth Sulfate (SLES):

Found in most shampoos (including "health" varieties). Also in toothpaste, soap, perfume, deodorants. Both silently boost cancer rates in children and adults. They cause carcinogenic nitrates / dioxins to form in shampoos and cleansers by reacting with other product ingredients. Cancer is the #1 cause of death of American children and #2 cause of adult death. Large amounts of nitrates enter the blood system from just one shampooing. SLS is a harsh detergent and wetting agent used in garage floor cleaners, engine degreasers, and auto cleaning products. SLS is a skin irritant. It is rapidly absorbed and retained in the eyes, brain, heart, and liver, which results in harmful long-term effects. It retards healing, cause cataracts in adults, and keep children's eyes from developing properly. In fact, this carcinogen is the #1 cause of eyesight degeneration in children. SLES is the alcohol form (ethoxylated) of SLS.

Murderous mercury in your mouth.

The mercury in dental fillings is a serious health threat. It is largely mercury that makes pesticides so deadly. Some 200 million Americans have mercury fillings in their mouths. Amalgam fillings are typically composed of about 50% mercury and 35% silver, with the balance consisting of tin, copper and zinc. Mercury vapor is released from fillings during chewing or grinding or brushing teeth and is the most common source of mercury found in humans. **Reduced kidney function / kidney impairment** is one of the health problems caused by mercury. Mercury is retained in the kidneys, liver, and certain regions of the brain.[1]

Murderous fluoride in your toothpaste and water.

Most toothpastes contains fluoride, a lethal chemical sold as rat poison, responsible for over 45, 000 deaths each year. Tap water is a toxic, medicated, chemical soup which contains fluoride. Fluoride and its derivatives harms your health, making people more susceptible to cancer. Since fluoride increases dental problems, thus profits, the American Dental Association promotes the use of fluoride toothpastes!

The druglord-chemical corporations are killing us with their poisons and heavily charging us for it!

They reap phenomenal profits from our misfortunes, drugging us to death with an estimated 3.2 billion tons of deadly chemicals they collectively make each year in the U.S. alone. Examples: Ciba-Geigy does a $10 billion dollar a year business. And **the 4th leading cause of death in America is "adverse reactions" from prescription drugs**. An estimated 100 million Americans suffer a form of chronic illness – increasingly found to be caused by exposure to or ingestion of some chemical substance in food. Testing by the World Health Organization implicated environmental chemicals in 60-80% of all cancers. Read the chapter, "*America the Poisoned*" in John Robbin's *Diet for a New America* and learn the truth about your so-called food (and personal-care products). Ignorance of this information is not bliss but eventual death. This is how serious the problem is. If you are reading this, you are still alive and likely have a chance to save yourself. Just because these toxins have not accumulated in sufficient quantity to kill you now does not mean they won't get you eventually...unless you take protective counter-actions (detailed in the other two volumes of this book). **The top *drug* companies are also *chemical* companies** which manufacture lethal chemicals /drugs /pesticides /hormones /toxins that are killing everything including the planet. Yet the owners, presidents, staff and workers are never arrested or convicted for their ongoing deadly, mega, killer crimes against Humanity, including their own kind (Albinos). They are not even

1) Valerian, 0162.

restricted from making banned toxins. The biggest corporations include **Merck, Dupont, Bayer, Monsanto** (makers of DDT and parathion), **Ciba-Geigy** (makers of Ritalin), **Hoeschst, ICI**, and **Dow** (makers of Prozac – an anti-depressant, and styrofoam/styrene, which is produced with CFCs, a main gas destroying Earth's vital ozone layer. Styrofoam is a major source of styrene, a plastic chemical found in the flesh of literally in every American,[1] and is linked with a wide range of disorders; cancer, nervousness, nerve damage, fatigue, memory-loss).

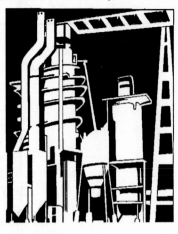

People of Color are specially targeted (covertly attacked) by these Killer Khemical Korporations (all Albinos)

Albinos have historically used drugs as key weapons in subduing, controlling, and exploiting Colored People around the world (crack against Blacks, alcohol against Native Americans, opium against Chinese...). And they haven't stopped, as proven by the CIA Crack-Cocaine exposé in the San Jose Mercury News (Aug. 18-20, 1996). These mega druglord-corporations continue making the most lethal of banned chemicals and sell them by the millions of pounds to the so-called "Third World" (Afrikans, People of Color). This is covert genocide (as noted on page 22). U.S. shipping records show that *"more than 58 million pounds of banned, suspended, never-registered, and restricted-use pesticides were exported in 1991 –a rate of nearly 80 tons per day."*[2] The U.S. company, **Vesicol**, sold and exported 3 million pounds of *Phosvel*, a lethal banned pesticide, to 30 Thirdworld countries, where it caused extensive damage to the nervous system in humans who consumed food that had been treated with it.[3] **Pfizer** *"withheld information from the FDA about Feldene...despite deaths and harmful side effects that occurred in other countries."* **Hoechst** marketed an analgesic, *chloromycetin*, found to cause anemia. It *"was banned in the U. S. so it was then sold in Latin America and Asia."*[4] And when white America sells toxic products like cigarettes /alcohol, to Thirdworld countries, the percentage of toxins in them are typically much higher than in the same brands sold in the U.S. As noted earlier, this also applies to Black neighborhoods (see page 44).

We are all under continuous assault from all directions

Commenting on his people's toxic society, the late Dr. Paavo Airola, a well known nutritionist, wrote: "We are all subjected to radioactive substances and hundreds of poisons and toxic chemicals every day of our lives. The air we breath, the foods we eat, the water we drink– even the clothes we wear and the beds we sleep on – all are filled with poisons that none of us can possibly avoid. Even those who most conscientiously and meticulously attempt to live poison-

---

1)Steinman, LH, 111. 2)FASE Reports, vl. 11 No. 1 Spring 93. 3)Rappoport, 53; Valerian, 0282. 4)Ibid., 0279.

free lives and eat only organically grown foods, are nevertheless subjected to many poisons. Even organically grown foods are grown in polluted air and are watered with polluted, chemicalized water. And the air, just about *anywhere* in the United States, is now seriously contaminated."[1]

How to protect ourselves from toxins?

This is detailed in the other two volumes of this book: *Unfood By The UnPeople*, and *Don't Worry, Be Healthy!* –a manual for achieving optimum health on a toxic planet. Additional details addressing other vital areas will be in the last volume (7) of *Blacked Out Through Whitewash.*

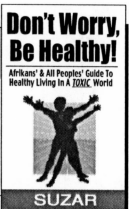

Don't Worry, Be Healthy!

Afrikans' & All Peoples' Guide To Healthy Living In A *TOXIC* World

SUZAR

All poisons, drugs, and drugfood "trap" your blood-proteins

You yell or cuss, having just bashed your big toe. Now it's swelling, besides being in agony. What makes bruises swell? If you can explain what causes fluid-retention (swelling) in smashed toes you are able to explain the cause of pain, loss of energy, and every disease known to humanity. *Simply*, the explanation is *"trapped blood proteins."* Lemme explain. Blood-proteins belong only in your blood stream. Like a powerful magnet, they attract and hold sodium and water in your bloodstream. All negative substances and conditions –in other words, anything harmful to the Body, Mind, Heart– (toxins, drugs, drugfood, smoking, holding a grudge, stress, resentment, fear, etc.) cause the tiny pores of your blood capillaries to dilate.[2] As a result, blood-proteins leak out into the spaces between your cells, where they become "trapped," pulling with them excess sodium and water from your bloodstream –literally flooding the spaces between your cells. They remain "trapped" until removed by your lymph system or some health-promoting means like exercise, fasting, deep breathing, massage, herbs, a big raise in your salary, etc. Normally, cells are snug and close to the capillaries in order to draw the nutrients and oxygen they need from the blood. This is called the "dry state." This is the state of HEALTH.

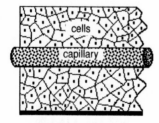

Dry State, Healthy

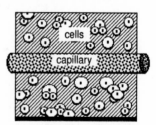

Flooded State, Unhealthy

1) Airola HG, 177.   2) West, GS, 8.

But when the space around /between the cells become flooded (due to trapped blood-proteins), the cells become too far from the capillaries. Then they can't get the nourishment they need, especially oxygen (hence, you feel *pain*). Then their energy-fields reduce because their "energy generators" (or "sodium-potassium pump") slow down or even stop working. Then they cluster or stick together (which makes them difficult to be removed by your lymph system). Then they start dying... by the thousands or millions depending on the severity of the condition.

Dr. Samuel West thoroughly documents this subject in his book, <u>The Golden Seven Plus One</u>. Death due to shock is really death due to trapped blood-proteins on a sudden massive scale (because shock dilates the capillary-pores, allowing the blood proteins /water to leave the bloodstream so fast that it causes collapse of the circulatory system). Trapped blood-proteins are the cause of death which results from traumatic or surgical shock following operations, severe burns and injuries.

Back to your aching swollen toe, or swollen insect-bite, swollen ankles, hurting back, joints, cut. Poisons from the damaged or killed cells of bruised tissues (anywhere in your body) attack the capillaries and dilate the tiny pores, producing a sudden shock-like effect in that area, resulting in trapped blood-proteins, hence "swelling." This is why yo po toe swelled! This also explains why gargling with salt water relieves a "sore" throat; or why ice reduces or prevents swelling of bruises. Or why vacations, fun, exercise, or that which bring you joy also improves your health. Like blood-proteins, salt attracts water. The gargled saltwater pulls excess fluids from your swollen tissues, restoring it to the "dry state" (=health). That icepack on your bruise prevents the capillaries from dilating, hence blood-proteins can't leak out. Therefore swelling goes down or is even prevented if caught early. As a result of trapped blood-protein and resulting fluid retention, people with a loose cellular structure can gain 20-90 or more pounds very quickly. Trapped or clustered proteins can be dissipated or removed to relieve pain, reverse injury, and speed up healing through goodies like fasting, a regenerative diet of raw fruit & veggies, fun, exercise, herbs, deep breathing, vacations, laughter, accupressure, rest, massage, and so on.

Anything that damages a cell causes trapped proteins, hence <u>loss of energy, sickness, and death</u> in (or to) your body. Water in the bloodstream follows the blood proteins. A sudden loss of protein and water from the blood stream, as in shock, will cause thirst. Trapped proteins pull water out of the bloodstream and make you thirsty. Thus, low energy (tiredness, fatigue) and thirst are two signs of trapped blood proteins. Stress causes a shock-like effect on the body, as do drugs, drugfood. This is why stress and the so-called "foods" (*Drugs Masquerading As Foods*) that cause thirst are directly related to loss of energy,

What's done to the Produce, Farm Animals, & Us is being done to the Planet!

That's heavy. Think about that. The whole planet is being poisoned on all levels: Earth, Water, Air, Light. Continuously saturated with artificially produced incredibly lethal poisons, directly added to the soil, water, air. Encapsulated in a gridwork of deadly artificial radiations. Plus, denied the full amount of full-spectrum sunlight it should be getting but cannot because heavy air pollution thwarts this. Earth's natural resources and minerals are ruthlessly mined out. Nuclear bombs are "tested" within the Earth and her oceans. **Earth is being turned into one vast graveyard as she herself is being killed, along with all the lifeforms she bears.**

Things have come to a quantum crisis. Earth is a living, sentient, conscious being like ourselves. When any healthy organism is infected, it defends itself; purges itself, else succumb and die. All life moves towards healing (maintaining balance) when it becomes imbalanced. The organism called Planet Earth IS moving to purge herself. This is exactly what the "Earth Changes" are about! **The people (and lifeforms) that do not get back in balance with Nature are toxins which will be purged from the Planet.** Thus if Humans want to survive, they need to get back in balance with Nature. Since our whole way of living (the white "western" way of living) is in fact, a disguised *Way of Dying,* this means we need to drastically change our way of life, else we will arrive where we are rushing to: Death.

In the wink of an eye, Mother Earth, *Mother Nature* could easily rid herself of the *Great Disease* infecting her and threatening her life. If necessary, *She* WILL do this. The only reason She hasn't is because of Her Love.

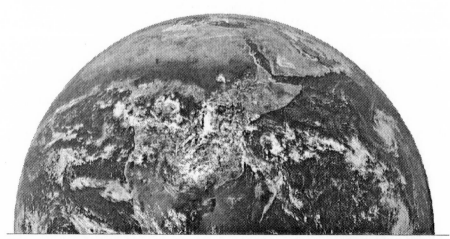

The Top Drugfood-Weapons Killing Us Slowly & Deliciously

*They look so innocent,
they taste so good,
they are attractively packaged,
they are gloriously advertised,
they are deceptively
presented to us as food.
We buy them and eat them,
believing they are food.
They are not food.
They are deadly
highly addictive*

Drugs Masquerading as Foods.

*Filling our supermarkets,
crowding our cabinets,
dominating our refrigerators.
We eat the so-called food
but really, the food is eating us,
killing us by degrees,
little by little
with each delicious bite.*

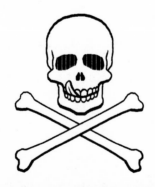

DRUG # 1 *Wicked White Sugar*

Drug addition initiated the Afrikan Slave Trade:
–Albinos' addiction to a drug called *Sugar*.

Sugar (and spices) were the drugs of earlier cultures. Sugar was worth its weight in gold at one time in early Europe. Afrikans were primarily enslaved to grow sugar on Albino plantations. Albinos are still addicted to sugar. And American-Afrikans are equally addicted to the same sugar that their great-great-grandparents were brutally enslaved to grow –to satisfy the Albino demand (addiction). Virtually all Americans are addicted to sugar, regardless of ethnic roots. In fact, this pathological condition is global. **White sugar is the world's #1 drug addiction.** White sugar is a legal drug, hence is poison. White sugar is as addictive as nicotine and heroin – and as poisonous, responsible for plagues ranging from depression to coronary thrombosis to diabetes.

White sugar <u>penetrates through the walls of your stomach and small intestines without being digested</u>, giving you a quick high followed by a later crash.

When you eat white sugar or sugar-sweetened food, the sugar bypasses digestion and enters your bloodstream within three minutes, yanking up your bloodsugar level. This results in an "instant high," –that is, the perception of having more energy and a feeling of well being. This is shortly followed by a crash in bloodsugar levels (due to release of insulin from the pancreas) and a depression and drop in energy that tends to be corrected with another dose of sugar. This becomes a dangerous habit, subjecting the body to a yoyo of stimulation, depression, restimulation which results in damage and diseases.

(Natural sugars from fruits and vegetables undergo the digestion process and enter the bloodstream gradually without disrupting bloodsugar balance.)

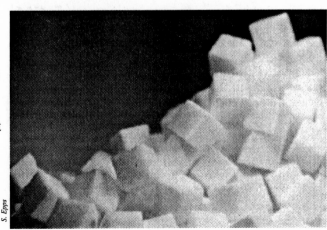

S. Epps

> **We eat as much sugar in a *week* as the average American ate in a *year* during the 1700s. This is a 4500% increase in sugar consumption since that time.** This means we are consuming a carbohydrate load that is several thousand percent above that which was ever consumed by people in history. Our bodies cannot tolerate this kind of abuse without dire health results!

Sugar is added to <u>almost all</u> foods in supermarkets,

including common table salt! You can prove this by reading the labels the next time you go shopping, keeping in mind that syrup, corn syrup, dextrose, sucrose, maltose, fructose and any other kind of "ose" is sugar. **Sugar is consumed at the rate of nearly 180 pounds per American each year**, according to the USDA (U.S. Department of Agriculture). This is almost a half pound per day – or the equivalent of eating 8 pounds of sugar cane or sugar beets per day. The average healthy digestive system can only eliminate 2-4 teaspoons of sugar daily. One 12-ounce cola contains 11 teaspoons of sugar.

Sugar is NOT FOOD: it provides absolutely no nutrition

In fact, it causes deficiency by robbing your minerals and vitamins. Sugar starts out as the dark juice of sugar cane or sugar beets and is "refined" (bastardized / debased) until it becomes sucrose, a white granulated chemical that is totally void of nutrition, having no vitamins, enzymes, fiber or minerals. It only has calories.

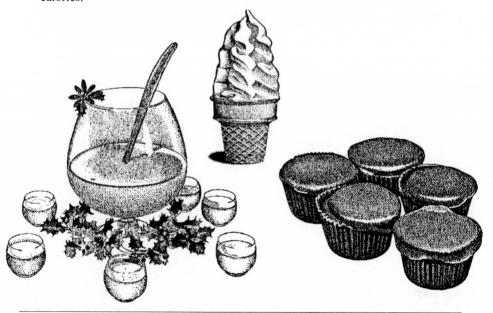

Sugar causes "cross linking," making your flesh and skin stiff and leathery

Cross-linkage explains why leather and plastic become hard, stiff and brittle. A high-sugar diet causes your flesh to "cross link." Cross-linking is a condition wherein the cellular membranes become so damaged that they become hardened, stiff, and stick together, –and their protein strands get entangled in each other. When this happens they can no longer perform their normal function. Thus, sugar is stiffening human tissues from the inside out and speeding up aging. Sugar damages cell protein. Sugar wreaks havoc upon the cell proteins and membranes, altering them from their flexible fluid-like state to a stiffened and therefore, malfunctioning one.[1] Cross-linkage is largely why skin becomes leathery. In essence, the cell membranes and proteins become functionally incompetent as a result of a high-sugar diet.

Sugar outright kills your cells

Sugar addicts often have high uric acid levels in their blood. Uric acid is a breakdown product of cellular nuclear material. The implication is that sugar is killing human cells[2]...sweetly. The next paragraph explains why.

White sugar is almost PURE CARBON! –breaking down your cells

The oxidation of white sugar in the body produces carbonic acid. Why? Because white sugar is almost pure carbon! [3] Because since it has no nutrients or organic salts, white sugar breaks down cells in order to furnish the blood with the necessary alkaline elements to neutralize the carbonic acid (formed by the oxidation of the carbon called sugar).

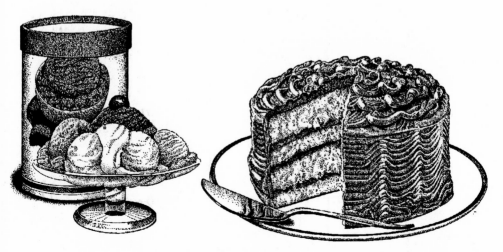

1) Igram, STN, 155.   2) Ibid.   3) Doctor's Health Review, July 1989, page 2.

White sugar is loaded with bleached PIG BLOOD and *STUFF*

An article in the July 1989 issue of *Doctor's Health Review*, educates us about this horror: Commercial sugar is made from sugar cane and sugar beets. At one phase of the (beet) sugar "refining" process, *"blood albumin from the slaughter house is used" (to flush protein particles out of sugar beets/ sugar cane). "Also purchased from the slaughter house is bone-black or animal charcoal, which comes from low-grade animals used as a filter to 'purify' this mixture called sugar. ...It is then bleached with a strong bleaching agent referred to as blue water. ....sixty-five percent of the animals slaughtered for the markets are swine. Therefore, the slaughter house products being used in processing sugar are derivatives of pork."*

Mold and Yeast loves sugar too.
Eat sugar and you feed / encourage molds in your body

Molds and yeasts thrive instantly in the presence of sugar. Sugar is their favorite food. Eating sugared food proliferates yeast disorders (fluid retention, yeast infections, athlete's feet, ear infections, candida...).

All sugars are not created equal

- **Brown sugar** is white sugar with molasses added.
- **Molasses** (blackstrap or otherwise), is claimed to be healthy but this is questionable since it is the overcooked waste product of sugar manufacturing.
- **Honey** is bee vomit. Despite its touted virtues, honey –whether pasteurized or raw– is basically as devastating as sugar. Like sugar, it enters the blood stream too rapidly. Honey also contains harmful acids. Its manite acid makes its combination with other foods even more harmful than cane sugar. Honey is harmful to digestion, the teeth, and nervous system. It is also a stimulant, hence damaging to humans. <u>Plus, commercial bees are fed refined sugar and drugs!</u>[1] This practice results in diseased bees and inferior honey. Commercial honey has toxic residues from the toxins used in its production (benzaldehyde, carbolic acid, propionic anhydride, nitrous oxide, sulfa drugs, antibiotics, hydrocyanic gas, and moth balls).[2] Honey also has ergot-mold pollution.
- **Pure maple syrup**, being a complex sugar, is supposed to be healthier than white sugar and honey because it enters the bloodstream more slowly. However, it's healthfulness is compromised because it is *cooked*; it is created by *boiling* down the sweet watery sap from maple trees. Also, maple syrup is usually contaminated with mold toxins. And it is additionally toxic because paraformaldehyde pellets are put in the maple trees to increase the tree's syrup production.[3] All things considered though, maple syrup is still considerably less harmful than sugar and honey.

1) Nelson, MY, 82. 2) Afrika, AH, 91. 3) Ibid.

Artificial sweeteners are more lethal than refined sugars

No artificial sweeteners are safe! They're just sweet deadly chemical poisons. They all are highly injurious drug-chemicals providing zero nutrition as they wreck your health. And there is little proof that they are useful for weight loss! Humans are not designed to digest artificial sweeteners such as **saccharin (Sweet' N Low)** and **aspartame (NutraSweet, Equal, Spoonful)**, all produced from petro-chemical waste, coal tar. Even small amounts are toxic. **Saccharin** is a carcinogen linked to causing bladder cancer; and it interferes with blood sugar level, blood coagulation, and digestive functions. **Aspartame** causes brain lesions, brain tumors, nerve damage, nerve disorders, memory loss, blurred vision, blindness, birth defects, seizures, mood disorders, behavioral disorders, digestive disturbances, joint pains, hives, migraine headaches, plus 92 other "official" side effects.[1] Aspartame also stops the pancreas from producing enzymes. After only a few doses of NutraSweet –as found in 6 cans of pop, enzyme production comes to a halt.[2]

Once aspartame is consumed, it turns to 4 chemicals in your body which rapidly enter your bloodstream: phenylalanine (50%), aspartic acid (40%), methanol (10%), and formaldehyde. Methanol (wood alcohol), a deadly narcotic metabolic poison, is first to be separated. Methanol can cause serious tissue damage including blindness and even death. The body lacks the enzymes to destroy it. For aspartame to be eliminated at all, the body must first convert it to formaldehyde, then to formic acid and lastly to carbon dioxide. One 12-ounce can of most aspartame-sweetened soft drinks contains about 10 mg. of methanol. Methanol is used in wood strippers, Sterno fuel, anti-freeze compounds, paints, shellacs, varnishes, as an octane booster for gasoline, and as raw material for making formaldehyde. Such has no business being in our bodies! Aspartame is found in over 6000 items including baked goods, cereals, vitamins, drugs, and especially diet soft drinks.

Other deadly synthetic sweeteners include <u>glycine</u>, <u>mannitol</u>, and <u>xylitol</u>. Intravenous injections of these substances have been associated with many disorders (especially around metabolism), such as acidosis, dehydration, kidney stones, kidney failure, confusion, unconsciousness and death. They lurk in sugarless gum, mints, breath fresheners, toffee, antiacid tablets, cough-cold medicine, children's aspirins, and dietary candy/ marmalades /jams.

<u>STEVIA</u>, a healthy sweet alternative
A healthy alternative to synthetic sweeteners is the juice from the Brazilian shrub, <u>STEVIA</u>, 30 to 40 times sweeter than sucrose. Stevia has been used in South America for several hundred years and has no adverse reactions. Stevia has other great reported benefits: helps normalize blood sugar, helps people with hypoglycemia & diabetes, inhibits bad bacteria growth, speeds healing when applied to wounds, cuts and skin problems.

1) Steinman, LH, 89, 90; Igram, ST, 12.   2) Ibid., 163.

Why are refined sugars deadly?

- **Causes, develops, promotes, or is directly linked to:**

hypoglycemia	diabetes	cancers	schizophrenia
heart disease	stroke	gallstones	depression
atherosclerosis	arthritis	migraines	mental illness
hypertension	asthma	cavities	behavioral disorders
hyperactivity	infertility	obesity	criminal behavior
kidney damage	emphysema	senility	multiple sclerosis
yeast infections	hemorrhoids	blindness	DNA impairment

- **Outright kills cells. Destroys** *essential fatty acids*, a cell component.
- **Yanks up blood sugar levels,** stresses the pancreas and liver.
- **Overstimulates the pancreas** (to produce insulin) and "wears it out."
- **Causes hypoglycemia and diabetes** by overstimulating the pancreas.
- **Are acidifying.** Overstimulates production of alkaline digestive juices.
- **Raises triglycerides** (blood fats) & artery-clogging cholesterol since sugar rapidly converts to fatty acids, triglycerides, cholesterol.
- **Hardens arteries,** damages arterial linings, elevates blood pressure.
- **Elevates blood pressure** by increasing adrenaline production resulting in increased blood vessel constriction and increased sodium retention.
- **Populations consuming the highest amounts of sugar** have the highest levels of cardiovascular disease.
- **Leading cause of stress. Causes fatigue** (is a downer, not a pick up).
- **Causes mental illness,** memory loss, depression, psychotic behavior. Mental patients /criminals often have low bloodsugar caused by white sugar.[1]
- **Causes children to have** memory lapses, delinquency, laziness, hyperactivity, crankiness, difficulty concentrating, anxiety, etc.
- **Irritates kidneys,** disrupts adrenal function, agitates nervous system.[2]
- **Robs the body of oxygen**; consumes oxygen at an alarming rate.[3]
- **Depletes enzymes, minerals, vitamins (especially B) & chromium** (involved in metabolism of sugars/fats). For sugar to be used by your body, it must be supported by minerals, vitamins, enzymes. Since it lacks these, your body robs them from its tissues.
- **Interferes with absorption of protein, calcium, minerals.**
- **Imbalances the calcium-phosphorous relationship.** Calcium and phosphorus work in optimal relationship only when their ratio is 10:4 in the blood. Even two teaspoons of sugar is enough to mess this up.[4]
- **Leaches calcium from the blood, bones, teeth.** Causes calcium loss which leads to osteoporosis (porous bones).[5] After you eat sugar, much more calcium is in your urine. **Causes cavities** (osteoporosis of the teeth). Is turning America into a toothless nation. 99% of Americans have bad teeth.
- **Weakens, damages immune system.** Inhibits white-cell functions.[6]

Continued >>

1) Afrika, AH, 80.   2) Igram, STN, 208   3) Law, 121.   4) David, NW, 164.   5) Ibid., 163.   6) Murray, 468.

Continued:

Why are refined sugars deadly?

- **Has bleached PIG BLOOD:** *"White Sugar is a psychotic mixture of pig blood, bleach, acids, antibiotics, carbon dioxide and sugar crystals. A combination of cheap diseased scrap meat (TB, Cancer, etc) of pigs and cattle is used to get Blood Albumin."* [1]
- **Has propyl alcohol pollution.** [2]
- **Causes "cross-linking"** /hardening of cells. Damages cell protein.
- **Weakens eyesight.** Promotes eye disorders, cataracts, blindness.
- **Causes infertility.** Contributes to major birth defects. Slowly deteriorates the reproductive organs. Can impair DNA structure.
- **Are acidifying. Plus, the combination of sugar & starch ferments** in your gut, producing many toxic substances including alcohol.
- **Restrains the growth of friendly intestinal bacteria.**
- **Overstimulates the thyroid**, causing mood swings, weight problems.
- **Upsets gland-balance** and produces a hyper-secretion of hormones comparable to what you get with taking drugs and artificial hormones.
- **All artificial sweeteners are chemical poisons**, very injurious to health.

1) Afrika, N, 265. 2) Clark CAD, 475.

Recommendations for Better Health

Avoid or Reduce Eating:	Healthier Replacements:
• white sugar	**Best:**
• brown sugar, date sugar	• ripe bananas, pureed sweet fruit
• raw sugar, turbinado sugar	• frozen fruit, blended (instead of ice cream)
• all refined sugars	• *fresh* fruit juice
• fructose, dextrose, maltose, "oses"	(not bottled juice because all *bottled*
• molasses, blackstrap molasses	juices and beverages have solvent-
• all syrups, corn /barley syrup	pollution from sterilization)
• ice cream, frozen desserts	
• all honey (raw or refined)	**Good:**
• fruit juice concentrates	• Sucanat (dried, dark, unprocessed
• pasteurized fruit juices	sugarcane juice or powder)
• jelly, jam, Jell-O (is 60% sugar)	• Stevia (a near no-calorie, safe, herbal
• candy, chewing gum	sweetener. 2 drops of Stevia extract = 1
• soft drinks, pop	T. of sugar; 1 T. of Stevia powder = 1
• ketchup (is 1/3 sugar)	cup of sugar)
• fudge, cake, "sweets"	• dates
• sugary cereal/granola (are 40% sugar)	• unsulfured dried fruit, raisins ("de-
• foods containing sugar	mold" it as later described)
(practically all foods in supermarkets!)	
• all artificial sweeteners	**Improvement:**
• commercial toothpaste	• 100% pure maple syrup, organic
	("de-mold" it as described on pg 140)

DRUG
2
Constipating, Ossifying
Wretched White Flour

Also labeled *enriched flour,* *wheat flour,* and just *flour.* White flour is so white because it is **bleached** white. White flour is an ultra-refined (i.e., ultra-*bastardized*), inert product, so devoid of any life giving properties that in embarrassment, the government requires the milling industry to put back a few of the nutrients it takes out. This so-called "enriched flour" has 4 of more than the 20 vitamins and minerals (removed in the "refining" process) put back into it. These added vitamins are synthetic, made from coal-tar. This white no-good stuff is the basis from which breads, cookies, pastries, and pasta are made.

Any "refined" grain is harmful as white flour
- white rice
- white grits
- white starch
- pasta
- cereals
- flours from such

White flour turns into deadly sugar when eaten
White flour is pure starch. Molecularly, it consists of sugar molecules attached by chemical bonds. Once eaten, this starch is rapidly broken down into glucose. Thus, Wretched White Flour is a twin of Wicked White Sugar, even becoming sugar, causing the same health assaults as sugar, in addition to dis-eases of its own. **One slice of bread equals about 5 heaping teaspoons of sugar.** Feeding cooked white-flour and grain products to babies, children, and adults promotes and develops diabetes in the same. The human digestive processes were never intended by Mother Nature to be (ab)used to convert such unnatural drugfood into (mal)nourishment for the cells and tissues of our body.

White flour is the king of constipation! –helping to glue us up inside
It is the most constipating of foods. Bookbinder's paste is often made of white flour. Being devoid of fiber, white flour causes bowel disorders (constipation, colitis, diverticulitis...). 90% of Americans suffer from clogged colons – impacted with 2-30 or more pounds of hardened feces that never come out except via special programs. No wonder colon cancer is the #2 cancer killer.

1) Ehret, RF, 160.

Why is refined starch deadly?

- **Turns to sugar during digestion, hence, causes the same dis-eases as sugar, plus other problems.**
- **Regular consumption hardens the tissues & joints, resulting in:**[1]

arthritis	heart problems	varicose veins	hardened arteries
tumors	diabetes	hemorrhoids	gall /kidney stones

- **The reason for the above:** When any starch (or calcium-containing food) is cooked, its calcium becomes insoluble inorganic calcium (as in concrete), unusable by your body; clogs your system. If your body is not able to excrete it, it dumps it wherever convenient, such as the gallbladder (gallstones); kidneys (kidney stones); dead-ends of blood vessels in the abdomen /anus (resulting in tumors /hemorrhoids).
- Overworks the liver, causing cirrhosis or the liver tissues to harden.[1]
- **Promotes colon cancer,** the #2 cancer killer in America.
- **The most constipating of all foods is white flour** (and starches in general). 90% of Americans suffer from constipated, clogged colons.
- **Intoxicates us:** Cooked starches quickly ferment in your body in the presence of heat /moisture, producing **alcohol**, carbonic acid gas, and other poisons, especially if eaten with sugars or proteins (pastries /sandwiches). Starch /grain food, a "complex carbohydrate," must be cooked before eating; heating dextrinizes starches. Dextrinized starches especially ferment in the gut. People who eat lots of starches (almost everyone) have made their body into a distillery, constantly producing alcohol.
- **Is very mucus forming. Forms acids in the body** which cannot be neutralized by the body's secretions.
- **Mold is common in grains**, producing mycotoxins (mold poisons). All packaged breads /starches/pasta contain harmful mycotoxins.
- **Promotes calcium deficiency** and tooth decay.
- **Many experiments of feeding animals on white bread** have established that it will not sustain life. Cows fed on refined grain die of heart failure.[2]
- **Cooked cereals/starch cause nervous afflictions** [3] and arteriosclerosis due to its high content of inorganic sulfur and phosphorous.
- **Baked flour products** are made with baking powder, usually containing aluminum potassium sulfate. 40 million pounds are used yearly. Aluminum is toxic and causes Alzheimer's disease.[4] The residues left in bread by baking powders & baking soda also retard protein/gastric digestion.
- **White flour & foods made with it cause "inorganic iron toxicity"** for its heavy consumers (nearly entire American population). How? All white flour is fortified with iron as *iron sulfate*, a chemical form hardly different from iron filings. When ingested over a long period, inorganic iron may cause liver damage and increase the risk for heart disease and cancer.[5]

1) Walker, FV, 33-34, 47, 131   2) Bragg, AV, 76.   3) Walker, FV, 60.   4) Valerian, 0144.   5) Igram, 196.

Recommendations for Better Health

Avoid or Reduce Eating:	Healthier Replacements:

• Starchfoods <u>made with white flour or any "refined" grains</u>:
 – bread, buns, rolls
 – creamed soups, gravies
 – bread dressing, croutons
 – cereals, grits, rice
 – pancakes, waffles
 – pasta, noodles
 – macaroni, spaghetti
 – dumplings, pot pies
 – pizza, pretzels, crackers
 – cookies, cakes, donuts
 – egg rolls, crepes
 – malt, malted milk
• White rice, grits, etc.
• So-called "wheat bread" or multi-grain bread made with a <u>combination of white flour /whole wheat flour</u>.
• baking powder containing aluminum
	NONE!
	All grains /starchfoods are harmful to humans in the long run. Limit eating them.
	
	Almost OK
	("almost" because grains are <u>cooked</u> to make them edible, which also renders them more harmful. Cooked *wholegrains* are less harmful)
	• Wholegrains:
	  – kamut – amaranth
	  – quinoa – buckwheat
	  – wild rice – spelt
	• Breads, pastas, etc. made with the above
	• (best to limit eating wheat, rye, oats, barley and brown rice)
	• Millet (least mucus-forming of grains)
	• Essene-type, sprouted-grain breads
	• Wholegrain breads you make yourself!
	• *RED potatoes* are a good grain substitute (white potatoes are unsafe)
	• Agar-agar, flaxseed meal, etc. (see Tips)

Tips

Healthy non-starch thickeners: Arrowroot, slippery elm, agar-agar, flaxseed meal. They can be used in (or to make) gravies, soups, salad dressings, breads, candies, smoothies, etc. Flaxseed meal has a satisfying nut-like flavor. Agar-agar, a sea plant product, can also be used (instead of gelatin) to make congealed fruit & vegetable salads..

Baked Spaghetti Squash: excellent, healthier substitute for pasta spaghetti.

Psyllium fiber: The constipating effects of starch foods can be reduced / eliminated by taking psyllium seed powder or husks. Mix a couple of teaspoons in water or juice and drink immediately since it thickens quickly, then drink another glass of water. Do this 1-3 or more times a day. This is a safe, non-laxative way to eliminate constipation if you insist on having your bread and eating it too. Psyllium expands to about 10 times its volume in your colon when you take it with fluid, acting as an effective intestinal broom.

All packaged breads, pasta, including health varieties are ontaminated with mold-toxins (according to Dr. Hulda Clark). Best to make your own; it's fun.

Mold-detoxing is possible by cooking with vitamin C (see page 140). The best way to avoid mold toxins is to make your own bread /pasta. However, bakery breads in paper bags are usually mold-free.

DRUG # 3
White Fatal Fats

Heart attacks & cancer were rare until hydrogenated vegetable oils were invented in 1913 and unleashed upon the population

Now, heart disease is the Number 1 killer in America and cancer is Number 2. To become a target for both, help yourself to foods made with "refined" oils. Most Americans do, as evidenced by the epidemic of heart attacks and cancer. Over a billion pounds are used each year according to government statistics. 54% of Americans die of heart disease. Over 50 million Americans suffer from severe heart disease. Autopsies show that almost every child over the age of 4 already has incipient to severe cardiac problem. Heart specialists say everyone over 30 has some form of heart disease.

The danger of fats /oils is from being fractionated, cooked, hydrogenated, refined, and even "cold pressed"

Cooked, heat-processed oils are generally impossible to metabolize. Such oils are corrupted at the molecular level and deadly. Vegetable oils are processed with gasoline solvent, sodium hydroxide (Draino, caustic soda), phosphoric acid, bleach and other toxins. They contain residues of these deadly chemicals along with abnormal, mis-shapen, manmade oil molecules ("trans-fat"). In extracting and processing, oils are exposed to light, oxygen, heat, and (as with supermarket oils) chemical solvents. All these degrade the oil. When oils are overheated (cooked/fried) and used for too long, as the case with oils at fastfood restaurants, they become oxidized, loaded with damaging free radicals.

Gunk-Plaque, turning your soft arteries into hard ceramic pipes

If your diet is loaded with fatty, greasy foods, and high in salt, sugar, and hydrogenated oils, you can bet you got plaque accumulated on the inside of your arteries, making them as hard and inflexible as ceramic pipes. "Plaque" is created when ions of minerals get trapped in a sticky, gooey "gunk." The gunk is the fatty, fried and hydrogenated oils. You now have a brick of mineral particles cemented together with pieces of grease. The cement is the cholesterol and triglycerides that bind together. Plaque restricts circulation, raises blood pressure. A **heart attack** or **stroke** results when those fragments get caught by plaque already formed along the arterial walls, and completely blocks the flow of blood and oxygen. Fortunately, plaque can be safely dissolved through natural nutritional programs (see *Don't Worry, Be Healthy!*).

Your body needs oil (fats, "fatty acids," lipids)

The Brain, when the weight of water is removed, consists mainly of fat! –in the form of *lecithin,* a phosphorized fat. The pineal gland is richer in lecithin than any other part of the body. Lecithin-fat is also the chief constituent of nerve tissue and semen. Fat is found in all the body cells and especially the cell *membranes.* It soothes the nerves, coating them with a protective shield. It lubricates the arteries. It combines with protein to compose your hair. Fats gives us a full satisfied feeling after a meal since they stay long in the gut. *Essential fatty acids* are involved in moisture-retention in the brain cells. "Essential fatty acids" (vitamin F) are called such because the body can't make them, hence your diet must supply them. They include omega-3 (alpha-linolenic) and omega-6 (linoleic, arachidonic). In the American diet, linoleic is abundant but linolenic acid is scarce. Hemp /flax seed are rich *wholefood-*sources of both. Other rich sources are nuts and *extracted* (hence unnaturally concentrated) "supplement oils" like hemp, flax, primrose, wheatgerm and fish oil (unsafe). All dark green leafy vegetables have omega-3.

There are mainly three types of fats: **monounsaturated, polyunsaturated,** and **saturated.** All three in varying proportions compose all fats. If fat is *unsaturated,* there are points in its molecular structure where it can combine with other nutrients within the cell and thus nourish the cell. If fat is *saturated,* it is chemically inert and the body deposits it as excess blubber, arteriosclerosis, etc.

Monounsaturated Fats	Polyunsaturated Fats	Saturated Fats
Have molecules with a single "kink," making them fluid and reactive. Are liquids. Lower bad cholesterol (LDL) while maintaining good cholesterol (HDL). Thickens when refrigerated; returns to fluidity at room temperature. OK for diets of those with cholesterol problems. Have linolenic and linoleic acids.	Have molecules with two kinks, making them more reactive. Are liquids. Lower both bad & good cholesterol (LDL & HDL). Have linolenic and linoleic acids. Some extracted oils cause cancer and massive free-radical activity. The rare *"super-unsaturated"* fatty acid molecules have 3 kinks.	Solid at room temperature. Have molecules shaped like a straight line (so they easily stack in a compact mass) & are "saturated" with hydrogen atoms. Resist changes; slow to spoil. Found in all animal products. Raise cholesterol in the blood. Cause heart disorders, arteriosclerosis.
Better olive oil avocado oil sesame	safflower hemp, walnut sunflower wheatgerm flaxseed primrose	whole milk (raw) cream (from raw milk)
Bad canola oil peanut oil	corn oil cottonseed oil soybean oil mayonnaise	margarine animal fat shortening lard butter coconut oil cheese palm oil palm kernal oil peanut butter (commercial) hydrogenated vegetable oil

Edible plastic oil: deadly "trans-fats"

Refining and hydrogenating oils are deadly. Hydrogenation of oils converts 40% to 60% of the oil into **unnatural** *trans-fats*, a major cause of heart disease, cancer, immune system breakdown, and obesity, etc. Margarines in healthfood stores often claim they contain no hydrogenated oils, but they are made from refined oils, which are 25-40% trans-fats. Margarine can contain up to 47% trans-fatty acids. "**Refining**" of oils converts 25-40% trans-fats in the oils.

Shocking Experiment

Take an egg-poaching pan. Put *butter* into one of the egg cups; *margarine* in the other. Bring the water under the cups to a boil. The butter melts almost instantly; the margarine will not fully melt even after being in the heat of boiling water for a full 10 minutes!

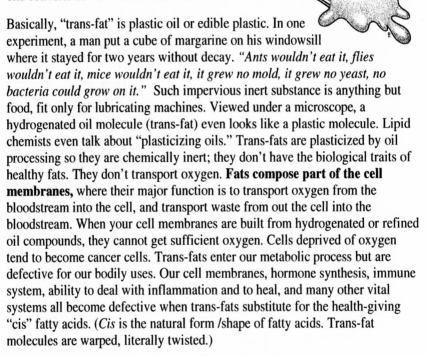

Basically, "trans-fat" is plastic oil or edible plastic. In one experiment, a man put a cube of margarine on his windowsill where it stayed for two years without decay. *"Ants wouldn't eat it, flies wouldn't eat it, mice wouldn't eat it, it grew no mold, it grew no yeast, no bacteria could grow on it."* Such impervious inert substance is anything but food, fit only for lubricating machines. Viewed under a microscope, a hydrogenated oil molecule (trans-fat) even looks like a plastic molecule. Lipid chemists even talk about "plasticizing oils." Trans-fats are plasticized by oil processing so they are chemically inert; they don't have the biological traits of healthy fats. They don't transport oxygen. **Fats compose part of the cell membranes,** where their major function is to transport oxygen from the bloodstream into the cell, and transport waste from out the cell into the bloodstream. When your cell membranes are built from hydrogenated or refined oil compounds, they cannot get sufficient oxygen. Cells deprived of oxygen tend to become cancer cells. Trans-fats enter our metabolic process but are defective for our bodily uses. Our cell membranes, hormone synthesis, immune system, ability to deal with inflammation and to heal, and many other vital systems all become defective when trans-fats substitute for the health-giving "cis" fatty acids. (*Cis* is the natural form /shape of fatty acids. Trans-fat molecules are warped, literally twisted.)

FAT content of some foods

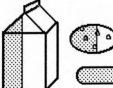
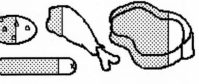

2% Milk **35%**
Chocolate chip cookie **54%**
Beef frank **82%**

Chicken w/o skin **24%**
Beef steak, untrimmed **74%**

Mayonnaise **99%**
Potato chips **60%**
Cheddar cheese **74%**

Heart Snatching, Cell-Suffocating Hydrogenated Oils

Hydrogenated oils include **shortening, margarine, and "partially hydrogenated vegetable oil."** Hydrogenated oils are **saturated fats** (solid). They cause platelets (blood clotting elements in the blood) to stick together, forming clumps that slow down the flow of blood. **These clumpings cause the blood pressure to rise sharply within hours of a meal rich in saturated fat, and account for the many heart attacks that occur within hours of rich meals.**[1] Plant oil is "partially hydrogenated" to make it partially hard at room temperature because completely hydrogenated oil would be too hard to work. When oil is hydrogenated, it is pressure-cooked at about 400° F with hydrogen gas and a metal catalyst for about 7 hours.

The end result is empty snow-white grease, ready to sit beside its other empty vile cousins: wicked White Sugar and wretched White Flour –a deathly trio typically found together in pastries and breads. This white grease of death is sold as *shortening*, **or flavored/dyed and sold as** *margarine*. Hydrogenated oils are massively found in mayonnaise, peanut butter, dressings, chocolate candy (to make it hard), fried foods at restaurants. Naturally saturated fats include butter, lard, coconut oil.

Cancer-Triggering Polyunsaturated Oils

When researchers want to ensure that lab animals gets cancer, they feed them high amounts of **corn oil**. Numerous studies show that heat-processed, polyunsaturated fats –**especially corn oil**– cause cancers. Research reported in the March 1971 issue of *Lancet* shows that heat-processed, polyunsaturated, fatty acids, although linked to decreased heart disease to some extent, **have been associated with the near doubling of cancer rates** as compared to control people in the study who were on a low intake of polyunsaturated fatty acids.

Polyunsaturated oils suppress the immune system (killer T-cells) more than saturated oils like butter or lard, leaving us vulnerable to the *100 million cancer cells that are formed inside humans every day*. **Hydrogenated oils and** *isolated* **polyunsaturated oils are unnatural;** they did not exist as part of our diet until a few decades ago. We don't have enough antioxidant enzymes / nutrients in our body to handle the massive amount of peroxidation and free radical activity they introduce into our body.

---

1) Robbins, DNA, 297.

What you don't know about <u>CANOLA oil and SOY oil</u> is killing you

Allegedly coined from "Canada oil," the term *Canola* is the oil of genetically mucked-with rape seed turned into "canola" via genetic engineering and irradiation.[1] Canola oil is a common ingredient in many foods in supermarket and "healthfood" stores. An article informs us that *Canola* oil:[2]

- **Comes from the rape seed** (of the mustard family of plants). It's not called "rape" for nothing. Rape is the most toxic of all food-oil plants. Like soy, rape is a weed. Insects won't eat it; it is deadly poisonous. Rape seed oil is a hundred times more toxic than soy oil.

- **Is an industrial oil** which does not belong in the body.

- **Is a semi-drying oil** used as a lubricant, fuel, soap, synthetic rubber base.

- Canola & Soy oil forms **latex-like substances** that agglutinate the red blood corpuscles, congesting bloodflow through out body.

- *"Rape (canola) oil causes emphysema, respiratory distress, anemia, constipation, irritability and blindness in animals and humans. ..is also the source of the infamous chemical-warfare agent, mustard gas, which was banned after blistering the lungs and skin of hundred of thousands of soldiers and civilians during WWI."*

- **Contains large amounts of isothio-cyanates** (cyanide-containing compounds), a mucus membrane irritant which inhibit the mitochondrial production of ATP (Adenosine Triphosphate), the energy molecule that fuels the bio-electric body and keeps us young.

- **Canola oil's claim to fame** is that it's higher in unsaturates than any other oil, making it the most "heart-healthy" oil on the market. While there's some truth to this, there is more to the story: **Polyunsaturated oil lowers cholesterol by driving it out the blood –but WHERE does the cholesterol go? Into the colon where it increases risk of colon cancer** [3] **(#2 cancer killer). This is why vegetable oils are the most "cancer-unhealthy" (cancer causing) oils on the market.**

- A medical study (on ABC news broadcast, 2/15/94) showed a definite link between Canola/Soy oils and the development of **prostrate cancer** in men.

- Canola /Soy contain **organic alcohols which depress the immune system** by causing T-cells to go into a stupor (get drunk?) and fall asleep on the job. Alcohols in Canola are extremely "pure," far more toxic than hard liquors.

- An article by Amal Kumar Maj,[4] related that smoke from rapeseed oil used for stir frying in China was found to emit **carcinogenic chemicals,** increasing the incidence of lung cancer in China.

---

1) *California Sun*, vol. 21, March 1997, 10-11.   2) Ibid.   3) Ibid., June, 1998.   4) Wall Street Journal, 6/7/95.

And COTTONSEED oil is not a food, nor a vegetable

Hence is inedible. Cottonseed oil is a waste product of cotton harvesting, sold only to stretch profit dollars reaped by the cotton industry.[1] It is contaminated with large amounts of pesticide /herbicide residues, more so than any other type of oil. It has gossypol, which contains benzene rings and is toxic to the liver and gall bladder. Cottonseed oil may cause shortness of breath and water retention in the lungs. Look on the ingredient list of your potato chips and you will likely see that it is fried in cottonseed (or canola) oil.

Aren't "cold-pressed" and "expeller pressed" oils good to eat?

Learn this about many so-called "cold-pressed" and "expeller pressed" oils: Tremendous heat (300-500 degrees Fahrenheit) is generated by expeller presses used in making "expeller pressed" oil. In the oil-extracting process, first the seed or germ meal is **cooked for about two hours at 30 degrees above boiling**. The cooked seed mash is then pressed to squeeze out the oil. The friction in this process produces temperatures between 200–250 degrees, unless nitrogen is used as a coolant; then the temperature is around 140–150 degrees.[2] *"If this is to be a premium grade oil sold in health food stores as 'raw, unrefined, cold pressed oil' it will now be filtered and bottled."* [3] How can this be called "cold-pressed" with all this heat?! Oh, I guess you didn't know that *"the oil industry is allowed to use the term 'cold-pressed' as long as they are not applying external heat during the pressing process."* (*Deception*, by any other name!) The seed mash is then **recooked** for several hours at 150°F with **hexane solvent** to extract any remaining oil. Then it is heated to 250° to evaporate the solvent, which is reused. Residues of the solvent remain in this second extract of oil. Incredibly, such oil is often mixed with the originally pressed oil and then bottled and sold as "unrefined oil." [4]

On the positive side, some companies, like *Spectrum Naturals*, say that their oil-processing temperatures are kept below 120°F.

"All types of processing of oils tends to destroy the lipase [a fat-digesting enzyme in raw fats/oils], **not just cooking them. For example, olives and coconuts have plenty of lipase, but their oils have none. In general, oils as they occur naturally in plants, as in sunflower seeds and avocados, have all their nutrients and enzymes intact, whereas the extracted oils, even if cold pressed, are missing many nutrients and their associated enzymes."**[5]

Therefore, __ALL__ extracted oils are generally unsafe! They are all drugfoods, including the oils in healthfood stores.

---

1) Igram, STN, 189. 2) Kulvinskas, LTC, 224. 3) Healthiatry Course II, 10. 4) Ibid. 5) Cousens, CE, 287.

Why is hydrogenated fat deadly?

- **Causes, develops, promotes, or is linked to:**

heart disease	stroke	lethargy	multiple sclerosis
atherosclerosis	obesity	gallstones	bloodsugar problems
hypertension	cellulite	malnutrition	hypoglycemia

- **Causes heart disease** –the #1 killer of Afrikans & all Americans.
- **Builds plaque in the arteries,** hardening them. This hinders circulation & passage of nutrients to cells. **Builds up fat around the heart.**
- **Destroys** *essential fatty acids.*
- **Melanin shows extreme affinity** for binding with the fat compounds.[1]
- **Raises cholesterol and triglycerides** (blood fats) to dangerous levels.
- **Causes /worsens bloodsugar problems.** Diabetics nearly heal when saturated fats /oils are removed from their diets.[2]
- **Partially blocks respiration function of cell membranes.**
- **Cooked fats and fried food** are the most common cause of disorganized gall bladder function.[3] **Fried fats** are highly carcinogenic.
- **The more fat a person eats, the shorter their life span.**[4]
- **Fats combine with oxygen** to speed up the free radical deterioration process. (Free radicals are incomplete molecules that attach to & rob parts of other molecules, causing damage to DNA and other cell components.)
- **Is loaded with nickel,**[5] a carcinogen and one of the most toxic metals.
- **Even in small amounts,** causes cell damage via "lipid peroxidation" (rancid fats within tissues) signified by skin aging and liver spots.[6]
- **Refined oils /fats cause immune disorders** because it destroys vitamin A, essential for maintaining optimal immunity. [7]
- **Stresses gall bladder & liver,** resulting in heartburn and indigestion.
- **All extracted oils** are fractionated /concentrated, hence drugfoods.

Why are heat-processed & many "cold pressed" polyunsaturated oils deadly?

- **Outstanding cancer trigger.** Cancer is the #2 killer in America. Studies show that polyunsaturated oils increase the tendency to form tumors.
- **Causes massive free radical activity** in our tissues which accelerates aging. May lead to a deficiency of essential fatty acids.
- **Suppresses the immune system.**
- **Canola, soy, corn, & cottonseed oils are deadly.** (details on earlier pages)
- **So-called "cold pressed" oil is still cooked,** hence hazardous.

1) Barnes, MCK, 32-33.   2) Robbins, DNA, 277.   3) Walker, FV,137.
4) Kulvinskas, STC, 14.   5) Clark, CAD, 372, 420.   6) Igram, STN, 187.   7) Ibid., 77.

Recommendations for Better Health

Avoid or Reduce Eating:	Healthier Replacements:

• all types /brands of margarine
• shortening (will shorten your life)
• baking sprays
• expeller pressed oil
• most "cold pressed" oils
• canola oil (totally avoid!)
• corn oil, soy oil
• peanut oil (has aflatoxin)
• peanut butter (hydrogenated)
• chocolate candy
• coconut oil
• palm & palm kernel oil
• cottonseed oil
• *pasteurized* butter
• lard, animal fat
• mayonnaise
• tartar sauce
• oil-based salad dressings
• cooked fatty /greasy foods:
  – ice cream, chocolate candy
  – fried foods, stir fry
  – donuts, corn dogs
  – "fries", onion rings
  – egg rolls, wontons, fondue
  – gravies, creamed sauces
• many granolas
  (loaded with fat /sugar)
	Best:
	• Meet your oil /fat needs with unprocessed raw oily wholefoods like avocados, nuts, and the seeds of hemp, sesame, sunflower, and flax (flax –very rich in rare linolenic acid).
	• Hemp seed (essential fatty acids & more)
	• Bee pollen (essential fatty acids & lecithin).
	
	Improvement:
	*Remember, ALL extracted oils are fractionated, hence drugfoods. **Best to choose "cold pressed" or "expeller-pressed" oils. Use sparingly):***
	• **olive oil** (Virgin /extra virgin, unfiltered. Does not become rancid without refrigeration. Least processed of oils. Virgin means from 1st pressing)
	• **sesame oil** (Lightest of veg oils. Has *sesamol*, a natural antioxidant that prevents the oil from spoiling. Is the most stable naturally-occurring veg oil, hence can be stored a long time without going rancid. Is one of the few oils that can be made without refining.)
	• **tahini** (ground sesame seed spread)
	• **safflower** or **sunflower oil**
	• **these "supplement" polyunsaturated oils**:
	  – flaxseed oil – hemp seed oil (best if greenish)
	  – primrose oil – wheatgerm oil
	• **raw butter or cream** (From organic goats / cows. Better to use butter than margarine; butter is *real;* all margarines are unnatural)

Tips

- **Olive or sesame oils**, good for salad dressings. Flaxseed oil, a good butter replacement.
- **Avoid a high-salt diet** because it creates a craving for fats.
- **Avoid all rancid (spoiled) oils.** You can identify a rancid unrefined oil by its unusually strong odor and sharp or bitter flavor. The off-odors are gases produced by the reactive fatty acid molecules. Spoilage in refined oils is harder to detect because such oils have their odor-bodies removed. **Dispose of older oils,** especially if they have been opened but have sat unused for long periods.
- **Lipase, a fat-digesting enzyme,** is recommended for people with poor fat-assimilation.
- **Fried fats are highly carcinogenic.** If you plan on cooking with oils anyway, don't let oils heat to smoking. Never re-use oil that has been used for frying.
- **Safflower oil is good for frying /hi-temp cooking.**
- **Fish oil is risky, likely toxic,** since almost all fish are living in polluted waters.
- **Ground flaxseed** may be used as generous toppings on food or mixed in beverages.
- **Primrose oil, lecithin, and ground flaxseed** helps drive toxic oils out the tissues.

DRUG # 4

White Refined
Insidious Salt

If the average person's weekly intake of white salt were eaten all at once, they would quickly die! [1]

The "western diet" is spiked with 20 times the salt that occurs in natural food; and this is 20 times the salt required for optimal health! For health requirements, the average person only needs about 2–5 grams a day but consumes 10–20 grams or more each day. Just as there is white refined sugar ravaged from natural dark sugar cane, there is white refined salt ravaged from gray ocean salt. Out of the richest spectrum of 92 essential minerals found in the ocean, refined white salt retains only two! It's about 40% sodium and 58% chloride. The remaining 2.5% is various poisons called "additives."

Refined white salt is protoplasmic poison.

Pure salt (sodium chloride), whether mined from the earth or sea is an _in_organic, poisonous mineral compound with no nutritive value. It passes through the body _without undergoing any change._ It is not metabolized as are organic salts. Though sodium and chlorine are important nutrients, your body needs them as they exist _organically_ in plants, and moist, never-dried, whole ocean salt. It is admitted everywhere that sodium chloride is an _"irritant poison."_ This is why you become thirsty after eating salty food – your body is making you drink water to dilute the harmful, irritating salt from its delicate tissues. Refined salt wreaks havoc with all the body's tissues. Thus salt has been termed a "protoplasmic" poison, meaning it's poisonous to all organic life. **Fish and marine life will <u>die</u> in a solution of refined salt (pure sodium chloride) and water in the same ratio as found in seawater.**[2]

Celtic sea salt. This _moist, never-dried_, genuine "gray whole ocean salt" is actually healthy!

It actually _normalizes blood pressure!_ Doctors in Europe regularly prescribe it for many diseases, for it is full of assimilable minerals, and supplies a substantial part of the trace elements missing from today's supermarket produce. Oceans are the lifeblood of Earth. Our blood and body fluids are similar to ocean water in their chemical composition. All of ocean-salt's trace and macro-elements _stay within the crystal only as long as the moisture of that salt is retained._[3] Applying artificial heat destroys the riches of the ocean while removing that moisture. This water-retaining part of seasalt is called the **"mother liquor"** or _bitterns_, and is centered around magnesium salt. Mother liquor restores hydro-electrolytic imbalance (a disorder causing many health problems). Its marvelous healing powers are still used by Europe's medical profession, as by the Celts hundreds of years ago.

"Celtic sea salt... can help in correcting excess acidity; restoring good digestions; relieving allergies and skin diseases; and preventing many forms of cancer." Natural moist whole grey salt provides a steady boost in cellular energy and gives the body a heightened resistance to infections and bacterial diseases. [1] Chronic disease is caused by the acidification of the blood and the cellular tissues. **Acidosis can be corrected by using whole salt (Celtic salt) in the diet.**[2] French scientist Dr. Alexis Carrel kept a chicken heart alive for over 37 years by having the pulsating heart in a solution of whole sea salt. He voluntarily ended the experiment, having proved that living cells can have physical immortality. For this, he won the Nobel prize.

"Sea Salt" is an impostor! The term is misleading and deceptive. *Sea salt* and *refined salt* are the same.

The "sea salt" offered as natural in healthfood stores comes from the same refineries as the commercial salt.[3] In fact, refined salt is often labeled "sea salt" in supermarkets and "natural sea salt" in healthfood stores.[4] *"The salt sold in health food stores, even that which is labelled 'sea salt,' must conform to the same regulations [U.S. Codex] and comes from the same refinery that produces toxic industrialized salt. Such sea salts as Lima, Si-salt and others have been purged [refined] of their minerals down to the 2% of macro-nutrients spelled out in the U.S. Codex."*[5] Thus "sea salt" and refined white salt are equally toxic. **Such salt has not seen the sea for billions of years but comes from dried-up inland seas, dead salt lakes or long buried salt mines.** Refined salt has lost its ionic, electrolytic, positive/negative charge properties, which are only found in whole, never-dried, gray salt such as Celtic ocean salt.

Refining turns ocean salt into a poisonous drug.

When moist, gray ocean salt is "refined," dried out /superheated, the minerals are striped away, its molecular structure is rearranged, and it becomes a poisonous, highly addictive drug. After the moisture is removed, to prevent any moisture from being reabsorbed, salt refiners add alumino-silicate of sodium or yellow prussiate of soda as desiccants, plus different bleaches to the final salt formula. *"But since table salt, chemically treated this way, will no longer combine with human body fluids, it invariably causes severe problems of edema (water retentions) and several other health disturbances."*[6] Edema and water-logged joints disappear with the use of Celtic salt because it contains all three magnesium salts in the correct quantity (all 3 salts make up 3/4 of 1% of the solids in Celtic seasalt).

Trace elements are properly absorbed and used safely only when they occur in <u>parts per million</u> concentration. Here, concentration of these elements in excess of micro doses would cause clumping and provoke malabsorption in the living cells.[7] *"[T]oo great a concentration of trace elements in an organism increases the risk of forming strong aggregations –clumping– of similar elements that cannot easily be freed from the solid mass, in order to serve as truly useful linkages with others on the outside."*[8]

1) de Langre, 58. 2) Ibid., 34. 3) Ibid., 11. 4) Ibid., 25. 5) Ibid., 28 6) Ibid., 14. 7) Ibid., 16. 8) Ibid., 24.

Refined white salt causes internal drowning

In an article, *"Body Fluids-A Major Medical Problem,"* J.D. Ratcliff wrote: *"This year some 200,000 Americans will drown, –not in oceans, streams or pools, but in their own body fluids. The cause is often congestive heart failure..."*

Heart failure is often the result of excess fluids (water) which the body retains to reduce the concentration of poisonous salt in the tissues and bloodstream. When diseased hearts are unable to pump enough blood to the kidneys, those organs fail to excrete the body's surplus fluid and it congests tissues. Feet, leg and ankles swell with retained water, a gallon or more may accumulate in the abdomen or chest. **An ounce of salt in the body will trap and hold three quarts of water.** In *Seasalt's Hidden Powers*, Dr. Jacques de Langre wrote:

"Biology states that excess salt collects in tissues and body fluids. However, only refined salt will cause this problem. Natural Celtic salt does not accumulate in the tissues; the magnesium salts will eliminate sodium chloride after it has performed its important jobs of acid-base balance, cell permeability and muscle contractibility."[1]

Our kidneys are designed to handle 5-10 grams of mineral salts daily.

But the average American consumes 10 to 20 grams of salt each day. Even if we do not salt our food, salt shows up in hidden ways put there by the criminal food-processing industry. Most foods in supermarkets are salted; salt is a cheap preservative. As our age increases, the function of our kidneys decreases, – reducing our ability to handle these excess salts, causing them to backup in our bloodstream where they negatively affect our blood colloids. Over time, excess salts are stored in various parts of our bodies as the elimination system cannot handle them. The end result: obesity, high blood pressure, kidney/heart diseases.

Celtic Salt Composition (Complete Analysis[2])

Chloride	51%	Zinc	0.87%	Manganese	0.026%
Sodium	32%	Magnesium	0.50%	Copper	0.018%
Water	7%	Iron	0.38%	Calcium	0.012%
Sulfur	1.12%	Potassium	0.26%	Silicon	0.011%

Plus trace amounts of these 61 elements:

Carbon:	0.034%	Strontium:	0.009%	Boron:	0.004%	Hydrogen:	0.003%
Fluorine:	0.001%	Nitrogen:	0.0008%	Argon:	0.0005%	Lithium:	0.0002%
Rubidium:	0.00014%	Phosphorus:	0.000112%	Iodine:	0.00007%	Barium:	0.00002%
Molybdenum:	0.000012%	Nickel:	0.000008%	Arsenic:	0.0000037%	Uranium:	0.0000038%
Antimony:	0.00000035%	Vanadium:	0.0000024%	Tin:	0.0000009%	Cobalt:	0.00000045%
Mercury:	0.0000002%	Silver:	0.00000032%	Krypton:	0.00000024%	Chromium:	0.0000002%
Germanium:	0.00000007%	Neon:	0.00000012%	Cadmium:	0.000000112%	Selenium:	0.0000001%
Zirconium:	0.00000003%	Xenon:	0.00000006%	Scandium:	0.0000005%	Gallium:	0.000000035%
Thallium:	0.000000022%	Lead:	0.000000026%	Bismuth:	0.000000024%	Niobium:	0.000000023%
Gold:	0.000000019%						

And Pico-Traces Of :

Helium	Lanthanum	Neodymium	Thorium	Cerium	Cesium	Terbium	Yttrium
Dysprosium	Erbium	Ytterbium	Hafnium	Gadolinium	Prasodymium	Beryllium	Samarium
Holmium	Lutecium	Tantalum	Thulium	Europium	Tungsten	Protactinium	Radium

1) de Langre, 57.   2) Analysis by Nantes University, France.

Why is refined salt harmful?

- **Fish and marine life will die in a solution of refined salt** (pure sodium chloride) and water in the same ratio as found in seawater.
- **Is a highly addictive poisonous drug.**
- **Major cause of cardio-vascular stress,** leading to heart attacks.
- **Considered leading cause of high blood pressure** (hypertension), the #3 killer in America. About 42 million Americans suffer high blood pressure. **Afrikans suffer the highest rates of hypertension. High blood pressure was never a problem for us in Afrika,** where the traditional diet was low in sodium and high in potassium. Salt increases blood pressure by drawing water into the blood, increasing the pressure on the arterial walls.
- **Many Afrikans have "salt sensitivity."** Their system retains salt under stress, rather than excrete it as most people do, making them far more prone to hypertension.
- **Waterlogs your system**; an ounce of salt in the body holds 3 quarts of water (6 pounds).
- **Too much salt overworks and weakens the kidneys.** This also causes fluid retention. (Taking diuretics further weakens the kidneys).
- **Causes kidney disease. Produces pain, aches or tightness in the back**, indicating a problem in kidney function.
- **Overstimulates your nervous system** and adrenal glands.
- **Is a potent adrenal stimulant**, urging body to increase its blood levels of adrenal hormones, creating a feeling of well being –a drug in other words! Adrenal exhaustion often results in asthma or hay fever.
- **High salt diet causes loss of blood potassium**, which leads to drop of blood sugar.[1] Depletes the potassium reserve of the body.
- **Hardens your cells, tissues, blood vessels, liver and arteries.**
- **Impedes the elimination of uric acid**, which paves the way for gout, sciatica, rheumatism, and lumbago.
- **Disturbs your cell mineral balance** which can lead to cancer.
- **Greatly upsets the normal balance between the electrolytes** and solutions within/without the cells.
- **Commercial salt contains aluminum** compounds to keep it from caking. Aluminum causes gradual brain damage.
- **Dulls your taste buds and weakens sense of taste.** To salt eaters, unsalted food taste "flat." Creates a craving for fats.
- **Preserves you just like it preserves plums**.
- **Dries out your skin, scalp, and hair.**
- **Promotes wrinkling and accelerated aging.**
- **Increases frequency of stomach cancer.**

Continued >>

1) Airola, HGW, 113.

Continued:

Why is white refined salt harmful?

- **Curtails the secretions of the adrenals and pituitary gland.**
  "Vasopressin or ADH and the hormone cortisol that are vital to assure optimum sexual functions are no longer secreted when white table salt is the condiment. These <u>sexual malfunctions</u>....can create a combination that <u>destroys sexual functions</u> and sensitive response."[1]
- **Robs the bones.** The sodium overload inhibits normal calcium metabolism in complex ways, all of which harm a wide range of bodily functions, including blood pressure and bone formation.[2]
- **A high-salt diet diminishes the zeta potential** (free energy) of our blood and other biological fluids.

1) de Langre, 54. 2) Colgan, NN, 59.

Recommendations for Better Health

Avoid or Reduce Eating:	Healthier Replacements:
• **refined white salt** • **"sea salt"** • **salty foods:** – cheese – potato chips, pretzels – salted nuts /crackers – soy sauce, teriyaki sauce – ketchup, spaghetti sauce – pickles, relish, sauerkraut – mayonnaise, dressings – bacon, jerky, hot dogs • all foods containing added salt	• **Celtic salt** If used for <u>cooking</u>, add the Celtic salt near the end of the cooking process, or dissolve it in a little fluid and pour this in the food after it's been cooked. This way, the food will absorb the nutrient-gases. <u>If the Celtic salt is not heated above 250 degrees</u>, its chemical consistency and balance will remain fairly unchanged. • **filtered, unheated seawater** (not from inland seas) • **seaweed** (kelp & dulse are mineral-rich) • **herbal seasoning** (salt-free) • **raw celery/spinach/beets** (high in sodium)

Guidelines for determining if a salt is whole, truly natural seasalt
To determine a salt that is truly a whole product of natural crystallization of the ocean, uses these guidelines. Only truly natural whole seasalt will have these characteristics (de Langre, 17):
1. Light grey in color.
2. Moist to the touch; retains moisture even when kept a long time.
3. Formed of very small, precisely cubic crystals.

Only natural sea salt will have these traits. Each of these traits proclaims the natural sea salt's integrity and wholeness. Also guarantees its effectiveness as an outstanding food/condiment/medicine that helps maintain health.

Where to find Celtic Salt? Contact the *Grain and Salt Society*, 273 Fairway Drive, Asheville NC, 28805 • (800) 867-7258.

DRUG
5

Waters of Woe

Are you drinking rat poison?

Contrary to what you've been led to believe, fluoride (in fluoridated tap water) and its derivatives are deadly to your health. Fluoride makes people more susceptible to cancer and causes 30,000 to 50,000 deaths each year.[1] Medical authorities state that fluoride can cause kidney disorders, bone diseases, impotency, Mongoloid births, and even madness. Fluoride is derived from *fluorine*, a deadly chemical to humans. While seemingly not dangerous in small amounts, the government investigations of 156 cancer deaths indicates that fluorine accumulates in the human body and eventually causes cancer or other fatal illnesses. A dictionary defined fluorine as: "A pale-yellow, highly corrosive, poisonous, gaseous halogen element, the most electronegative and most reactive of all the elements, used in a wide variety of industrially important compounds." *Tap water* is the largest source of fluoride, *toothpaste* is the second largest source. *Drugs* are another source; for example, fluoride is the trigger ingredient in Prozac, one of the biggest-selling psychotropic drugs.

But isn't Fluoride good for teeth?

Dr. Paavo Airola wrote: "...there is *no positive, conclusive, scientific proof* that the addition of this inorganic toxic chemical [sodium fluoride] does the least bit of good, even to the teeth of children between ages 7 and 12. But there are dozens of reliable studies made around the world that show that the fluoridation of the water causes fluorosis (mottling of tooth enamel), mongolism in infants, kidney damage, and other harmful effects to the body...These studies are however, suppressed; researchers are persecuted; and their findings are not published in medical journals."[2] Another doctor wrote: "Medical and scientific 'peer reviewed' journals have routinely suppressed the publication of articles and research opposing fluoridation."[3] Those promoting fluoride in toothpaste are the trade association called *The American Dental Association*, who derive royalties from toothpaste-manufacturers who recommend fluoridated toothpaste![4] Fluoridation may harden some people's teeth, but it also hardens the arteries and brain, and it is the same compound that is used as a rat poison. Yet 88 million pounds of rat poison shipped to our water systems for human consumption are not colored blue or marked poison. Only fluoride which goes to exterminators must be colored blue or the supplier goes to prison.[5]

1) *Fluoride: The Aging Factor*, by Dr. J. Yiamouyiannis.
2) Airola, AYC, 149. 3) Williams, S, 19. 4) Info-pak by *Citizens For Safe Drinking Water.* 5) Banik, CC, 28.

Fluoride weakens your immune system.

In an article by Dr. Thomas Levy, *Fluoridation: Paving the Road to the Final Solution* (published in *Extraordinary Science Magazine* Jan-Mar 94), we learn that as little as 0.1 ppm fluoride retards white cell migration, an important component in the immune system. In addition, fluoride interferes with the process of phagocytosis, one of the mechanisms by which white cells attack foreign agents (e.g. bacteria).

Are you drinking recycled sewage water?

A recent study of a major city's tap water shows that the main ingredient is water. The second major ingredient is shredded toilet tissue![1] Today's tap / faucet water is yesterday's toilet water. Raw sewage water is often recycled as drinking water. Some 40,000 or so carcinogens have been found in tap water.[2] So many chemicals are added to tap water that it is a toxic, complex chemical soup. Plus, it often contains microorganisms and parasites which cause sickness. More than 700 contaminants have been found in water supplies nationwide and 200 are toxic chemicals, including lethal *fluoride* and *aluminum* which cause disease and death. Pesticides and agricultural chemicals also invade our nation's water supply. The body stores the chemicals found in tap water in our arteries, veins, joints, tissues and vital organs. Clearly, tap water is not clean enough for consumption. It is one of the top menaces to public health.

Is your water turning you into stone?

Tap water, mineral water, spring and well water are loaded with inorganic minerals your body cannot assimilate. This is why such water is called "hard." And "soft water" is only soft in comparison with water that is harder. These inorganic minerals leave water-spots on your glasses, a stony coating in your kettle, and lime deposits around your faucet-nozzles. They also leave the same deposits in your body! –hardening your soft tissues over time, turning you into a living rock. The cumulative effect is witnessed with the bodies of elderly people. At birth, a baby's body is over 90% water; by adulthood, the body is about 75% water, and even less than this as it ages. Where does the water go? It is displaced by accumulation of precipitated, inorganic minerals. Were it not for the activity of the eliminative organs, most people would become statues of themselves by age 40. **You can consume about 450 pounds of inorganic minerals from tap /spring /mineral /well water in your lifetime.** If our bodies are not capable of excreting them, these inorganic minerals settle in our soft tissues, veins, organs, and bones, causing mineral deposits. The cumulative results include kidney stones, gallstones, glaucoma, arthritis (cemented joints), enlarged joints, ossification of the tissues, and other problems. Therefore, water containing high levels of inorganic minerals –especially *cationic* minerals– is usually unhealthy for drinking. Inorganic minerals are not nutrients but unusable toxic material to the body. <u>However, if these minerals are mainly *anionic* minerals, such as potassium or sodium sulfate, the water is much healthier and even beneficial</u>.[3] But this type of water is rare. Most mineral,

1) Flanagan, 61.   2) Ibid., 62.   3) Ibid.

spring, and well waters are cationic. Most bottled mineral /spring waters are cationic. *Volvic Water* from France is favorably anionic. **A superhealthy, mineral water is the water of the Hunza people in the mountains of India.** They live beyond 150 years and their women birth children after age 100. They attribute their great vitality mainly to their water. What makes their water so special? It is **"liquid crystal water"** – also known as *structured water.* A form of this very healing, rejuvenating water can be made from "Willard Water concentrate" available from healthstores (see *Tips*, page 102). It is described in *"Miracle Cures –Catalyst Altered Water"* by Russ Michael, and, among other important things, *"Elixir of the Ageless"* by Drs. Gael & Patrick Flanagan.

How to remove these deposits & resoften our harden tissues?

To remove these deposits from our tissues and organs, drink distilled water or clean rain water. Distilled water is the greatest solvent known. Its continued use flushes out mineral deposits, acid crystals, and other hard deposits from the body. It passes directly into the blood, increasing the blood's solvent properties.

But doesn't distilled water leach minerals from the body?

Though distilled water is accused of leaching minerals, it allegedly only leaches inorganic minerals which your body cannot use.[1] Any leaching tendency is only slight. Some health experts say it does not leach organic usable minerals.

If you are concerned about leaching you can prevent it by:
- adding a bit of filtered, unheated *seawater* to it (4 teaspoons of seawater to a half gallon of distilled water [2]) or
- exposing the distilled water to sunlight for a few hours or
- soak dried or fresh fruit /vegetables, seed (alfalfa, wheat, fenugreek), or crushed grass in it overnight to introduce nutrients into it and convert it to live juice.[3]

Organic Apple Cider Vinegar also softens your hardness

In *Apple Cider Vinegar Health System* (page 10), Dr. Paul Bragg shows that hardened tissues /arteries and premature old joints can be softened over a few months by drinking the "apple cider vinegar and honey cocktail" once or twice daily. Use only **unpasteurized, unfiltered, organic apple cider**. His formula is 2 teaspoons of apple cider vinegar and 1 heaped teaspoon of [raw] honey in a glass of water. (Honey is *not* necessary [4] in order for it to work; you may leave out the honey –it's harmful.) This works mainly because of the potassium content. "Potassium is to the soft tissues of the body what calcium is to the hard structures of the body... Potassium might be called the great detergent of the arteries." Many old, senile, degenerated people can be restored to useful lives again if the toxic poison can be flushed from their bodies and their deficiencies corrected. Dr. Bragg says the cocktail speeds this process. It is a great tonic with many other regenerating effects upon the whole body. It also helps heals a variety of ailments such as sore throats, bladder infections, and prostrate disorders. Besides potassium, it contains phosphorus, chlorine, organic sodium, magnesium, sulphur, iron, copper, silicon, other minerals, and malic acid.

1) Banik, CC, 32.   2) Clark, KYN, 203.   3) Kulvinskas, STC, 31.   4) Cousens, CE, 146.

Is your water damaging your irreplaceable brain cells?

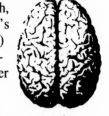

Besides fluoride, your tap water likely contains aluminum. Both, fluoride & aluminum muck with your brain, affecting the brain's neurotransmitters.[1] The Nazis (Albinos) and Russians (Albinos) used fluoride / fluoride-laced water as effective means of mind-controlling the population. Now you know the real reason water is fluoridated in America. Water companies treat water with aluminum sulfate.[2] Aluminum is a metal deadly to humans.
Aluminum causes permanent deterioration of brain cells and nerve connections. This damage is progressive and not responsive to any known treatment. In fact, aluminum accumulates in the brain, causing Alzheimer's disease, which kills over 100,000 Americans each year. Seven percent of Americans over 65 have been diagnosed with Alzheimer's. Aluminum is a neuro-toxin also associated with dementia and seizures; it is carcinogenic in laboratory mice and is added to vaccines to "promote antibody response." [3] ALCOA (Aluminum Company of America) is the main source of fluoride *and* aluminum. In fact, fluoride is usually extracted from aluminum waste.[4] Sodium fluoride is a by-product of aluminum-manufacture and is largely the waste disposal of ALCOA.

"Water yourself" more and you'll get healthier.

Your body is about 75% water. Like Mother Earth. Water carries oxygen and nutrients to your cells through the blood. Water regulates body temperature through perspiration, keeping us from burning up; it keeps us cool like it keeps our car engine-radiator cool by removing extra heat resulting from our daily average 3000-ish calorie-intake. Water bathes our eyes, mouth. Helps maintain proper pH balance. Provides traction, lubrication. Even lubricates our joints. Water is essential for digestion and all our body functions including breathing, for the lungs must be moistened by water for oxygen intake and carbon dioxide removal. We lose about a pint of water daily from exhaling. Most of us are constantly dehydrated. No wonder we have dry skin, frequent constipation and infections, clouded minds. For good health, we need to drink water. Not juice, not tea, not soda, but pure water. Nothing substitutes for pure plain water. (An *almost-exception* is eating plenty of juicy fruits). **What color is your pee? If it's yellah /amber /pungent then you ain't drinking enough water!** It's supposed to be *clear*...like *water*. By just drinking more water you'd be amazed at how health problems may diminish until gone. Even obesity and "fluid retention." If one does not drink enough water, the body cannot metabolize fat, and water is retained –adding to one's weight. Water flushes impurities out your system. Keeps you internally purified. Without water, we'd poison ourselves with our own metabolic waste. Drinking a simple full glass of water can relieve anxiety attacks, headaches, hot flashes, food intolerance reaction, acid burning in the stomach, colitis pain, etc. Yes, this greatest-of-solvents is also the greatest-of-Healers, for *Water* is a form of... *Love*. A precious gift from The Great Mother.

1) Valerian, 0142.   2) Ibid., 0143 .   3) Awadu, E, 10.   4) Law, 96.

Why is tap water & mineral-loaded water harmful?

Pollutants in tap water:
- Some 40,000 carcinogens have been found in tap water.[1]
- More than 700 contaminants have been found in water supplies nationwide and 200 are toxic chemicals.

Bacteria, Parasites in tap water:
- Tap water often contains microorganisms and parasites which can cause sickness. Over 20,000 cases of giardiasis, caused by an intestinal parasite from drinking water, have been reported in the U.S.
- More than 900,000 people get sick in the U.S. annually from bacteria contamination of drinking water.

Minerals in spring /mineral /well /tap water:
- The **inorganic** minerals in tap, spring, mineral, and well water settle in our soft tissues, veins, organs, and bones. The cumulative results over time include:
  - kidney & gallstones
  - hardened arteries
  - brain ossification
  - bunions
  - enlarged joints
  - accelerated aging
  - arthritis (cemented joints)
  - ossification of tissues & veins

Fluoride in tap water:
- Causes from 30,000 to 50,000 deaths each year.
- Cancer rates increase 5% in cities using fluoridation.[2]
- Causes or intensifies allergies.
- Promotes free radical formation and has been shown to inhibit the normal use of oxygen by the body. Is an enzyme inhibitor.
- Weakens immune system by damaging the thyroid or interfering with thyroid function (causing hypothyroidism leading to obesity problems and even a weakening of the immune system.[3]
- Affects the neurotransmitters of the brain, causing docility.[4]
- Is toxic to bone cells /promotes osteoporosis (bone mass reduction).[5]
- Causes or has been directly linked to:
  - kidney /bladder disorders
  - arthritis
  - skin disease
  - liver damage
  - impotency
  - fluorosis (mottling of teeth)
  - calcified deposits in the aorta
  - mongolism in infants
  - bone diseases, bone cancer
  - madness

1) Flangan, 62.   2) Williams, S, 19.   3) Ibid., 18.   4) Valerian, 0142.   5) Burton, AM, 775.

Continued:

Chlorine (bleach) in tap water:

- Linked to heart attacks. Heart attacks became epidemic when chlorine was added to the nation's water supplies.[1] Combines with animal fats in the diet to form a gummy chemical amalgam in the arteries, creating atherosclerosis which brings on heart attacks and angina pectoris attacks.
- Linked to cancer. Can combine with organic compounds in water to form toxic VOC's (volatile organic compounds) and THM's (thrihalo-methanes) which can increase risk of gastrointestinal cancer 50-100%.
- Chlorine and its by-products are linked to diabetes, kidney stones, gout and possibly multiple sclerosis and muscular dystrophy.
- Destroys cells, attacks the lungs, accelerates aging. Destroys vitamin E.
- Chlorine is a lethal gas used in making bleaches, solvents, pesticides, plastics, disinfectants. Chlorine often contains carcinogenic carbon tetrachloride, a contaminant formed during production. Carbon tetrachloride is poisonous by inhalation, ingestion, or skin absorption. Acute poisoning causes nausea, diarrhea, headache, stupor, kidney damage and death. Chronic poisoning involves liver and kidney damage.[2]
- Chlorination has also been found to sometimes form toluene, xylene and styrene, all lethal "ring" compounds.[3]

Aluminum in tap water:

- Causes Alzheimer's disease, which kills over 100,000 Americans each year and is the 5th leading cause of adult death in the U.S. Seven percent of all Americans over 65 have now been diagnosed with Alzheimer's.
- Causes permanent deterioration of brain cells and nerve connections. This damage is progressive and not responsive to any known treatment.
- Affects the neuro-transmitters in the brain.[4]

Why is all bottled water harmful?

- **Solvents!** All bottled water of any type is harmful because they all contain solvent contamination from the bottle-sterilizing equipment. Solvents dissolve fats and are life threatening, because fats form the membrane wall around each of our cells, especially our nerve cells. Solvents also kill liver cells /tissue.
- Solvents in bottled water (including distilled water) are benzene, propyl alcohol, carbon tetrachloride and wood alcohol.
- Toxic plastic gases (hormone disruptors /impostors) from the plastic containers leach into the water. (see pages 45-46 for effects)
- By law, bottled "spring water" need only be 50% spring water; the rest can be regular tap water.

1) Valerian, 0135. 2) Winter, FA, 110.. 3) Ibid., 120. 4) Ibid., 0142.

Recommendations for Better Health

Avoid or Reduce Consuming:	Healthier Replacements:

• tap water
• drinks made with tap water
• food made with tap water
• ice cubes made with tap water
• purchased ice
• carbonated water
• limit use of all bottled water because of solvent contamination
• limit use of mineral water, well water, and spring water
	• reverse osmosis mineral-free water
	• purified water from water-dispensers
	• filtered tap water, depending on the type of filter system used
	• clean rain water
	• distilled water:
	  – plain or mixed with any of the above waters (in order to take advantage of distilled water's ability to expel inorganic minerals deposits from the tissues)
	  – mixed with seawater (4 teaspoons of *filtered, unheated seawater* to a half gallon of distilled water in order to prevent distilled water from removing *any* minerals, organic or inorganic, from body)
	• "Liquid crystal water" (see *Tips* below)

Tips

- (See "distilled water" in the above right column)
- *Liquid crystal water*: why does it cure health problems and diseases (so quickly at that), plus increases our vitality and well being when regularly consumed? It has these properties: has a polymer nature that neutralizes the alkaline or acid nature of humans, animals, plants & soil. Balances the pH, allowing body's enzymes to work far better. Makes body's enzymes work 10 times more effectively, thus producing a 10-fold increase in body's own natural healing power. The enzyme action of our bodies is accelerated when the pH is neutralized. Super penetrating. Penetrates the skin, tissues, cells, organs, muscles and even bones, like no other penetrant (great for arthritis). Since it has a polymer base, breaks up fatty deposits, kidney stones, toxins. Cleanses the tissues. Also called "catalyst altered water," it can be made by adding one ounce of "Willard Water Concentrate" (available from healthstores) to a gallon of water, preferably *distilled* water.
- **Best to store your water in *glass* containers.** Avoid plastic if possible; definitely avoid storing water in metal, especially aluminum.
- **If you keep a (preferably clear) quartz crystal/s** in your drinking water, the crystal improves the taste. It doesn't matter if the crystal is broken or dinged. Before using, first "purify" the crystal of any possible negative vibrations by burying it in plain salt for a week or leaving it in direct sunlight for several days (this is very important!). Then thoroughly wash it. To test its effect on water, leave water in two glasses overnight; one with a crystal in it and the other without. Next day remove the crystal and try it on friends to see if they taste a difference.
- **A yogi method of improving and oxidating water:** Get two glasses. Fill one with water, then pour it into the other empty glass, then pour it back. Do this several times. It not only improves the taste but it charges the water with "prana" from the air, as well as oxygenates it.

DRUG # 6

DIE-ry Dairy, Mucus-Heaven, Hormony,
Murder-Us Milk

Farmers know if you feed <u>pasteurized</u> milk to a calf, it will die within 6 weeks due to malnutrition.
In one study, animals died within 5 weeks of respiratory complications (mucus) when placed on a diet of pasteurized milk and orange juice.[1] When raw milk is pasteurized, it is corrupted at the molecular level (like any food that's cooked) and loses most of its nutrition. It also loses *phosphatase*, an enzyme important for assimilating minerals, including calcium in the milk. Pasteurized milk is inferior and lacks the enzymes, vitamins and minerals required to maintain good health.

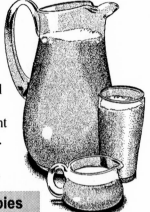

It is child-abuse to feed cows' milk to our babies

It is abuse to feed *pasteurized* milk to any creature.

● **Cows' milk raises babies' deathrate.** In a study of over 20,000 babies, the rate of illness was compared between completely breast-fed babies and bottle-fed babies. Pasteurized milk-fed babies had a mortality rate 56 times greater than breast milk-fed babies. The general rate of sickness was nearly double for the pasteurized milk-fed babies.[2]

● **Cows' milk makes babies /children diabetic.** At a Finland university, Dr. S. Virtanen discovered that feeding cows' milk to babies 3 months old and younger, often results in complete insulin deficiency.[3] Bovine milk-protein destroys the insulin-producing beta cells of the pancreas and causes diabetes.

● **In children, milk is responsible for allergies,** colic, colitis, earaches, colds, sore throats, congestion, respiratory illness and is linked to asthma.

● **Children who are fed cows' milk formulas** grow up into adults with a higher susceptibility to multiple sclerosis than breast-fed children.

● **The BGH hormone** in milk is linked to rapid, unnatural growth in children.

● **The human baby develops its brain first while the calf develops its bone structure first.** Thus, human milk is high in *phosphorus* and the amino acid *taurine*, both important to *brain* development; while cows' milk is high in calcium –for bone structure, and deficient in phosphorus and taurine. Cows' milk has 300% more casein than human milk. Casein furnishes a number of amino acids for supplying the protein molecules to build bone structure that will carry the calf's body weight. A baby human develops twice its weight in 7 *months* whereas a baby cow develops twice its weight in 7 *weeks*.

1) Kulvinskas, STC 30.   2) Cousens, CE 346.   3) Cohen, MDP, 264, 219, 220

Dairy is DIE-ry: Milk is the top Heart-Attack-producing food

As shown by many studies, dairy products are a top cause heart attacks, strokes and atherosclerosis. Worse than pasteurized milk is *homogenized* milk, wherein all the fat is in microscopic pieces evenly distributed. This is a lethal heart hazard. In examining the deathrate from atherosclerosis (clogged arteries) in 13 nations, Dr. Kurt Oster[1] found it correlated directly to the drinking of homogenized milk in that nation. Finland, a country with one of the highest rates of dairy consumption, also has the world's highest death rate from heart-disease. A 10-year study proved cooked milk is a primary contributor to all heart disorders. Heart disease is the #1 killer of Americans. 40% of America's diet is dairy, according to the USDA. These two facts are directly related.

Got Milk? Got Mucus!

Milk wins first place as the most mucus-forming of all foods. Drinking a cup of milk is like drinking a cup of mucus. Cheese has this quality 100-fold, being concentrated milk. It takes about 4-5 quarts of milk to make a pound of cheese. People that drink milk and eat dairy products are always full of snot, coughs, colds, congestion. This is why babies fed mostly on cow's milk have constantly running noses. CASEIN, the dominant protein in milk, is the main cause of mucus. Casein causes histamines in your body which create mucus, congestion. If you must have your cheese *fix* (you drugfood addict you), cut up a small amount in a big salad. This will counteract some of its clogging effects. And commercial **ice cream** is totally unfit and unsafe for consumption. Whether pasteurized or raw, dairy products from cows' milk are the most mucus-forming of all foods. This includes milk, cream, cottage cheese, cream cheese, yogurt, ice cream, skim milk, whey, butter, kefir and ghee. Robert Gray observed: *"Every one of these is a pernicious mucoidformer. Goats' milk, however, is substantially less mucoidforming than cow's milk."*[2]

IN ESSENCE:
Milk =
mucus

Cream =
snot

Cheese =
boogies

..and Got Glue!

80% of the protein in milk is CASEIN, a tenacious glue. Casein from cow's milk makes one of the strongest water-resistant glues. It holds together the wood in your furniture. It will glue you too! The main ingredient in Elmer's glue is casein. Casein is also found in some artificial "cheeses" at health stores.

1) Chief of Cardiology, Park City Hospital, Bridgeport, CT.   2) Gray, CHH, 33.

Is milk giving Asthma, Heart-Attacks & Genocide to Afrikans?

Asthma is three times higher in Afrikans than in whites. The same Afrikans lead the nation in heart attack rates. Asthma and heart attacks are both directly linked to diary consumption. 80% of all milk protein is CASEIN, the most allergenic substance found in our foods. Casein is also a tenacious glue used to hold furniture together. Casein causes histamines in your body which create mucus. This mucus fills the lungs, making breathing difficult, if not impossible. In asthma, the muscular spasms, together with increased mucus, are brought on by histamine produced by the body's immune system during an allergic response. In just New York half a million children have asthma and most of them are Black and poor. Courtesy of the USDA they get free breakfast and lunch. A major part of that meal program is casein-containing milk-&-dairy. Thus, these freefood programs are largely harmful to Afrikan children. The government / USDA know that Blacks can't digest dairy. 90% of Blacks do not produce *lactase*, the enzyme necessary to digest *lactose*, the sugar in all milk products.

4000 Colored Babies die from cows' milk every 24 hours

A more effective program of apparent *Genocide-Disguised-As-Benevolence-from-Albinos* is rampant in Afrika and the "Thirdworld," causing the eventual death of 4000 Babies of Color each day. These mentally colonized people have been well conditioned by their colonizers to highly regard anything from Albinos. Mothers are the victims of vast campaigns selling western infant form-ulas. Shortly after birth in a maternity hospital, their babies are fed free milk formula from western corporations. As mothers leave the hospital they are given more free samples of infant formulas. They assume it's the best food for their babies since it's from the hospital. Worse, they believe their own breastmilk is inferior. *"They think that in using the formulas they are feeding their children the modern way. They think bottle feeding is 'glamorous, convenient, highly scientific and nutritionally superior.' That's what the advertisements have told them."*[1] The formulas lack the immunological protection their own milk would provide. Further, these illiterate mothers cannot read the directions to sterilize the baby bottles /water; and pure water is not usually available anyway. Now their babies will be subjected to diseases they would not have gotten otherwise. Soon their babies get sick. At the same time, the mothers can't afford the high cost of the formulas. If they try to go back to breast feeding they can't because their milk has dried up. To stretch the formula they can afford to buy, they add water to it. They watch helplessly as their babies get diarrhea so severe that all they can do is cry in pain –deprived of adequate nutrition, growing weaker each day, and wracked by parasitic and infectious diseases. They love their babies and would do anything to help them. In desperation they go without food themselves to save money to buy more formula. Over 1.5 million Colored Babies die yearly from this "Bottle Baby Disease." For Thirdworld babies exclusively breastfed, the deathrate *drops* 95%.

1) Robbins, May All Be Fed, 129.

> **Thus, Nature's perfect food for baby cows is definately not Nature's perfect food for Afrikans...or any people.**

Cancer proliferates from the IGF hormones in milk

The most powerful growth hormone in the human body is identical to the growth hormone in cows! [1] It is called IGF-1 (Insulin-like Growth Factor). Whenever you consume milk /cheese, you are ingesting this hormone, found in commercial cows' milk. **The same hormone in milk is the key factor in every human cancer.** As noted by Robert Cohen in _MILK The Deadly Poison_, his exposé book on milk and the dairy industry:

> _"There are studies that the dairy industry refuses to release...Thousands of things cause cancer, but one hormone that you naturally produce is the key factor in the growth of each human cancer, particularly breast cancer. There are millions of hormones in the animal kingdom, but only one hormone that is exactly alike between two species. That hormone is called insulin-like growth factor (IGF-1) and is an exact match between humans and cows. When drinking a 12-oz. glass of milk, you double the amount of that hormone in your body —a hormone described by scientists and scientific journals as the key factor in cancer's growth and proliferation."_

IGF-1 levels are being artificially increased in much cows' milk sold in the U.S. IGF-1 in the blood is linked with higher risks for common cancers than any other factor discovered. Studies link this hormone with a 7-fold increase in risk of breast cancer and a 4-fold risk of prostate cancer.[2] Both are major killers of men and women in America and other industrialized countries.

Commercial milk causes many other diseases

Pasteurized milk is a poor source of calcium. Since it's cooked (pasteurized), its calcium is mostly inorganic, hence unusable. Also, its mineral/calcium-assimilating enzyme –_phosphatase_– is 100% destroyed. Furthermore, in order to absorb calcium, the body needs comparable amounts of another mineral, _magnesium_. Milk and dairy contains only small amounts of magnesium. Without *magnesium, the body only absorbs 25% of dairy calcium. The remainder of the calcium causes or contributes to **kidney stones, arthritis, atherosclerosis** (by building plaque on our artery walls), and **osteoporosis**. In fact, 25 million American women over age 40 have bone-crippling arthritis and osteoporosis. These women have been drinking about two pounds of milk per day for their entire adult lives. Osteoporosis results from calcium loss, not from a lack of calcium intake. The large amount of protein in milk results in a 50% loss of calcium in the urine.[3] Plant calcium (from leafy greens and vegetables) is far better absorbed than milk calcium.

---

1) Cohen, MDP, 70.   2) _Lancet_, May 98; JScience, Jan. 1998.   3) Cohen, MDP, 266.
* Magnesium itself requires vitamin B6 in order to be properly absorbed; and taking one B-vitamin instead of the B-complex creates other problems. All this reflects the importance of eating _wholefoods_, not _fractionated_ foods.

> ## Thus, the following common advertisement is a BIG *WHITE* LIE:
> ## "Milk Does A Body Good"

Milk is rich in drugs, pus, poisons & 'crack-hormones' fed to cows

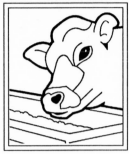

We learned in chapter 4 that mothers' milk is now unfit food for their babies because it is highly contaminated with toxins from her Standard American Drugfood Diet. Same thang applies to cows. Centuries ago, people often got poisoned from the milk of foraging animals because the natural toxins in the plants which animals ate were secreted in the animals' milk. Today, cows are literally fed poisons, drugs, pesticides (to keep flies away from their feces), antibiotics and often the flesh from dead diseased cows (and other animals). Cows are also regularly injected with unnatural synthetic hormones and subjected in other ways to lethal chemical toxins. Many of these toxins wind up in her milk and products made from such milk: cheese, yogurt, baked goods. Toxins absorbed through the animal's gut and skin are secreted in the milk. In fact, antibiotics no longer work for many people because they have been drinking milk and eating dairy products containing increased amounts of these powerful drugs, found in cows' milk. Since cows are often fed molded grains, their milk also often has mold-toxins, including aflatoxins (which kills liver cells). All this underscores the fact that commercial dairy milk is DIE-ry milk, killer milk, killer cheese, rich in killer toxins from the cows' poisoned DIE-t.

Feces-based artificial hormones in milk turn cows into hi-tech super MILK-Machines

50 years ago, the average cow produced 3000 pounds of milk per year. Today, the top producers yield 40,000 pounds or more! What makes this possible? The synthetic hormone "rBGH" (Recombinant Bovine Growth Hormone, also called Bovine Somatotropin or BST), plus drugs, antibiotics, specialized breeding, and forced feeding. Cows are being injected with genetically engineered versions of *their own* growth hormones. Bovine growth hormone (BGH) is a normal product of the pituitary gland of cows. The synthetic version, rBGH, is like "crack" for cows. It "revs" up their system, forcing them to overproduce milk. It makes cows sick and leads to increased pus, bacteria and saturated fat in milk. This unnatural rBGH is disgustingly made: Monsanto Agricultural Company of St. Louis, Missouri, isolated swarming E. Coli germs from human feces in the colon. They snip out a fraction of cow DNA that codes for this hormone, insert it into the DNA of the bacteria, grow the bacteria in vats, and extract large quantities of rBGH from the vats. In this way they created a strain able to recombine the natural cow-growth hormone into a new hormone more powerful than the natural cow hormone.[1] Injected every two weeks into cows, this hormone changes the cows' milk while boosting milk production –and boosting cancer rates in humans who consume the meat and milk from such animals.

No wonder most cows in America are sick and diseased

- 60% of America's dairy cows have leukemia virus.
- In America, *Mad Cow Disease* is called *Downer Cow Syndrome,* which kills at least 100,000 cows per year.[2] The dead diseased cows are made into feed which is fed back to cows or other animals, thus spreading the virus.[3]
- The artificial growth hormone, rBGH, makes cows sick with mastitis (infected udders, hence more pus in milk), persistent sores and lacerations, severe reproductive problems, food and leg ailments, and digestive disorders, thus the cows are given enormous doses of antibiotics.

PRION-infected milk, dissolving the brain of cows & humans

Feeding dead cows to cows results in diseased, unnatural **milk** and **meat** containing diabolical "prions" which can dissolve the brain in cows and in humans that drink the milk or eat the flesh of such cows. Horrible. Prions are tiny protein crystals; they are *twisted* variants of certain kinds of normal proteins. Prions are infective because when a twisted-prion comes in contact with normal-prion, it makes it twisted. The new twisted-prion has the same effect on any normal-prion protein it contacts, so the spread is like a domino effect. **Prions are *not* viruses and they are not considered to be living** because they do not have inputs /outputs, or respond to stimuli, or have DNA, or reproduce totally new copies of themselves. They slowly destroy the human brain until Alzheimer-like symptoms develop. In fact, **some cases of dementia, insanity and Alzheimer's are misdiagnosed prion-disease.** After the first exposure to a prion, the onset of disease might take up to 20 years to develop. As it dissolves brain tissue, prions pockmark the brain with holes, making it resemble Swiss cheese or a sponge (hence the term *spongiform*). The diseases called Mad Cow Disease, Downer Cow Syndrome, Bovine Spongiform Encephalopathy (BSE), Sheep Scrapie, –and in humans– the Creutzfeldt-Jakob Disease (CJD), Kuru Disease (produced from human cannibalism), and Gerstmann-Sträussler-Scheinker syndrome (GSS), are all really the same prion-disease.

1) Cohen, MTP, 192. 2) Ibid., 281. 3) Ibid.

Drugs Masquerading As Foods...

Thus, cows' milk is unnatural because

• Synthetic hormones injected into the cows make them produce unnatural, cancer-proliferating milk. • Feeding cows to cows results in diseased, unnatural milk containing "prions" which cause brain-dissolving diseases in cows and in humans that consume the milk /cheese /flesh of infected cows. • Dairy cows themselves are unnatural animals, created through crossbreeding. The modern dairy cow (Holstein Frisian) has only been developed over the last 50 years.

Milk is only for newborns anyway

Milk is a maternal secretion intended as shorterm nutrient for newborns

Humans are the only animals that continue drinking milk after they are weaned. Lactase is the enzyme needed in order to digest milk –with its high content of *lactose*, milk sugar. The ability to produce lactase declines as babies grow into adults. Most (3/4) of Earth's human population (i.e., People of Color) cannot tolerate lactose. Blacks should not drink milk or eat cheese; 70-90% of Black adults do not produce lactase; 90-95% of whites do produce lactase.

Milk is a "hormone delivery system"

Milk is appropriate for newborns who must gain weight quickly. But milk is inappropriate for adults. The purpose of milk is to enable infants to receive nourishment, including hormones, that will direct and regulate growth. Newborn humans and animals double their weight within weeks or months. Baby cows will gain 500 pounds in 6 months. **Hormones in cows' milk include:**

– Pituitary hormones (PRL, GH, TSH, FSH, LH ACTH Oxytocin)
– Steroid hormones (Estradiol, Estriol, Progesterone,
    Testosterone, 17-Ketosteroids, Corticosterone, vitamin D)
– Hypothalamic hormones (TRH, LHRH, Somatostatin,
    PRL-inhibiting factor, PRL-releasing factor, GnRH, GRH)
– Thyroid & Parathyroid hormones (T3, T4, Calcitonin, Parathormone, PTH peptide)

Breast-milk is for baby-cows; Cow milk is for baby-humans

Yes, I know that's bass ackward. So let's feed our babies the milk from horses, hogs and hippopotamuses instead –and get them off to a bad start right at the beginning so that they grow up into weak, compromised adults. This practice is "normal" and prevalent in this society. You see how inappropriate it is to cross-feed species? *Milk is perfect food only for the species it belongs to.*

Healthy milk-substitutes for human babies

Freshly made juice of ripe, raw organic fruit /leafy greens. And fig juice, hemp seed milk, nut /seed milk (avoid soy). Hemp protein globulin resembles human blood globulin. Afrikans used fig juice as a substitute for human milk. Figs are similar in chemical composition to human milk. In six months, it can double an infant's size.[1] For babes being nursed, fresh raw fruit /veggie juices may be given between nursing periods after two months. Other "Natural Blender Formulas for the Growing Baby" are offered by Dick Gregory.[2]

1) Afrika, AH 89.   2) Dick Gregory's Natural Diet for Folks Who Eat...130-132.

Why is pasteurized, homogenized milk deadly?

- **Causes, develops, promotes, or is linked to:**

heart attacks	asthma	gout	mad cow disease
osteoporosis	diabetes	allergies	arterial degeneration
atherosclerosis	cancers	breast cancer	rheumatoid arthritis
kidney stones	pyorrhea	prostate cancer	mucus congestion
allergies	cataracts	neuro diseases	respiratory disorders

- **Cows' milk is for baby cows.** Goat milk is for baby goats. Zebra milk is for baby zebras. The milk of cows, goats and zebras is perfect food for its respective species but is not fit as food for humans, let alone human babies and children. Any wonder milk allergies are so common?

- **Milk increases the death rate of babies (& grownups).** Also causes sore throats, colds, earaches, colitis, and other health problems in children.

- **Pasteurized & homogenized milk is a *grave* danger to the heart** and the primary contributor to all heart disorders. Also increases blood cholesterol.

- **Is a chemical & hormonal solution** rich with hundreds of different toxins including pus, drugs, antibiotics, pesticides, mold-toxins, bacteria, viruses, hormones and other poisons fed to cows. Each toxin has the potential to exert a powerful biological effect when taken independently of the others. Together, they keep America in a perpetual state of subhealth & disease.

- **Milk boosts cancer rates,** especially for breast and prostate cancer.

- **70-90% of Blacks do not produce lactase,** the enzyme necessary to digest lactose, a sugar present in all milk products.

- **Is the most mucus-forming of all foods,** due to its abundant Casein, which makes an effective glue. Congests body with mucus, impeding its ability to operate efficiently. Casein causes thyroid dysfunctions.[1]

- **Promotes a calcium deficiency.** Causes deposits of unusable calcium.

- **Most cows are sick,** hence their milk is sick. 60% of cows have leukemia.

- **Coats the stomach** and thus cause poor digestion.

- **Makes ulcers worse** (though easing pain). Increases acid production which further erodes the linings of the duodenum & stomach.

- **Children who are fed cow's milk formulas** grow up into adults with a higher susceptibility to M.S. than children who are breast fed.

- **The synthetic vitamin D** added to milk is toxic, another drugfood.

- **Commercial milk used for cheese is bleached** (!) –like other bleached-white foods– with *hydrogen peroxide* or toxic *benzoyl peroxide*.[2]

- **Pasteurized milk is acid-forming.** Normally, raw milk is alkaline-forming. Since cows are being fed protein, even raw milk is acid forming.

1) Nelson, MN, 77.   2) Block, IA, 48, 99.

Each SIP of MILK & every
BITE of CHEESE provide you with:

- **PUS & COW BLOOD:** All cows' milk contains blood. USDA allows milk to contain 1 to 1 1/2 million white blood cells per milliliter (1/30 of an ounce).
- **GROWTH FACTORS:** IGF's (I and II), IGF binding proteins, Nerve growth factor, Epidermal growth factor and TGF alpha, TGF beta, Growth Inhibitors MDGI and MAF, and Platelet-derived growth factor.
- **COW HORMONES:** Pituitary hormones, Steroid hormones, Hypothalamic hormones, Thyroid and Parathyroid hormones, and often synthetic rBGH.
- **MUCUS-MAKING GLUE:** Casein, used to hold wood together in furniture.
- **BACTERIA & VIRUSES:**
  — Even when milk is pasteurized, not all the microbes are killed. The acceptable standard for pasteurized milk is 100,000 bacteria per teaspoon (or 20,000 germs per milliliter). The Jan. 1974 *Consumer Reports* found that 1 out of 6 milk samples from stores had 130,000 bacteria per milliliter.
  — Antibiotic-resistant microbes. The antibiotic residue in milk standard was increased 100-fold. As a result, new strains of bacteria developed, immune to antibiotics in milk. Antibiotics no longer work because Americans have been eating dairy products containing increased amounts of these powerful drugs.
  — Milk drinkers become exposed to animal-borne diseases.
  — 60% of America's dairy cows have leukemia virus.
  — Viruses of bovine leukemia, bovine tuberculosis, cow immunodeficiency.
  — America's equivalent of *Mad Cow Disease* is called *Downer Cow Syndrome.* It kills at least 100,000 cows per year in the USA.
  — Dead diseased cows are fed to cows & other animals, spreading *Downer Cow Syndrome,* other viruses, and **brain-dissolving PRIONS.** (pg 108)
- **DRUGS & ANTIBIOTICS:**
  — 52 different antibiotics are found in commercial milk.
  — In 1990, the antibiotic residue in milk standard was increased 100-fold from 1 ppm to 100 ppm (part per million).
  — Authorities test for only 4 of 82 drugs that are given to dairy cows.[1]
- **"CIDES."** Because cows eat huge amounts of vegetable matter, their milk contains high concentrations of pesticides, herbicides and fungicides. A Congressional hearing admitted: *"No milk available on the market, today, in any part of the United States, is free of pesticide residues."*[2]
- **RADIOACTIVE PARTICLES:** Iodine 131, Cesium 134 and 137, and Strontium 90. Milk is the main carrier for Strontium-90.
- **GASTRO-INTESTINAL PEPTIDES:** Vasoactive intestinal peptide, Bombesin, Cholecystokinin, Gastrin, Gastrin inhibitory peptide, Pancreatic peptide, Y peptide, Substance P and Neurotensin.
- **OTHER STUFF:** Fat, Cholesterol, Delta sleep-inducing peptide, Transferrin, Lactoferrin, Casomorphin, Erythropoietin, PGE, PGF2 alpha, cAMP, cGMP.

1) Cohen, MDP, 216.   2) Cousens, CE, 337.

Recommendations for Better Health

Avoid or Reduce Eating:	Healthier Replacements:

• *pasteurized* cows' milk
• homogenized milk
• skim milk, evaporated milk
• babies' milk formulas
• powdered or dry milk
• ice cream, cream
• cheeses made with *pasteurized* milk and *rennet* (a coagulating enzyme made from calf/pig stomachs; all cheese is made with rennet unless otherwise noted)
• all dairy products made from *pasteurized* cows' milk:
  – butter – cream – ghee
  – whey – yogurt – kefir
  – cottage cheese – cream cheese
• nondairy creamers (Most "nondairy creamers" do contain milk products; sodium or calcium caseinate and lactose)
• yeast powders (have up to 50% whey)
• "milk" chocolate & foods made w/ milk
• fake cheeses made with casein
	Best:
	• seed or nut milk (see below)
	• coconut milk (fresh)
	• sesame seed milk (sesame has 1,125 milligrams of calcium per 100 grams [about 1/4 lb.], whereas a pint of milk has only 590 milligrams. Sesame seed also has lecithin and 19-28% more protein than most meat.)
	
	Improvement:
	• frozen ripe bananas or fruit (Instead of ice cream. You may put it through a juicer, grinder or blender)
	• RAW, unpasteurized milk (preferably from **GOATS** since goat milk is greatly less mucus-forming & closer in composition to humans' milk)
	• cheese made from raw milk
	• organic, rennetless cheese
	• artificial milk /cheese /ice creams (be careful; these are still drugfoods)

Making Nut Milks or Fruit Ice Cream

All nuts & edible seeds make nutritious milks. Generally to make a nut milk, put a few *soaked* nuts in a blender with water and *liquefy*. May be sweetened.

Sesame Seed Milk
- 1/2 cup sesame seeds (blends easier if presoaked a few hours)
- 2 cups water
- 1/2 teaspoon maple syrup or Sucanat (optional)
Blend sesame and 1 cup water. Add sweetener and remaining water, blend a few seconds and strain if desired. Makes 2 1/4 cups. White, dehulled sesame may be used for a milder more milk-like drink, but unhulled is more nutritious. Has more calcium than cow's milk.

Almond Milk
- 1/2 cup almonds, chopped
- 1 3/4 cups water
Blend 1/2 cup water with nuts for 1 minute. Add remaining liquid, blend, then strain out pulp if desired.
Makes 2 1/4 cups.

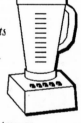

Banana Marble Ice Cream
- 6 large bananas, frozen on tray or in a cellophane bag
- 2 cups of any (frozen) berries
Feed the bananas, one at a time, in a grinder, with chilled dish to catch the ice cream. When the banana is nearly ground, add a few frozen raspberries or strawberries for marbling. Serve at once. Serves 6.

DRUG

7

Cancer-Yes Commercial Flesh

**That red meat in those nice supermarkets looks and feels so fresh.
This *illusion* is created by chemical poisons.**

When an animal is killed, the flesh immediately begins spoiling and starts to turn brownish-yellowish. Rigor-mortis sets in quickly, making the carcass stiff. No problem; that off-colored meat is dyed to look red and fresh; chemicals are added to make the flesh pliable – that's why your raw steak isn't stiff; cancer-causing nitrates /nitrites are added to camouflage the rotten smell and rotten taste! People that eat meat can become addicted to the drugs in the meat which are fed to the slaughtered animals.
Furthermore, the animals are filled with terror prior to and during their slaughter. This terror causes their adrenal glands to flood their bodies with adrenaline which poisons their already-poisoned flesh.

We are falsely led to believe we need to eat lots of flesh or protein-rich food to be healthy.

The opposite is true! Eating lots of flesh or any high-protein food invites cancer and other diseases, and contributes directly to our rapid degeneration. Have you wondered where cows get (or should get) their protein from? (hint: it's *green*) Note that the largest, strongest, and longest living animals on Earth are all plant-eaters. And many animals thrive on just eating nothing but grass or leaves. **Humans recycle 90% of their protein wastes** through the processes of pinocytosis and phagocytosis.[1] Only 16% of our body is protein. Our actual protein needs are only 20-30 grams per day.[2] The much touted 10-100 grams of protein a day is a meat-and-dairy-industry-fostered myth. Our daily protein (amino acid) requirement is easily met on a diet of organic fruit and vegetables. Human milk is only 1.1 % protein –for a growing human baby (on a mono-diet at that). Sufficient, high quality, assimilable protein is available from simply fruit and vegetables, uncooked. **Most meat is no more than 20-25% protein.**

1) Honiball/Fry, IL, 104.   2) Ibid.

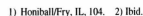

Flesh is the hardest food for humans to digest.

Meat takes long to digest (4-6 hours in the stomach) and 1-4 days to pass through the intestines –during which time undigested pieces rot in your colon, slowly poisoning you. Any food remaining in the colon over 8 hours spells future health problems. Retarded digestion always encourages putrefaction and fermentation. Protein is the most difficult food for humans to metabolize. Cooked animal protein coagulates, becoming virtually digestion-proof. Cooked animal protein feeds the Escherichia Coli bacteria in your colon. This bacteria produces large amounts of toxic, harmful waste products as it literally rots the cooked protein.[1] This applies to cooked eggs and pasteurized milk / cheese / yogurt. About 30-50% of your stool is colon bacteria; this percentage can be as high as 75% bacteria when you eat flesh! The waste products of protein metabolism (urea, uric acid, etc.) are non-oxidizable. Eliminating them greatly burdens and strains the liver, kidneys, and adrenal glands.

Flesh is the most putrefactive of all foods.
It literally rots in your colon and poisons your bloodstream.

Animal flesh begins decaying at the moment of death. When eaten by humans, it continues decaying in the guts, poisoning the blood. Putrefaction in meat eaters is evidenced by bad breath, heartburn, eructations, foul-smelling acid stool and foul emissions – absent in vegetarians. As it rots in your colon, flesh produces toxic waste which speeds the metabolism and causes degenerative diseases leading to premature death. Thanks to the help of scavenging Excherichia Coli bacteria (or E. Coli, the bacterial of putrefaction), up to 36 toxins are formed in your gut as flesh rots. Absorbed into your precious bloodstream to defile it, these toxins include:

- **Skatole** and **indole** which largely gives feces its characteristic stench, and a foul odor to breath. Skatole depresses circulation and the central nervous system. Indole affects the brain and causes headaches and lassisitude. It also affects the liver, causing it to become sluggish and ineffective in the removal of toxic substances from the blood.[2]
- **Phenol** (carbolic acid) is so poisonous that it is used as an antimicrobial agent. It is both a local corrosive and systemic poison which can cause necrosis of gastrointestinal mucosa, kidney and liver cells.
- **Hydrogen sulfide gas,** (giving "farts" a rotten egg odor) in concentration is as toxic as cyanide. Poisoning by this gas causes weakness, nausea, clammy skin, rapid pulse and cyanosis.[3]
- **"Sepsin,** a poison so virulent that a minute dose given to a large dog caused death in a few hours, is always present in the bowels of persons who eat flesh, and is always found in putrid flesh."[4]
- **Ammonia.** "Rich protein decomposes in the stomach into poisonous ammonia, which in turn produces nitrosamines. Biochemist, Dr. Lijinsky said: '...they are among the most potent cancer causing chemicals known.' "[5]

1) Preston, 110. 2) Ibid., 135. 3) Kulvinskas, LTC, 304. 4) Clements, 159. 5) Kulvinskas, STC, 26.

The corpse of a flesh eater putrefies more rapidly than that of a vegetarian, and will have an intolerably offensive odor.

The vegetarian corpse will remain two or three times as long as the flesh-eater's corpse.[1] This reflects the difference between flesh and plants; flesh spoils immediately, plants take a much longer time to spoil.

Yes, meat *seems* to make you strong, but you won't last very long. Meat is a *stimulant*, at the expense of our vitality.

There are many examples of heavy meat diet producing robust and apparently healthy individuals. Dr. L. H. Newberg of Ann Arbor University found that when he fed large quantities of meat to test animals, they grew bigger and more alert than other animals on a vegetarian diet. But three months later, these animals contracted kidney damage and died while the vegetarian animals lived healthily and happily.[2] People may feel strong after eating meat, not because it gives them energy but because meat is a stimulant, speeding the body's metabolism –because the body is trying to evict this poison as rapidly as possible, at the expense of its own vitality. All this excess exertion depletes vitality over time. This is also the same reason for the "stimulating" effects of caffeine, amphetamines, drugs, drugfood, and poisons. Eating meat actually robs the body of energy, for it takes more energy to digest it than what you get back. It's like paying $100.00 to get $60.00

Tryptophane, an essential amino acid, causes growth & aging. It is about 20 times more concentrated in meat than in fruit.

In one study, by excluding tryptophane from the diet, animals were kept youthful and active with out any signs of aging in excess of normal lifespan. Introducing tryptophane resulted in the appearance of normal aging.[3] The formula for tryptophane is very close to that of indole-acetic acid, which is a growth hormone in plants. This hormone can be produced by plants from tryptophane.[4] Tryptophane is carcinogenic in the urinary tract, especially when flesh is eaten often over a period of time.[5]

Flesh shortens your lifespan.

During World War I, when Denmark drastically reduced its population's intake of fleshfood, the death rate decreased 40%. Additionally, diseases declined, and when Europe suffered an epidemic of influenza, Denmark was not affected.[6]

Hot dogs and sausages are made of garbage meat.

They contain the diseased and rejected parts of animals: cut off tumors and cancers, lungs, testes, hog blood, fat, worms, detergents, sodium sulfide to hide the rotten smell, meat "by products," filth, and extenders such as cereals, coal-tar, insect scales. This also goes for salami, luncheon meat and bologna.

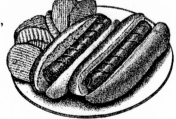

1) Hotema, 96. 2) Kulvinskas, STC, 28. 3) Ibid., 26. 4) Ibid. 5) Ibid., 26, 27. 6) Nelson, MYN, 64.

Are you consuming cow urine & manure-germs unknowingly?

Uric acid (a chief component of urine), manure germs, pus, blood, and putrefied flesh are what gives red meat its delicious flavor! If you doubt this, try eating kosher-style meat before it's spiced! As the blood is drained out, so is most of the uric acid. Now about those manure germs: When the animal is alive, the osmotic process in its colon keeps the putrefactive colon bacteria from spreading to its other tissues. When the animal is dead the osmotic process is gone and the putrefactive manure germs swarm through the walls of the colon and into the flesh, tenderizing the meat. Meat has to age. What ages or softens the flesh are the putrefactive colon germs. Experts say the bacteria in meats are identical with those of manure and more numerous in some meats than in fresh manure. Is that what you want to eat?

Schizophrenia in meat

More people in America are hospitalized and treated for the condition of "schizophrenia" than for the total cases of cancer, diabetes and heart disorders! Dr. Yuri Nikolayev of Moscow Research Institute of Psychiatry showed that "schizophrenia" and numerous other diseases are forms of protein toxemia. In his "starvation therapy," psychiatric patients suffering from "schizophrenia" and other diseases go on a cleansing diet, then a 20-40 day fast. Afterwards, the patients followed a vegetarian diet if they did not want the sickness to return.[1]

Commercial eggs of "Eggribusiness" are toxic and cruel

First of all, the chickens are all diseased or cancerous, literally insane, and abominably abused. They are fed insecticides, antibiotics, and other poisons. Their yolks are dyed to make them a "healthy yellow." Billions of hens, turkeys, etc., are raised in utterly cruel, disease-ridden conditions. 8 billion are killed each year for American caskets, I mean stomachs. To reduce cannibalism, hens are "debeaked," a painful procedure whereby their sensitive upper beak is sliced off with a hot blade. Many die from shock during the process. Over 200 million male chicks are destroyed each year as commercially useless. They are thrown into plastic bags to suffocate slowly under the weight of chicks dumped on top. Others are ground into animal feed – while *still alive*. Thus, cholesterol in eggs ain't nothing compared to the other stuff not talked about.

Do your flesh smell of death?

Wild animals run away from humans that eat animals because they can smell the smell of death exuding from these people –from the dead animals eaten which has become a part of the person's flesh.

Charcoal-cooked flesh has the toxic equivalent of 600 cigarettes.

Benzopyrene, a powerful carcinogen, is produced when flesh (or any food) is cooked over charcoal fire or direct flameheat. This substance goes up in the smoke from the charcoal and coats the flesh. It's been estimated that in 1 kg. (2.2 lbs.) of charcoal broiled steak, there is as much benzopyrene as in the smoke from 600 cigarettes.[2] As the thymus deteriorates from its benzene burden, so does your immune system.

1) Kulvinskas, STC, 27. 2) Nelson, MYN, 72

Our Disguised Cannibalism!

Human genes are being added to livestock (and produce), making Americans *Unknowing Cannibals!* (see page 34) This further increases our risk of PRIONS (see page 108) and other unknown horrible dis-eases /insanity.

Too much protein causes cell starvation and cellular rotting

Only a limited amount of protein excess can be excreted in the urine each day. The rest float through the blood, thickening and congesting it. As the chain-like amino acid molecules work their way like snakes into the tiny capillaries they finally come to a halt. Now they begin to line the wall of the capillaries. According to Professor Lother Wendt of Frankfurt Germany, they build up layer upon layer, thickening the capillary walls until they are 2–3 times as thick as normal.[1] Capillaries are the tiny vessels that feed nutrients to the cell. But as the excess amino acids thickens the capillaries, they prevent the proper transmission of nutrients through the capillary walls into the cells. As a result, the cells begin to starve, then they degenerate, then they rot and die.

Too much protein interferes with lymph flow

The molecules of amino acids (protein) are long chains. As excess amino acids build up in the capillaries, the pressure eventually breaks some of these chains into smaller pieces and they slip through the capillary walls. They slither in between the cells since they cannot enter the cells. If the body is in balance and protein excess is not too great, these acid chains make it to the lymph to be discarded. But if the body is nutritionally unbalanced and the salt content is high, then trouble. These acid chains have a *negative* electrical charge so they attract and hold *positive* sodium ions. This <u>attracts and holds water in the tissues</u>.[2] This upsets osmotic balance in the tissues, causing a collapse of lymph vessels. Results: cell-metabolism waste is unable to properly escape. In effect, the sewer is backing up. Hence, cellular contamination rapidly increases.

Too much protein produces too much Urea Salt

Most amino acids are *di-basic*. This means that upon contact with a base (alkali), they give up two hydrogen atoms and combine with the base to form two salts. With too much protein in our diet, the body converts much of it into urea salts /mineral salts to get it out the way.[3, 4] These unneeded salts usually end up being stored in our connective /fibrous tissues; ligaments, tendons, cartilage, tissue supporting the nerves, arteries. Results: soft tissue becoming rigid, stiff painful joints, clogged arteries, high blood pressure. Excess urea salts overstimulates the heart making it beat much harder, putting it in danger of a pectoris heart attack.[4] Signs of too much urea salt: being tired upon awaking in the morning, fatigue, tension, forehead wrinkles. Drinking *distilled water* (especially with fresh lemon or lime juice in it) greatly reduces urea salts.[5]

The average American, in their lifetime, consumes:

– 12 cows	– 3000 chickens / birds	– 18,000 eggs
– 6 hogs	– 3000 sea-creatures	– 30,000 quarts of milk

---

1) Preston, 111.   2) Ibid., 112   3) Ibid., 119.   4) Kirban, 166, 169.   5) Ibid., 90, 168.

Pick your favorite cancer:
Delivery 99% guaranteed on a HIGH-flesh diet

Colon & Rectum Cancer

Researchers reported in the *Journal of the National Cancer Institute* that there is not a single population in the world with a high meat intake which does not have a high rate of colon cancer.[1] Heavy beef eating is related to the high incidence of colon and rectum cancer.[2]

Breast Cancer

The more fat, especially animal fat in a woman's diet, the greater her risk of breast cancer. Those who eat meat daily are 4 times as likely of getting breast cancer than those who eat little or no meat. The more meat /eggs /cheese /butter eaten, the greater the risk of breast cancer.

Urinary Cancer

Tryptophane is about 20 times more concentrated in meat than in fruit. Tryptophane is carcinogenic in the urinary tract, especially when flesh is eaten often over a period of time.[3]

Prostate Cancer

Is highly related to fat consumption. 25% of all men –with high consumption of animal fat– develop latent prostate cancer by their old age.[4]

Leukemia

Promotes leukemia due to its high content of uric acid. Leukemia is always associated with an extremely high amount of uric acid in the blood.

Uterine Cancer / Cervical Cancer

Is highest among women who consume diets high in fat, especially animal fat.

Ovarian Cancer

Rises with egg consumption and animal fat.

Commercial Flesh & Produce has much cancer-causing Nitrates.

The drugfood of the Standard American Diet is grown with excessive nitrate fertilizers which end up in the produce and fleshfoods. Results: proliferating cancer. One doctor summarized it:

"The nitrate problems caused by the enormous application of synthetic nitrogen fertilizer to our soils, and the addition of nitrates and nitrites to our bacon, hot dogs, and lunch meats is a primary cause of the cancer epidemic that threatens the survival of this nation."[6]

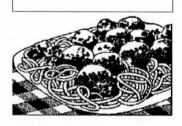

Cooked flesh selectively feeds (and causes) cancer.
Each year, 900,000 Americans learn they have cancer. 460,000 die of it.
In *Cancer Research*, Dr. Ronald Phillips reported that the evidence is now overwhelming: vegetarian diets strongly reduce the incidence of breast, uterine, ovarian, colon, and many other cancers."[5]

Putting the dead bodies of animals into our dying bodies speeds our demise.

1) Robbins, DN, 253.   2) Kulvinskas, STC, 26.   3) Ibid., 26, 27.   4) Robbins, DN, 270.   5) Ibid.   6) Preston, 60.

Five special reasons to stop or limit eating animals

Eating dead animals is an acquired habit. Humans are not natural killers. The sight of ripped, bloody flesh does not whet our appetites. The flesh of dead animals is made acceptable to us only after extensive preparation, cooking and seasoning.

Your gut & teeth are like those of the fruitarian gorilla.

We do not have the digestive system and teeth of flesh-eating animals. Not a single tooth in their mouths resembles ours. Our digestive tract looks like that of a gorilla, a fruitarian animal. Our bodies aren't made to handle eating flesh, as hereby shown:

Natural Flesh-Eaters	Natural Plant-Eaters
The flesh of animals begins decomposing at the moment of death. Dead flesh *putrefies so rapidly* that Nature provides natural carnivorous animals (cats, dogs, etc.) with *short guts* so that the toxic substance can be quickly eliminated. Flesh-eating animals secrete 5-10 times the quantity of hydrochloric acid (HCl) into the stomach than humans. Their acid is vastly stronger than ours (dogs have 5 times more HCl at 100 times the strength of a human's HCl). This allows them to digest bone, flesh, feathers, fur, hair and sinews, since true meat eaters eat the whole body of the prey. Their gastric juice is super acidic to prevent putrefaction while flesh digests. Carnivores and omnivores secret the enzyme *uricase* that breaks down uric acid (found abundantly in flesh food). Humans do not. Flesh-eating animals have a different type of intestinal bacterial flora than non-meat eaters. Guts of carnivores are smooth (to allow the quick passage of their toxic flesh diet), and 3 times the length of their body. Carnivores have dagger-like, <u>SHARP</u> long, round, slender canines /fangs. Their jaws only move up & down.	Fruit and vegetables *spoil slowly*, so Nature provides natural plant eaters (cows, gorillas, humans...) with *long guts*. This enables plant nutrients to be slowly absorbed & assimilated. Also our guts are corrugated to hold food as long as possible so nutrients may be extracted. This is the worst possible condition for digesting and processing flesh! Our guts are also 12 times the length of our body (4 times that of carnivores). Big strong bodies are built from fruit protein, as any gorilla proves. Humans do not secrete *uricase* (for digesting uric acid of meat). In humans, uric acid is poison, causing osteoporosis, dental cavities (=osteoporosis of the teeth) and arthritic /rheumatic complaints. Our short, stout, flat, <u>DULL</u> teeth are just like those of the gorilla. We can "grind" our jaws; carnivores can't. We suck our liquids; carnivores all lap theirs.

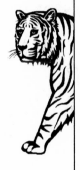

2.

Flesh-toxins overload, strain, and damage your liver and kidneys

Your liver and kidneys buckle under the toxic overload of fleshfood. Flesh-eating places unnatural stress on our organs of detoxification and elimination. For example, uric acid and urea are two poisonous compounds produced in the animal body by waste and decay. The amount varies with change of diet. A test of the urine of a man living for some time on an exclusive vegetable diet, showed only *1.3 grains of uric acid*, and *181.29 grains of urea* excreted in 24 hours. A similar test of a man living for some days on a strictly flesh diet, showed *22.64 grains of uric acid*, and *819.2 grains of urea*.[1] From this it is clear that eating flesh imposes a labor upon the kidneys that is many times the amount Nature that intended. Hence, some uric acid will remain in the body from any one meat meal which will accumulate to produce gout, kidney gravel, rheumatism, or complications of arthritis. Over time, the strain of handling flesh toxins weakens the liver and kidneys, causing them to grow sluggish and malfunction. Then they are not able to remove all the toxins they should. These toxins then remain in the body to sabotage our health and even kill us.

Liver:

The chief function of the liver (body's largest gland) is to neutralize and destroy toxins in the blood and toxins entering the blood from digested food. Carnivores (flesh-eating animals like dogs & cats) have *huge* livers to aid in detoxifying their blood and generate massive bile secretion. But humans have a comparatively smaller liver. As a result, we cannot detoxify the poisonous products in flesh. Flesh-eating places a great strain on our small livers, impairing its function over time. **ANIMAL FAT (including fish oil, butter, cheese) contains high levels of cholesterol.** Cholesterol clogs the honeycomb structures in the liver, interfering with or blocking the liver's functions. This can lead to serious liver diseases. The cholesterol also collects in the blood vessels, causing heart problems. Toxins also concentrate in fat. *Beef fat* is the worst kind of animal fat. It will only break down when heated to temperatures of over 600 degrees. That's why it is used in heavy industries to lubricate machines.

Kidneys:

A lion's kidney is twice the size of a bull's and hardly smaller than that of an elephant's. This lets the lion handle large amounts of protein and nitrogenous waste contained in its flesh-diet. Our kidneys are smaller and become diseased from overwork caused by a diet high in flesh.

1) Clements, LLH, 156-157.

Commercial animals are raised in horrible cruelty. To eat them is to eat their agonizing pain and support murderous brutality.

The painful gory details are eloquently addressed in John Robbin's *Diet for a New America*. The truth may make you cry. Americans are not informed of the truth; they do not know that they eat the bodies and embryos (eggs) of enslaved, tortured, brutally murdered creatures who have suffered severely from day one of their life. To buy such meat is to support and perpetuate abominable cruelty to animals. To eat such meat is to take in the vibrations of the animals' pain into your own body and reap a continuing harvest of pain, mental unease, psychosis, and disease. It is bad karma. I once saw a documentary on a slaughter-house. The cows were not formally killed. Instead, secured to a conveyor belt, they died in the process of getting processed; as the conveyor belt moved forward, heartless mechanical hands/devices simultaneously made incisions at predetermined areas, pulled off the cows' skin, pulled out their organs, dismembered them, etc. The cows died in the process of getting dismembered by machines.

Animals destined for Americans' stomachs are usually totally confined.
They are packed so tightly in their metal cages, they can hardly move at all, let alone turn around. This is nearly identical to the way Afrikan captives were treated on slave ships. And the cages are stacked 3 stories high! These suffering, diseased, drugged, deranged, literally insane animals live in their feces and filth. Often they live their entire lives in total darkness. There is absolutely no regard for their natural urges, only more confinement, more drugs, more farming by automation and technology, and more assembly-line *beef, broilers, pork, veal*; deceptive formless terms hiding the fact that a real, feeling animal is /was there. Sows are enslaved to continuously produce litters of pigs through artificial methods until it kills them. Black slave women suffered similar fates. Chickens are kept in artificial light 24 hours a day so that they lay eggs continuously, since they only lay eggs in the light or daytime. The living conditions of chickens are so horrible, all of them are literally insane. Referring to the Albino practice of mechanized mass-brutality to animals, John Robbins wrote:
"Animals have been treated cruelly before, and in some cases sadistically – but the process has never before been institutionalized on such an overwhelming scale. And never before has the cold expertise of modern [=*Albino*] technology and pharmacology been employed to this end."[1]

1) Robbins, DNA, 95.

If you had a live cow, calf, chicken, or kitten, could you kill it yourself with your own hands and then eat it? If we had to kill the animals we eat, most people would probably become vegetarians. Can we be ever happy, peaceful, and healthy while making our stomachs the graves of tortured, brutally killed animals?

Are we reaping bad karma from the animals' suffering? Exactly what humans are doing unto the animals is karmically being done unto them.

There is a direct connection between the suffering of people and the way they unknowingly support the brutalization of helpless animals. When we eat any food, we also eat the essence of the food and essence of what was done to it.

<u>**Would you eat an animal from Hell? These animals are raised in Hell; the *Torture Chambers* of *Factory-Farms.***</u> Millions of Americans die tortured deaths each year from diseases caused from eating tortured, brutally killed animals. There are many cures for cancer, heart diseases, and other so-called "incurable" diseases. These cures are suppressed in this country. Cancer cures like Laetrile, CanCell, Cantron, Essiac, Shark Cartilage, the Rife machine, etc., are suppressed. This insensitivity is a direct reflection of people's insensitivity to the plight of the suffering animals they consume. We reap what we sow.

It isn't flesh-eating per se that I'm against; it's the unnatural horrible suffering inflicted upon the animals; – they suffer their <u>entire</u> lives in unspeakable cruelty. Can any flesh from such creatures be wholesome to eat? The Native Americans ate flesh. Ancient Afrikans also ate flesh. These and other indigenous cultures around the world honored the connectedness of all life and gave due respect to the spirit of the animal and to *The Great Spirit.* They ate meat because plant food was scarce or unavailable. Around the world, ancient cultures have consumed the flesh of killed animals, but never in Earth's history has such abominable cruelty been practiced towards animals, especially on the quantum scale it is today. Though this horrible practice was began and developed by the Albinos, all flesh-eaters are guilty of perpetuating it. **Can't we see that we are only a half step away from treating ourselves this way?** In fact, many humans *are* being this way in many parts of the world.

If you love meat and want to eat it too, go out of your way and find *organically* grown, *naturally* (= humanely) grown animals.

Your hamburgers are eating Earth's rainforests.

Every time you eat that burger, you are participating in destroying the *planet* and thus yourself, for if we kill our planet, we die too.

Eating flesh, especially "BEEF," is destroying planet Earth.

Albino culture and technology have placed Earth and her atmosphere in *grave* trouble. About 30% of the oxygen in the air comes from the rain forests in South America. Every few minutes, forest area the size of several stadium football fields are burned so that cattle may be raised to satisfy the fast food chains in the USA and Europe. **A quarter-pound hamburger requires the destruction of 55 square feet of rain forest.**[1] In his exposé book and video *Diet for a New America*, John Robbins details how your food choices affect your health and future of life on Earth.

There are billions more cows in America than people!

Over two billion cattle exist in the U.S.! And 80% to 90% of the fresh WATER supply and GRAIN grown in America goes to these cows! The chemical pollution from maintaining them is disrupting Nature's balance. The massive volume of methane gas (16 million metric tons per year –from bacteria in their guts) they belch out is the third largest contributor to the greenhouse effect.[2] Due to the chemicals in their diet, their feces is unnatural –inert, undissolvable (it doesn't decompose into the soil). No wonder the literal "mountains of feces" from these cattle has become a serious threat to American ecology.

● Studies show that to grow one pound of grain you need 60 pounds of water, and the major consumer of that grain is animals raised for their flesh.

● 4,000 pounds of water is needed to produce 1 pound of flesh!

● Just one large chickenhouse uses 100 million gallons of water every day! This water would supply a city of 25,000 people with fresh drinking water.[2]

● It takes 50 to 100 times more land to produce meat than it does to produce its equivalent in vegetarian food.

You can satisfy your craving (addiction!) for animal flesh by eating fake meats/hot dogs /sausages /eggs made from plant protein. **And *fasting* is the best way to rid yourself of the desire for meat since fasting removes most of the body's uric acid accumulation.**

1) Inglis, DG, 69.   2) Whole Life Times April 1991, page 17.

Is hormony meat making some people homosexual?

Upon learning that men can become *feminized* from eating hormoned meat, I wondered if the same drugmeat could make its faithful eaters incline towards or even become *homosexual*. According to another doctor, yes! In fact, Dr. Llaila Afrika said he has actually healed cases of homosexuality by detoxing his patients and changing their diet. His video, ***Understanding Homosexuality & Homosexual Detox***, addresses his treatment, plus social & chemical causes, and political purposes. (See *Afrika* in the Bibliography) In August 1998, Dr. Afrika and another brilliant Afrikan man, Cleo Manago, engaged in a debate on homosexuality entitled: ***How Homosexuality Originated in the Black Community.*** The program also included a panel of "gay" and "straight" American-Afrikans. (A video of this highly educational program is available; see *Talking Drum* in the Bibliography). So. **Hormoned, commercial animal flesh (and likely, hormoned *milk* as well) cause sex disorders. Men are becoming effeminized –and in some cases, homosexual,** from consuming the flesh (and milk?) of animals fed female hormones. Some men have even grown pendulous breasts as a result! Fastfood burgers are especially loaded with fake female hormones. Bombarding the male body with female hormones, thwarts the natural male hormones. **The same hormony drugmeat (& dairy?) masculinizes women** in that the body tries to balance the excess female hormones by creating more male hormones in women. Nor do our children escape. Fake hormones have caused children as young as 3 years to develop breasts and pubic hair. Why are DES and BGH hormones given to these animals in the first place? It's given to cows to vastly increase their milk production, and to cattle to make them grow big fast. It has the same effect on the people that eat these animals. This is why our children are so big so soon. They and ourselves are unnaturally large from eating hormoned drugmeat.

Another element, hardly considered: When you eat a food, you also eat the ESSENCE of whatever was *done* to that food. Most food of the "western diet" is made from produce /animals that are castrated, neutered, sterile. Seedless fruit. Infertile eggs. Neutered factory-farm animals. Castration is widespread in the cattle industry. The beef people eat is largely from STEERS (castrated bulls). Combine all this genital-defunct food with *xenohormones* in the environment (see pages 45-46) and we got a big problem. A chemical war on our reproductive system. Albinos, the white people –creators and perpetrators of this, got an even bigger problem. They are becoming sterile from the very toxins they continue to abundantly manufacture and eat. Their sperm rate /birthrate is decreasing. While Blacks' Melanin offer much protection, our diet-abuses (the "western diet") are catching up with us also. We have the highest infant-mortality rate. Can you see where all this is taking all of us?

Why is animal flesh deadly?

- **Causes, develops, promotes, or is linked to:**

heart disease	cancers	stroke	kidney damage
atherosclerosis	crib death	impotence	homosexuality
osteoporosis	parasites	liver damage	mad cow disease

- **Humans do not have the capability** to digest /metabolize flesh as efficiently as flesh-eating animals. We have guts like those of the fruitarian gorilla. Flesh digests incompletely in our system. The incompletely digested particles rot in our colon and flesh, defiling our tissues and also feeding bad colon bacteria. Results = diseases, death.
- **The younger they are, children cannot digest flesh** with their underdeveloped digestive system; grownups barely can. Children often fed flesh grow up with impaired digestive systems, fragile health.
- **Diets high in saturated fat/cholesterol clog arteries**, reduce flow of blood to our organs/hearts/brains –sometimes obstructing them (heart attacks, strokes); and to our genitals –producing impotence in men.
- **Flesh is the most putrefactive** of all foods. It rots in your colon and produces some of the deadliest toxins to poison your bloodstream.
- **A high-flesh diet is directly linked to all forms of cancer** and virtually guarantees eventual cancer of some form.
- **Nitrates added to fleshfood** combine with natural stomach and food chemicals to create *nitrosamines*, among the most potent cancer-causing agents known. Tiny doses cause cancer in animals.[1] Nitrates are used in cured meats, bacon, bologna, deviled/spiced ham, hotdogs, meat spread, Vienna sausages, smoke-cured fish /tuna.
- **Ammonia**, a by-product of meat-metabolism, is carcinogenic.
- **A high-flesh diet severely depletes** B6, calcium, magnesium, niacin.[2]
- **Causes osteoporosis** (bone softening) because it robs calcium from the bones –no matter how much calcium supplements you take.
- **Overburdens the liver and kidneys**, damaging them over time.
- Excess urea salts cause tissue hardening, stiff painful joints, thickened capillaries (causing cell starvation), fluid retention, hypertension, clogged arteries, makes heart beat harder (inviting pectoris heart attack).
- **Too much protein thickens and congests the blood**.
- **Meat is a stimulant** due to its large content of uric acid, similar in structure to caffeine. Uric acid accumulates and eventually precipitate in tissues as crystals. The body sacrifices its indispensable alkaline mineral reserves to neutralize fleshfood acids in the blood and tissues.
- **Excess nitrogen** in the blood accumulates and forms kinotoxin in the muscles, causing chronic fatigue.[3]
- **Causes menstrual problems.** Menstrual periods are heavier, longer, and more painful, with greater premenstrual difficulties.[4]

Continued >>

1) Winter, 74.   2) Cousens, CE, 282.   3) Nelson, MN, 42.   4) Robbins, DNA, 266.

Continued: # Why is animal flesh deadly?

- **Farm animals are being fed farm animals.** The flesh of such *cannibal-ed* animals has freak-protein-poison ("**prions**") causing brain-degeneration (Mad Cow Disease) in animals and humans who eat them.
- Farm animals are **hybrid, mostly** *albinos* (white), and **gene-raped**. Their meat is inferior & dangerous! They are usually sterile, neutered, castrated. Human genes are being added to livestock, making us *Unknowing Cannibals!*, more susceptible to Prions, insanity, etc. (seepages 34, 108, 117)
- **Shortens lifespan.** Promotes premature aging and early degeneration.
- <u>**Fish and seafood are no longer safe to eat**</u> because the deepest farthest oceans are now as contaminated as the lakes and rivers. In fact, seafood is as toxic or more toxic than commercial red meat.
- **Fleshfood has the highest concentration of pesticides**. Of all the toxic pesticide residues in the American diet, 95% to 99%, comes from meat, fish, dairy products and eggs.[1]
- **Since animals are at the top of the food chain**, environmental pollution & radiation is most concentrated in their flesh.[2]
- **Toxins are concentrated in the FAT** (and livers) of animals.
- **The continued eating of antibiotics** in animal corpses causes human resistance to medicines and immunity to penicillin.
- **Is high urea a chief cause of "unknown" crib death in babies?** (killing 10,000 infants annually)*"Too often, nursing mothers are eating too much meat. Therefore, there is too much urea –undigested protein– in the mother's milk. When the infant nurses, it gets that urea and its heart is so little and weak that it just can't handle it."[3]* (Urea is undigested protein, according to Dr. Carey Reams, made of nitrate nitrogen & ammonical nitrogen.[3])
- **An outstanding medium for growing cancer is pig intestine.** Raymond Rife *"discovered that pig meat and mushrooms were a natural cause of cancer in which the cancer virus liked to grow."[4]*
- **Parasites abound in almost all Americans** (and humans on Earth). Animal flesh (especially pigs /hogs), being full of such, is the major source of parasites. Many parasites in pigmeat survive cooking.
- **Schizophrenia** is a form of protein toxemia.
- **Pork, catfish, tuna & the scavengers –skinfish /shellfish** (lobsters, scallops, oysters, shrimp, crabs, clams): *"These unclean meats release energy too quickly for the body to make use of them. They digest so fast that you cannot use the proteins, which turn into urea and dump into the bloodstream so fast that the kidneys cannot eliminate them. A urea build-up in the body ensues and excessive urea leads to many health problems."[5]*
- **Factory-farm animals are being fed their own feces**.
- **Modern meat-eating with its grossly anti-Nature production methods** is destroying the planet, causing deforestation, accelerating the global greenhouse effect, and other serious ecological disasters.
- <u>**Men are becoming effeminized and even homosexual**</u> from eating the flesh (& milk?) of animals fed female hormones. Some men have even grown pendulous breasts. **The same food masculinizes women.**

1) Robbins, DNA, 315.   2) Cousens, SN, 113.   3) Kirban, 89, 166.   4) Lynes, 51, 52.   5) Kirban, 48.

Recommendations for Better Health

Avoid or Reduce Eating:	Healthier Replacements:
• commercially grown flesh (chicken, beef, veal, etc.) • cured meats • pork, ham, pigmeat • hotdogs, spam, jerky • liver (poison-detoxifier of body; has several times more poison than other flesh from the same body) • organ meats • animal FAT • chicken skin (too fatty) • all shellfish, shrimp, lobsters • all fish, seafood, tuna (unless you know it's from uncontaminated water) • fish with skin instead of scales • infertile commercial eggs • gelatin (made from boiled down hooves, bones, animal-parts) • cheese made with rennet (animal coagulant) • white sugar (has bleached pigblood) • mono & di-glycerides (of fatty acids derived from slaughterhouse byproducts like tallow. Food additive) • "animal crackers" to children (promotes, condones meat-eating)	**Best:** • **fruit, leafy green vegetables** (humans recycle 90% of their protein wastes) • **nuts, seeds, nut butters** • **spirulina powder** (Has more high-quality assimilable protein than lean meat) • **bee pollen** (Has 5-7 times more protein than meat, eggs or cheese. Pollen protein is predigested, easy to assimilate. Highest source of nutrients we require) • **sesame seeds** (Have 19-28% more protein than many meats. Is also rich in oil, lecithin and calcium. *Tahini* is ground sesame spread.) **Improvement:** • **beans** (have as much or more protein than meat, but have other problems) • **fake fleshfood, veggie burgers** (from vegetable sources; note these are still firstclass drugfoods) • **organic, fertile eggs** (raw or lightly poached) • **fish with scales** (from uncontaminated water) • **meat from range-fed, hormone-free, additive-free animals** (at health stores, quality meat markets)

Tips

- **Preparing meat (especially beef, pork):**
  - choose the *leanest* meat; trim off all fat before cooking; slice meat very thin.
  - to reduce toxins: soak the thinly sliced raw meat in water for several hours, changing water often. This draws out toxin-filled blood.
  - optional: marinate meat for 30 minutes in any strong alcoholic beverage like whisky, vodka, gin, to kill parasites (& germs) which survive cooking. re-rinse.
  - cook well-done on high heat, letting fat drain off as it cooks; discard fat.
- **To ensure more complete digestion when you eat fleshfoods:** take raw pineapple or raw papaya or other protein-digesting enzymes.
- **Best not to feed fleshfood to children**, especially young children. If you do, at least provide digestive enzymes with flesh-meals.
- *How Not To Eat Pork*, by Shahrazad Ali, identifies over 100 foods, medications, cosmetics, etc made from the pig.
- **Cancer Help Hotline:** Cancer Control Society. Info Pak /referrals /help. 2043 N. Berendo St.; Los Angeles, CA 90027; (213) 663-7801.

DRUG #	
8	# *Body-Bankrupting Beverages*

Suffocating, Oxy-thieving Carbonated Drinks

If you water your plants with carbonated water, they will grow vigorously because you are giving them an abundance of the gas they need in order to survive: carbon dioxide. In the human body however, this same gas is a deadly poison which we breathe out. Carbon dioxide is a deadly waste by-product of cellular metabolism. It is carried by the blood to the lungs where it is exchanged for incoming oxygen and then expelled with the outgoing breath. The average adult exhales enough carbon dioxide and other toxic products of metabolism in a 24 hour period to kill 12 adult elephants! [1] Carbon dioxide gas (CO_2) is added to water to produce "sparkling water," club soda type beverages, and pop or soft drinks. **Ingesting carbon dioxide robs your body of oxygen**, "Vitamin O," the most vital nutrition we require. When we drink carbonated beverages we increase the amount of CO_2 gas in our blood streams and place a heavy load on our gaseous waste handling system. The increased load of CO_2 decreases our ability to handle oxygen. Earth's atmosphere contains .04% of CO_2. If the content were increased up to only 3% all life on Earth would go unconscious. If the percentage were to go up to 4% all animal and insect life would die. For this reason it is extremely important to ventilate our homes and bedrooms.

Coffee, Tea, and Cola

Americans consume about 250 billion cups of coffee a year, and likely more than this in colas. Coffee contains no nutrients. Tea and colas aren't much better. All three generously contain <u>Caffeine</u>, a powerful, destructive, highly addictive toxin that is even listed as a drug. Caffeine creates a false sense of energy which forces the body to draw upon its nutrient reserves and deplete its strength. In lab animals, Caffeine promotes tumors caused by other substances, and also causes birth defects in animals tested at high doses. Hundreds of mutagenic (gene breaking/harming) substances have been found in coffee, including <u>Methyl Glyoxal</u>, a rat carcinogen. <u>Just one cup of coffee has 50 times the mutagenic activity of the smoke absorbed from smoking a single cigarette.</u> One cup of coffee has 0.5 mg of methyl glyoxal; instant coffee has 1/5 of this. Coffee also contains carcinogenic tannins, chlorogenic acid (a bacterial mutagen), toxic benzene, benzaldehyde, benzofurans, hydroquinone and small amounts of benzo(a)pyrene, a strong mutagen and carcinogen.

1) Flanagan, EA, 63.

Solvents, the unrecognized health-buster lurking in our drinks

We owe triple credit to Dr. Hulda Clark's research, for bringing to our awareness that, unknown to us: **1)** *SOLVENT residues* contaminate nearly all the bottled drinks, juices, water and beverages we buy, including health varieties. Powdered beverages /mixtures and other bottled foods, supplements, shampoos, are also contaminated with solvent residues. **2)** Solvents are wrecking our health, unsuspected by us. Solvents play a major role in setting the stage for common diseases and ills. The presence of solvents within us makes it easy for flukes, parasites, viruses and other micro-monsters to get a health-wrecking stronghold on us. **3)** Practical solutions to this epidemic problem. For example, you can build your own *Syncrometer* as instructed in her books, and test all your beverages /foods / personal-care items for solvents and other toxins; and build a *Zapper* (mini frequency generator) to kill those flukes, molds, viruses, etc. In *The Cure For All Diseases,* she wrote:

> **"Solvents are compounds that dissolve things. Water is a useful, life giving solvent. Most other solvents dissolve fats and are life <u>threatening</u>, because fats form the membrane wall around each of our cells, especially our nerve cells. ..The solvent that does the most harm is <u>benzene</u>. It goes to the thymus, ruins our immune system and causes AIDS. The next worst solvent is <u>propyl alcohol</u>. It goes to the liver and causes cancer in some distant organ. Other major culprits are xylene, toluene, wood alcohol.."** [1]

The solvents are residues from the sterilizing equipment. Solvents are used to sterilize the containers. There may only be a few parts per billion but a sick person trying to recover cannot afford any solvent intake.

- Coffee, decaffeinated beverages, soda pop and powdered drinks all contain very toxic solvents.[2]
- Solvents which are found in carbonated drinks are acetone, toluene, xylene, and wood alcohol (methanol).[3]
- Solvents which have been found in bottled water (including distilled water) are benzene, propyl alcohol, carbon tetrachloride, and wood alcohol.
- Solvents found in store-bought fruit juices including health varieties are benzene; methylene chloride in fruit juice, and propyl alcohol in commercial fruit juices.

And nasty DEP

The preservative (i.e., drug) called DEP (diethyl pyrocarbonate) is used in some fruit-based beverages (fruit drinks, –ades, nectars, punch), to permit "cold pasteurization," and inhibit fermentation. DEP reacts with ammonia to form urethan (ethyl carbamate), a carcinogen. Citrus juices contains ammonia, and since it is likely treated with DEP, it contains urethan.[4]

1) Clark H, CAD, 36.   2) Ibid., 421.   3) Ibid., 424.   4) Hunter, FA, 103, 104.

Why are soft drinks harmful?

- **Contains carbon dioxide (CO2 gas) which:**
  - robs your body of oxygen, the most vital nutrition we require.
  - enters your blood, increasing amount of CO2 gas already in your bloodstream. This places a heavy load on your gaseous waste handling system, decreasing body's ability to handle oxygen.
- **Phosphated beverages** dissolves bones, cause hardened arteries, joint disease, calcified tissues lacking flexibility, & kidney crystals that become stones.[1]
- **Increases heart action.** Can cause paralysis of the heart.
- **Contain large amounts of phosphoric and citric acids** which increases the acidity level of the entire body. Results often manifest as mouth canker sores and duodenal ulcers.
- **These acid-base soft drinks are in aluminum cans.** This ensures that brain-deteriorating aluminum will get into your system.
- **Contains as much neuro-toxin caffeine** as instant coffee (see next page).
- **Causes irritability. Causes insomnia.**
- **Contains very toxic solvents.** Solvents found in carbonated drinks include acetone, toluene, xylene, and wood alcohol (methanol).[2]
- **BVO (brominated vegetable oil)** is used as a clouding agent in many popular soft drinks. The main ingredient of BVO is bromate, a poison. Just 2-4 ounces of a 2% solution of BVO can severely poison a child.[3]

Why are all bottled drink/juices harmful?

- **Solvents!** All bottled drinks, juices (even health-variety fruit juices), and bottled water of any type are harmful because they all contain solvent contamination from the bottle-sterilizing equipment. (See previous page). Solvents dissolve fats and are life threatening because fats form the membrane wall around each of our cells, especially nerve cells. Solvents also kill liver cells /tissue.
  - Solvents in bottled water (including distilled water) are benzene, propyl alcohol, carbon tetrachloride, and wood alcohol.
  - Solvents in store-bought fruit juices including health varieties are benzene; methylene chloride, and propyl alcohol.
- **Mold toxins** (mycotoxins, especially aflatoxins) usually contaminate bottled and frozen fruit juice.[4]
- **Urethan:** preservative DEP, added to citrus juices, reacts with the ammonia in the juice, producing carcinogenic urethan.
- **High sugar/fructose content** (plus pasteurized/cooked, hence enzyme-deficient). Over-consumption may promote hypoglycemia, diabetes and other dis-eases produced by sugar.

1) Clark, CAD, 65-66. 2) Ibid., 424. 3) Burton, AM,, 169. 4) Clark, CAD, 38.

Why are coffee /tea /cola harmful?

- **Coffee is one of the greatest causes of low blood sugar**. It overstimulates pancreas, especially when no protein food is taken with it.[1]
- **Drinking over 5 cups of coffee or tea** daily doubles the daily intake of cadmium, a toxic metal.[2] Tea contains **theine**, another stimulant.
- **Phosphoric acid** in colas dissolves teeth enamel in animal studies.[3]
- **Among heavy coffee drinkers**, coffee "causes headaches, nervousness, indigestion, diarrhea, and worst of all, heart attacks," reports Dr. Lukash. [4]
- **The residue of coffee and tea combines with <u>uric acid</u>** and other colloids to precipitate as crystals (urates), which may deposit in our tissues to cause rheumatism, arthritis, and kidney stones.[5]
- **Coffee, taken in excess, causes a severe potassium deficiency**. Potassium is the foundation mineral of all muscular tissues.
- **Coffee has 100s of toxic, mutagenic, carcinogenic substances:** methyl glyoxal, tannins, chlorogenic acid, benzo(a)pyrene and solvents.[6]
- **Just 3 cups of coffee** (without sugar) is enough to cause the excretion of 45 milligrams of calcium.[7] This effect increases with sugar.
- **Taken with meals, tannic acid** in black tea blocks uptake of iron.[8]
- **Decaffeinated coffee** is a heart risk; it raises the bad LDL cholesterol.[9]
- **Decaf coffee is carcinogenic. Hexane, which causes nerve damage,** and methylene chloride, which causes cancer, are used to decaffeinate coffee.
- **Carcinogenic dioxin** leaches in coffee from bleached white coffee filters.
- **Styrene leaches into coffee** from polystyrene (styrofoam) cups.

They all contain <u>CAFFEINE</u>, a stimulant addicting drug which:

- **Is a neurotoxin.** Dr Paul Goss wrote: *"The long-term effect of coffee is nervous tension. When you see people with uncontrollable shaking of the hand and/or head, that is from coffee. ..That shaking is the effect the coffee is having on the nervous system."* [10]
- **Overstimulates the nervous system** and causes increased nervous symptoms. Creates a false sense of energy in the short run but exhausts the adrenal glands and endocrine system in the long run.
- **Causes release of adrenaline into the blood stream.**
- **Overstimulates and weakens your adrenal glands.**
- **Raises blood sugar levels** (by overstimulating adrenal glands which then release adrenaline substances that stimulate the liver to release excess glucose into the blood).
- **Aggravates heart and artery disorders.**
- **Causes cardiac stress and vascular disease.**
- **Stimulates the metabolism** and leads to depletion of nutrients.

Continued >>

1) Clark, NR, 183. 2) Ibid., 237. 3) Ibid., 277. 4) Ibid., 225 5) *Nutrition Almanac*, 178. 6) Clark, CAD, 42. 7) David, NW, 164. 8) Cousens, CE, 207. 9) Dixon, 170. 10) Goss, RG, 67.

Continued: # Why are coffee /tea /cola harmful?

● **Worsens premenstrual** symptoms, breast swelling, breast disease.
● **Irritates the lining of the stomach.**
● **May prevent iron from being properly utilized.**
● **May cause vitamins** to be pumped through and out of the body before they can be properly absorbed.
● **Causes loss of Vitamin B5** through the urine.

Recommendations for Better Health

Avoid or Reduce Drinking:	Healthier Replacements:
• carbonated drinks /water • colas, soda pop • coffee, decaf coffee, cappuccino • tea, iced tea, black or green tea • powdered beverages • bottled fruit & vegetable juice • bottled drinks & beverages	• pure water • fresh organic fruit juices • fresh organic vegetable juices • herbal teas in bulk or loose form (steeped, not boiled; and preferably unsweetened)

Tips

• Drink mo water (and less beverages /drinks /juices). You don't like the way your water tastes? **A simple slice (or squirt) of fresh lemon or lime delightfully improves the taste of water.**
• Make a *Syncrometer* and test your own beverages /water to determine which ones are solvent-free, hence safest. (Instructions are in *The Cure for All Diseases,* by Dr. Hulda Clark.)
• If you drink coffee, use unbleached coffee filters or buy a coffeemaker that uses none. To avoid toxic styrene, do not consume coffee (or any drinks / food) from styrofoam cups, containers.

How to Remove Caffeine from Tea in 30 seconds

Steep the tea in boiling water for 30 seconds. Remove the tea from your cup or teapot and discard the liquid. Then, using the same tea, make another cup or pot, allowing it to steep for a full minute or more. Since most caffeine is released in hot water during the first 30 seconds, you're now left with practically no caffeine in your tea.

How to Quit Coffee in Two Weeks

(Heavy users should taper off coffee gradually to minimize withdrawal reactions.) Select a malted-grain coffee substitute (such as **Pero** or **Teeccino**). Begin blending the substitute with your coffee. Start with 3/4 coffee to 1/4 substitute and gradually increase the amount of substitute until you are drinking 100% coffee-substitute.

DRUG # 9 — *Demented Fermented Fungus- Funky Foods*

Fermented and Fungused Foods include:

pickles	sauerkraut	yogurt	alcohol
pickled food	soured food	buttermilk	wine, beer, ale
marinated foods	sour dough bread	sour milk, kefir	malt liquor
relish	soy sauce	all cheeses	vinegar
ketchup	tempeh, miso	butter	baker's yeast
tamari sauce	pastry, crackers	dried fruit	brewer's yeast
	bread	raisins	mushrooms
		peanuts	

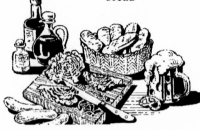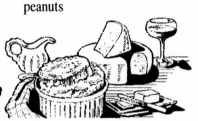

The "virtues" of some of these fermented foods are discussed in detail in many health books authored by Albinos. They sing praises to yogurt (for its "friendly bacteria"), brewer's yeast (for it's B-vitamins), sauerkraut (for its "natural lactic acid and fermentative enzymes") and so on. The evidence they present is convincing. That, however, is only a fraction of the whole picture. Let's look at the other parts of the picture and put things in proper perspective.

Eating half-spoiled food is a white-people-thang (European tradition)

A Caucasian admitted: *"Europeans [whites] eat lots of fermented foods, such as sauerkraut, sour pickles, sour bread, sour milk, etc."*[1] Bulgarians eat sour milk, sour vegetables and sour bread. Black sour bread is Russia's staple; the average Russian eats 2 pounds of it a day. Sauerkraut is an important part of the diet of Germans. "Kraut" is even a derogatory slang for a German. White people have as many varieties of cheeses as they have of brand names for those cheeses. Fermented foods may be good for Europeans but ain't necessarily appropriate for Afrikans. Along with scores of other harmful habits, Blacks acquired this habit from Albinos. Now we see that much so-called "soul food" (pickles, pickled pig meat) is "European."

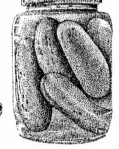

1) Airola, AUC, 192.

Fermented sour food is half-spoiled

"Fermented" is a euphemism for spoiled or half rotten. If the food is allowed to "ferment" all the way, it graduates to rottenhood. Yes the truth may "spoil" it for you but it's the same truth that may save your life. Fermented foods (cheese, yogurt, buttermilk, sauerkraut, beer, etc.) are processed with enzymes from bacteria, yeasts/molds that create chemical changes in the structure of the food.

- **Cheese, yogurt, butter, buttermilk** and other "cultured" dairy products are a class of fermented, hence half spoiled /rotten, typically moldy foods.
- **Butter** is made by adding a bacteria culture to cream to produce the typical flavor of butter, then churning the cream to separate the butterfat from the butter milk.[1]
- **Wine** is made from rotten grapes.
- **Beer** is made from rotten barley.
- **Brewer's yeast** is the waste product of the beer industry.
- **Supermarket pickled food** and **sauerkraut** is made with white vinegar which contains destructive acetic acid. (The word *vinegar* means *sour wine*)
- **SOY products.** The FU in *tofu* means curded (bean curd). *Tempeh* is half cooked, fermented soybeans. *Soy sauce* and *tamari* are fermented liquids made from soybeans, salt and wheat. *Miso,* a fermented paste is made of soybeans, salt and a grain, mixed together then left to ferment and produce bacteria by eating and digesting itself.

But it's "friendly" isn't it?

The *friendly* bacteria, "lactobacillus" is supposed to be able to suppress the growth of harmful microbes in the colon. However this same *Lactobacillus bulgaricus* cannot survive in the medium of the human intestines.[2] As evidence of the benefit of eating fermented food, Albino authors note that fermented food is a hefty part of the diet of many mountainous people that live long ages. What these authors don't tell you is that the yogurts made by such long-lived people were made from the milk of yaks, llamas and other creatures that roamed freely and lived natural active lives (like the people who consumed their yogurt). Their yogurt was not made from the milk of usually sick, drug-addicted inactive cows (unnatural animals to begin with) raised in slavery, captivity. Furthermore, such people lived in the mountains, in a poison-free, low-stress environment.

Molds, Yeasts & Mushrooms are one big happy Funky-Fungi Family

Mold and fungus are kin. Both are infamous for problems. Both grow on dead, rotting material. They can't grow on living cells. No fermented foods are living foods! All of them are dead. That's why "cultures" (germs, bacteria) can grow and thrive in them at all. Have you ever made yogurt? You had to boil the milk in order to kill any life in it so the "culture" you added could grow. Perhaps you are getting a sense of the bigger picture of what it means to be living on dead cooked food? Fungus loves it too! No, I'm not calling you a mushroom ...yet.

1) Block, IA, 84.   2) Gagne, 187.

Mold and Yeast belong to the Fungus family, consisting of over 200,000 species. They include yeast, mold, mildew, rots, smuts, and mushrooms. Like "air," mold (and bacteria) are everywhere, being part of the natural ecology. Fungi lack chlorophyll. Consequently, they can't perform photosynthesis and are parasitic and feed off dead organisms. Their precious function is to break down dead bodies into its basic elements and thereby recycle the ecology. This is what makes things *biodegradable*. However, yeast-overgrowth (that is, their toxins?) can also break down living organisms. Because yeast normally live on mucus membranes, modern lab tests usually fail to detect them.[1]

Fermented foods & beverages are a big source of Yeasts-Molds-Fungi, creating EPIDEMIC YEAST DISORDERS

Bacteria and molds are used to make cheese. You can actually see the mold in some cheeses. The blue spots in "blue cheese" is blue mold. It just doesn't seem or sound right to be eating mold, fungus, and bacteria. Eating yeasts, no matter what form, can add to the existing yeasts /molds in your body and exacerbate yeast disorders. Any wonder that eating cheese in excess can result in mold / yeast infections (among other problems)? Many women have reported that their vaginal yeast disorder flared up after eating Brewer's yeast for a few days. Yeast disorders are epidemic in western (i.e., white, Eurocentric) society, affecting "healthfood eaters" and standard drugfood eaters alike. And yeast /mold are also connected with flukes /parasites, as detailed in books by Dr. Hulda Clark.

Symptoms of probable yeast disorders include:

fluid retention	fatigue	white tongue	headaches
ear infections	eye problems	low immunity	yeast infections
candidiasis	athlete's foot	skin problems	hypoglycemia
anxiety attacks	depression	phobias	rashes
vaginitis	sore throats	asthma	colitis
bloating	painful joints	migraines	intestinal gas
schizophrenia	muscle aches	back pains	violence

'Yeast and fungal infections are a prominent plague of Western [= white] civilization. This is largely a consequence of the Western diet. Fungi utilize primarily sugars and starches as their food. Their favorite *dish* is sugar.' [2]

Books which show you how to resolve yeast problems and regain health include: *Breaking The Yeast Curse*, by Dr. Juliet Tien; *The Candida Epidemic*, by Norma Thompson Hollis; and Dr. Hulda Clark's book, *The Cure For All Diseases*. Dr. Clark believes that **the increase in violent crimes /violence (with almost no provocation) is due to the high level of mold consumption in the foods and beverages** of America's diet.[3]

1) Tien, 36.   2) Igram, 262.   3) Clark, CAD, 261.

Feast on Yeast

This is easy to do, since yeast is common in the truly SAD, Standard American Diet. **Yeasts are commonly used as starters for fermented foods,** or they may multiply within foods as a result of the fermentation process. Such foods include cheese, vinegar, wine, beer, and all baked goods you buy (breads, buns, doughnuts, cakes, pastry). Basically, if its raised or has a crust, it contains yeast. *(Yeast cells in bread die when the baking temperature reaches 140° F)* Terms indicating yeast additives on food labels include:

- autolyzed yeast protein
- hydrolyzed vegetable protein
- vegetable protein
- baker's yeast
- brewer's yeast
- torula yeast

Immune-system bashing mold-toxins in your starches

Mold is common in grains. Molds are in all packaged breads, pasta, brown rice, crackers, popcorn, corn chips, cold cereals, including and especially the health varieties, even when you can't see, smell or taste the molds. All these starchy foods contain mycotoxins, which are chemicals produced by molds. Mycotoxins are some of the most toxic chemicals known. **They disrupt immune function; they are so powerful that the immune response against the yeast/fungi is essentially neutralized.**[1] **Though mucus membranes are the main site of damage, chronic fungal infections of the organs may occur.** Mycotoxins include *aflatoxin* which reaches the liver and simply kill portions of it. Hepatitis and cirrhosis always reveal aflatoxin. *Sterigmato-cystin* is abundant in pasta (better to have *baked* pasta dishes). *Zearalenone* has immune-lowering effects and prevents you from detoxifying deadly benzene.[2] Main sources are commercial cereal grains, brown rice, popcorn and corn chips (but absent in fresh /canned corn, corn tortillas, white rice). Crackers are notoriously moldy and should be avoided completely.

Other inconspicuously very moldy foods

Dried fruit, raisins, honey, maple syrup, sorghum syrup, syrups, peanut butter (store-bought), tea (in bags), potato skins (grey parts, blemishes), nuts, peanuts, nut butters, vinegar and alcoholic beverages.

We eat the essence of a food when we consume it.

What are we eating when we eat fermented, pickled, soured, half-spoiled, half-rotten, fungus-filled foods, regardless of their touted virtues? Pickled foods will pickle you. Fermented foods will ferment you. Soured half-rotten foods like cheese will make you stink. Butter and all cheeses contribute to horrendous body odor.[3] And so on. You get the picture –unless you're already too "done." When spoiled or fermented food is eaten, the body rushes it to the nearest exit in an effort to protect itself. Sauerkraut, yogurt, pickles, etc., are hurried through the digestive tract where they are quickly expelled so as not to disrupt the body.[4]

---

1) Igram, 263.   2) Clark, CAD, 382.   3) Gagne, 188.   4) Baker, AS, 207.

Vinegar retards or stops digestion

As small a portion of vinegar as 1 in 5000, diminishes starch-digestion by inhibiting or destroying ptyalin (salivary amylase). One part in 1000 makes starch digestion very slow; twice this amount stops it completely. Thus, if you eat vinegar, vinegar-saturated salads, pickles, relish...with any starchy foods such as bread, cereals, potatoes, legumes... you won't be able to properly digest that food. Vinegar also contains alcohol, which impairs protein digestion. No wonder vinegar and pickles have been found useful in reducing weight; they cripple the first two stages of digestion!

And no one denies that (brain-killing) Alcohol is a harmful drug

You are born with all the brain cells you will ever have. **Every ounce of alcohol you consume kills brain cells; brains cells never grow back once lost.** Thus, alcohol diminishes your brain capacity. Alcohol also damages your liver, heart, kidneys, and negatively affects every cell in your body since it poisons your bloodstream. Alcohol coagulates colloid systems in our bodies. Alcoholic beverages abundantly contain *ergot* grain-fungus (a brain/liver poison) and also often contain deadly *aflatoxin* (which kills liver cells on contact).

WINE. The wine industry sometimes filters its wine through asbestos filters. Tiny particles of asbestos, a powerful carcinogen, may get into the wine.[1] "If you think you need to drink to have fun, you have a drinking problem."

BEER may be worse than other alcoholic drinks. Beer is extremely harmful to the system because it contains large amounts of cationic mineral electrolytes. The beer industry uses the hardest water it can find and then adds large quantities of cationic minerals to its brewing water.[2] Hops in beer can cause a hypnotic effect and can cause delirium tremens.[3] Beer manufacturers resist disclosing the ingredients of their products. They know you'd stop drinking them if only you knew. **Poisons in malt liquor and beer include:** [4]

- petroleum
- starch alcohol, sugar
- isobutenol (natural gas)
- alcohol
- wood alcohol
- gypsum (Plaster of Paris)[5]

These poisons deteriorate the brain, sex organs, liver, pancreas and lungs. They are highest in <u>**malt liquor**</u>, which is consumed heaviest by <u>**Black men**</u>.

Malt liquor and such, disguised weapons of Black Genocide?

As noted in chapter 4, the malt liquor and other alcoholic drinks sold in Black neighborhoods contain an anger-provoking agent not found in the drinks sold in white neighborhoods. And in the August 18, 1985 edition of the South African *Sunday Times*, former South African President P. W. Botha wrote: *"My scientists have come up with a drug that can be smuggled into their* [Black South Afrikans] *brews to effect slow poisoning results and fertility destruction."* Malt liquor has been shown to cause sperm-related fertility problems and genetic birth defects.[6] No wonder many Blacks believe it is being used as a weapon of genocide on Blacks. Well-deliberated marketing strategies target Blacks and other minorities. The "<u>**40 oz. malt**</u>" is the worse culprit.

1) Flanagan, EA. 2) Ibid. 3) Valerian, 0140.
4) Lecture, Dr. L. Afrika. 5) Valerian, 0140. 6) Awadu, PW, 26.

Why are fermented, moldy or yeasted foods harmful?

- **Causes abnormal amounts of decaying soil within the body** for bacteria to ferment and putrefy.[1]
- **White distilled vinegar** rapidly destroys red blood corpuscles, resulting in anemia.[2] **Vinegar also damages the kidneys.**[3] **Promotes fatigue.**
- **Vinegar** contributes to hardening of the liver (cirrhosis of the liver), duodenal and other intestinal ulcers.[4]
- **Most fermented foods (esp. cheese) have high amounts of salt,** an item that's destructive all by itself. **Pickled foods** fermented in salt-rich brine greatly injures the mucous membranes of the alimentary canal.[5]
- **The stimulating effect** of pickled foods on the digestive organs is very detrimental due to so much inorganic salt solution.[6]
- **Fermented /pickled foods** (pickles, relish, sauerkraut, yogurt, cheese, vinegar, alcohol) retard or suspend digestion, prevent proper assimilation of food.[7]
- **Ethyl Carbamate,** in small amounts (1 to 5 ppb) is found in naturally fermented foods and beverages, yogurt, soy sauce, beer, wine, bread. It produces tumors in rats whether given orally, by inhalation or injection.
- **Methyl glyoxal,** a mutagenic substance and rat carcinogen, is found in bourbon whiskey, wine, apple brandy, sake, roasted bread, soy sauce.
- **Fermented pickled food** promotes coarsened withered wrinkled skin.
- **White distilled vinegar & wine vinegar** contain destructive acetic acid. (But *apple cider vinegar* has **beneficial, constructive** *malic* **acid** which combines with alkaline elements/minerals to produce energy or be stored as glycogen for future use.[7])
- **Fermented foods, drinks, and yeast are very acid forming.**
- **Supermarket sauer kraut and pickles** are prepared with vinegars and cannot be considered natural lactic acid foods.
- **Mold toxins disrupt immune function.** (see page 136)
- **Being highly acidic, cheese** contributes its acidic bacteria to the bacterial pool of the intestines and, if eaten in large amounts, often results in onset of yeast infections, allergies, infections, other problems.[8]
- **Yogurt** is a "pernicious mucoidformer," just like milk, its mother, and all dairy products (cheese, kefir, buttermilk, butter, etc).[9]
- **Aged cheese** or hard cheese, when eaten in excess, 'hardens and tightens,' creates an aged, wrinkled appearance to the skin and contributes to kidney and gall stones.[10]
- **Butter** (especially) and cheese makes you stink. All cheeses and butter contributes to horrendous body odor.[11] Diacetyl, a bacterial mutagen, is found in butter (and coffee), giving butter its aroma.

Continued >>

1) Baker, AOS, 235.   2) Walker, FV, 84.   3) Nelson, MYN, 91.   4) Walker, FV, 84.
5) Ibid, 70.   6) Ibid.   7) Ibid., 84.   8) Gagne, 188.   9) Gray, CHH, 33. 10) Gagne, 188.   11) Ibid.

Continued:

Why is fermented /moldy / yeasted food harmful?

- **Cheese (especially high-fat cheese) and butter** (and milk) are major sources of saturated animal fat and cholesterol.
- **Mold is common in grains**, producing mycotoxins. All *packaged* breads /starches/pasta contain harmful mycotoxins. Further, yeast (another mold) is added to breads/pastries.
- **Many popular "yeast" powders** contain as much as 50% whey, hence are highly mucus-forming.[1]
- **Alcohol is a product of fermented grain, wheat, rice, grapes,** and other fruit. Fermentation requires yeast. Sugar is a by-product of fermentation. When drinking alcoholic beverages, you are taking in yeast, mold, sugar, and chemicals all at once.
- **Ergot is a grain fungus that is abundant in alcoholic beverages**, beer and wine.[2] These beverages also may contain deadly **aflatoxin**, another mold-poison. Ergot, a potent liver /brain toxin, produces **LSD**, the most potent hallucinogen known. Its by-products are used in making migraine medicine. Ergot and alcohol interact to make each more toxic. Alcohol seems to drive the toxins deeper into your tissues. Some of the bizarre behavior of intoxication may be due to mold-alcohol combination.
- **Alcohol encourages yeast overgrowth.**
- **Wine** may contain asbestos, a powerful carcinogen.
- **Because it can kill microbes, yeasts, and molds**, the preservative DEP (diethyl pyrocarbonate) is used in noncarbonated wines, beer, malt liquors, draft beer and some fruit-based beverages to permit "cold pasteurization," and inhibit fermentation and preserve drinks (DEP in wine prevents it from becoming vinegar). DEP reacts with ammonia to form urethan, a carcinogen. Wine and beer contains ammonia, and since they are likely treated with DEP, they contain urethan.[3]
- **Deadly poisons in beer and malt liquor** include petroleum, isobutenol (natural gas), sugar, alcohol, wood alcohol. They deteriorate the brain, sex organs, liver, pancreas and lungs.
- **Alcohol kills irreplaceable brain cells**, hence dims brain capacity.
- **Alcohol damages the liver, heart, kidney,** and negatively affects every cell in your body since it poisons the bloodstream.
- **Like sugar –its main mother, alcohol destroys** *essential fatty acids.*
- **As little as one alcohol drink** per day may severely reduce folic acid.
- **Alcohol dehydrates the body**, causes fluids to be lost from the system.
- **Wine /beer often contains high levels of histamine**,[4] which can trigger asthma, eczema, hives, sneezing, migraines, sinus problems, diarrhea.
- **Mushrooms** are carcinogenic. They are a natural cause of cancer and cancer cells thrive in a mushroom medium.[5]

---

1) Gray, CH 35. 2) Clark, CA 228, 384. 3) Hunter, FA 103, 104. 4) Williams, DW 34. 5) Lynes, 51, 52.

Recommendations for Better Health

Avoid or Reduce Eating:	Healthier Replacements:
• *(see whole list on page 133)* • vinegar; foods containing vinegar • pickled & soured foods • yeasted foods, mushrooms • fermented foods & drinks • all alcoholic beverages • cheese (from pasteurized milk) • dried fruit, raisins • peanuts, peanut butter (has aflatoxin) • some veggie burgers (mushroom-rich)	• unspoiled organic food: learn to enjoy their natural flavors • **organic apple cider vinegar** (Does not contain *acetic* acid; it contains beneficial *malic* acid. To it, add a little vitamin C to demold it) • **fresh lemon juice** • non-irritant **herbal seasoning**

Using Vitamin C to Remove Mold & Mold Toxins from Foods

Vitamin C destroys mold toxin molecules and also helps your body detoxify poisons. Along with the following, Dr. Hulda Clark recommends keeping vitamin C powder in a plastic container and use it like salt on all your food, from cereal to soup (1/8 tsp. is enough).

Dried peas, beans: Throw away imperfect ones, rinse well, add vitamin C to the water they are soaked in and cooked in.

Pasta, Rice: can be partly demolded by cooking and partly by adding vitamin C before or after cooking. No need to add so much it affects the flavor.

Bread, Baked Goods: Make your own (it's mold-free). If you add a bit of vitamin C to the dough, breads will be mold-free longer and rise higher.

Hot Cereals: Pick out all dark colored, shriveled bits before cooking. Add sweetener /salt during cooking to raise boiling temperature. After cooking, add a sprinkle of vitamin C powder.

Fresh Fruit: Patulin, the main fruit mold-toxin, is in common fruit if they are bruised. Choose fruit meticulously. Wash and peel everything so you can see and avoid every bruise. Cut out bruises, dark spots.

Dried Fruit: Soak them in vitamin C water. Rinse and bake on low heat to dry again; store in refrigerator or freezer.

Potatoes: Cut away the eyes, blemishes, gray /dark spots. Do not buy green-tinged potatoes (are poisonous). Best to choose RED potatoes.

Honey: Warm it slightly and add vitamin C (1/8 tsp. per cup, 1/4 tsp. per pint). Stir with wood or plastic.

Tea: is moldy if in bags. Buy from bulk.

Bottled Beverages: Add a little C to bottle.

Maple Syrup: (has aflatoxin and other molds). Add vitamin C. To get rid of stearig, etc., heat it to near boiling while in the original jar with the lid removed. Keep refrigerated afterwards.

Nuts & Roasted Nuts: Just sprinkling with C is not effective because molds have penetrated the surface. First rinse nuts well in water (this removes a lot of mold). Cover with water, add about 1/4 tsp. vitamin C powder for a pint of nuts and mix. Let stand for 5 minutes. Pour off the water & dry nuts in gas oven at low heat.

Peanut butter, Nut butters: can't be detoxified using vit. C. Make your own.

Vinegar: Add a little vitamin C, refrigerate.

Millet, Sorghum: Rinse in vitamin C water before cooking, or add vitamin C to the cooking water. Avoid sorghum syrup.

Alcoholic beverages: Make your own from pristine fruit. Or at least add vit. C (1/8 tsp. per cup) to store-bought container.

Boiling: Just heating food to the boiling point does not kill molds. Boiling for many minutes at a higher temperature or baking does kill them (but not ergot), and also destroys aflatoxin. For foods you can't heat that high (like nuts already roasted or vinegar), use vitamin C.

DRUG # 10 *Spiteful Spices, Conning Condiments*

Condiments and spices are not foods but stimulants, poisons. That's why we use them in small amounts! Imagine eating a bowl of pepper.

Most condiments /spices were originally used as drugs in earlier cultures before being used as food! Many wars have been fought over spices. Condiments and spices are *stimulants*. *Spice* itself is a variant of *spike*. Stimulants are any substances which speed the body's metabolism. These include coffee, chocolate, meat, alcohol and many herbs. Stimulants give no more energy than a whip applied to a tired work horse. Condiments are substances used to modify food flavor. These include salt, mustard, pepper, cayenne, MSG, salad dressing, hot sauce, horseradish, white vinegar, ginger, and other cooking spices. Condiments have little or no nutritional value. Instead, they actually disrupt nutrition by irritating the cells and tissues of the body. Any substance that does this, whether salt, spice or polluted air, causes the mucus membrane to excrete mucus for protection and creates a catarrhal condition in time.

Regular use of <u>GARLIC</u> messes you up, despite its touted virtues

Garlic, especially raw, causes extensive edema, bleeding and ulceration of the stomach mucosa, reduction of red-blood cell count, increase in reticulocytes (immature blood cells), harm to the pancreas and sugar-balance –thus promotes hypoglycemia and diabetes.[2] Garlic, onions, leeks, shallots, chives, radishes, and mustard all contain toxic non-metabolizable *mustard oil*, a very irritating and indigestible substance which contains deadly *isothio-cyanate*, a mucous membrane irritant which inhibits the mitochondrial production of ATP (Adenosine Triphosphate), the energy molecule that fuels the bio-electric body and keeps us young. The soporific oil irritates the kidneys, bladder. It makes the eyes and genital mucus membrane water. Cooking partly evaporates this oil.

<u>MSG</u> (monosodium glutamate) causes brain damage

Glutamate and closely related substances are neurotoxins that causes brain damage and neuro-degenerative diseases. Glutamate, a salt of the amino acid glutamic acid, is a potent, rapidly acting nerve toxin in laboratory cell cultures, causing nerve swelling after only 90 seconds of contact. Glutamate, in the form of MSG is the world's most widely used food additive; aspartate composes half of the aspartame (NutraSweet®) molecule.[1] MSG has caused brain damage in young rodents, and brain-damage effects in rabbits, chickens and monkeys. MSG is used to intensify flavorings in meats, condiments, pickles, soups, candies, and baked goods. The "Chinese restaurant syndrome" is believed to be caused by a sudden elevation of glutamate in the blood which produces a blood vessel response. *Disguised names* for MSG are "hydrolyzed vegetable protein," autolyzed yeast, modified food starch, and "natural" flavors.[3]

1) Winter, PYF, 84.   2) Health Freedom News, March 1992, p29.   3) Igram, ST 220.

Why are spices and condiments harmful?

- **They are stimulants**, substances which speeds body metabolism
- **Overstimulates** /weakens glands of the mouth, stomach, intestines.
- **Spices**, like other stimulants, whip the adrenal glands to produce a false feeling of energy – derived at the expense of your body's energy reserves. This causes the body to break down more quickly.
- **"Stimulants can create a desire for excessive sexual activity**, which increases production of sexual fluids, drawing minerals and other nutrients from teeth, bones and other tissues for their manufacture. **This speeds the aging process** and the eventual wasting away of teeth, hair, vital organs and reserve energy."[1]
- **Are indigestible. Retards and deranges digestion.** Irritates the digestive tract / membranes of the alimentary canal, causing these to thicken, toughen, harden. This impairs their functional powers.
- **Puts stress on gall bladder/liver,** resulting in heartburn, indigestion.
- **Stimulates increased flow of body fluids** and can effect sensations of false hunger. Eventually, they cause thickening of cell walls
- **Creates a false desire for food** and induces overeating.
- **Creates a false thirst** that is not satisfied with water.
- **Alkenylbenzenes,** including Estragole & Safrole –all of which are carcinogenic in rats, are found in many spices and herbs. Estragole is found in tarragon, basil and fennel. Safrole is a natural component of nutmeg, mace, star anise, cinnamon and black pepper. Causing liver cancer in rodents, Safrole is also found in sassafras tea and makes up 75% of oil of sassafras.
- **Black pepper** is considered more harmful to the liver than alcohol.[2] The pepper family (black /white pepper [not cayenne]) contains the toxin *piperine*; said to affect the knee. Black pepper contains piperine 10% by weight. Extracts of black pepper have caused cancer in mice.
- **Found in cayenne pepper**, the poisons *piperidin* and *capsaicin* irritate the body so severely that circulation is increased to quickly eliminate it. This defensive reaction is often misinterpreted as an energy boost, but energy and stimulation are not the same. Its use can damage the liver and kidneys.
- **Body outpours mucus** when cayenne & other hot peppers are used in order to protect itself from the peppers' harmful, irritating alkaloids. This defense response is misinterpreted as aiding the healing process.
- **Vanilla beans** contain nervous system stimulants from the same chemical family as the neurotoxin caffeine.[4]

1) Kulvinskas, STC, 31   2) Nelson, MYN, 88.   3) Clark, CAD, 83.   4) Igram, STN, 232.

Continued:
Why are spices & condiments harmful?

- **MSG causes brain damage** (see earlier page).
- **Nutmeg** and mace contains high concentrations of the toxin *myristicin*, which, while helpful in small amounts for toothaches, diarrhea, etc.; in large doses such as an ounce of nutmeg or 2 whole nutmeg nuts, may cause shock, stupor, acidosis, or other intoxicating symptoms with euphoria for up to 24 hours after ingestion.
- **Regular use of garlic is harmful.** Garlic causes extensive edema, bleeding & ulceration of the stomach mucosa, promotes hypoglycemia and diabetes, reduction of red-blood cell count.
- **Garlic, onions, leeks, shallots, chives, cress, radishes, and mustard** all contain toxic non-metabolizable *mustard oil*, a very irritating and indigestible substance which contains deadly *isothio-cyanate*, a mucous membrane irritant which inhibits the mitochondrial production of ATP, the energy molecule. The soporific oil irritates the kidneys and bladder, and makes the eyes and the genital mucus membrane water.
- **Desensitizes the taste buds.** Blunts & depraves sense of taste, so that natural food flavors are neither detected nor appreciated. As you get older, the flavor of food changes because using salt/spices/condiments dulls the tongue's delicate taste buds and weakens your sense of taste

Recommendations for Better Health

Avoid or Reduce Eating:	Healthier Replacements:
• condiments, spices	• herbs, herbal seasoning
• garlic, onions, leeks	(salt-free, non-irritating herbs)
• vanilla, vanilla waffers (foods with vanilla)	– sage, bay
• black & white pepper, cayenne pepper	– sweet basil, majoram
• vinegar (white, distilled, or pasteurized)	– celery, peppermint
• salt (all white salt including seasalt)	• seasoning seeds such as:
• mustard, relish, tartar sauce	– papaya (dried & ground)
• soy sauce, tamari sauce	– chia, celery, caraway
• hot sauce, barbecue sauce	– dill (rich in mineral salts)
• ketchup, tomato paste	• Celtic salt
• MSG (monosodium glutamate)	(see page 95 for proper usage)
• disguised (names for) MSG:	• lemon or lime juice (fresh)
hydrolyzed vegetable protein, autolyzed yeast, modified food starch, "natural" flavor	• seaweed (kelp, dulse)
• additives that always contain MSG:	• apple cider vinegar
textured protein, yeast extract, sodium caseinate, calcium caseinate	(organic, raw)

Learn to enjoy food's natural flavor. After a fast, your sense of taste is renewed.

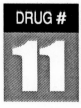

DRUG #

11

Nerve-Nocking
Chocolate

The sheer pleasure of chocolate may compensate for its negative effects. Chocolate also contains *phenylethylamine*, a chemical compound believed to mimic the physiological sensations of love. But unfortunately, chocolate also harms.

Why is chocolate/cocoa harmful?

- **Contains stimulants** (caffeine, theobromine, theophylline) which speed the heartbeat and stimulate the adrenal and central nervous system. (see page 131)
- **Overstimulates the adrenal glands**.
- **Raises blood sugar levels** (by overstimulating adrenal glands which then release adrenaline substances that stimulate the liver to release excess glucose into the blood).
- **Causes body to draw down energy reserves** at an accelerated rate
- **Contains oxalic acid**, which can interfere with calcium absorption
- **Contains wicked white sugar** in large quantities –real bad stuff.
- **Contains an abundance of hydrogenated oils** –heart attack stuff.
- **Contains actual filth**, rodent feces, insect parts and wax
- **Cocoa residue combines with uric acid** and other colloids to precipitate as crystals (urates), which may deposit in our tissues to cause rheumatism, arthritis, and kidney stones.

Recommendations for Better Health

Avoid or Reduce Eating:	Healthier Replacement:
Chocolate in all forms: cocoa, chocolate candy, milk chocolate, chocolate chips, dark chocolate, white chocolate, brownies, cake and other goodies (badies) baked with chocolate.	**Carob**. It's delicious, tastes similar to chocolate, and is dark brown like chocolate. Carob is a natural sweetener rich in B vitamins and minerals. It also contains protein, calcium and phosphorus.

DRUG # 12

Mutant, Malnourishing, Pesticided
Commercial Produce

No vitamin-C in commercial oranges?!!!

Commercial produce looks beautiful, for often it is cosmetically treated so that it looks good on the outside –however, it is nutritionally bad (deficient) on the inside. And it's displayed under special lighting to make it appear better looking than what it really is. What you can't see are its contaminating chemicals and pesticides, its mucked-with genes, and its woeful lack of nutrition. BIG example: fresh fruit at the supermarkets are hardly a vitamin-C source: citrus fruit is usually gas-ripened and consequently contains no measurable amounts of vitamin C! [1] (Proven by Dr. Michael Colgan at the Rockefeller Institute.) Most commercial oranges, tangerines and grapefruit are picked green and ripened in large warehouses. The ripening agent is bromine gas, which is such a noxious chemical that if inhaled in sufficient amounts, it can maim or kill.

Organic produce costs more but is worth it because it's richer

Commercial vegetables taste bland without condiments because they are so *deficient in minerals.* Organically grown produce taste richer because they have far more minerals and nutrients. An organically grown tomato may contain over 10 times more magnesium than a commercially grown one, plus three times the vitamin A and C. In one study, scientists spent two years comparing Chicago apples, pears, potatoes, corn, and wheat with their organic twins. The organic foods had about twice the nutritional elements![2] Organic wheat had 160% more copper than regular wheat. Pears had 40% more calcium. Potatoes, 60% more zinc. At best, supermarket vegetables supply a fraction of essential nutrients; when irradiated and cooked they supply even less. Organic produce is not available in most American regions. 99% of the food grown in the United States is produced on soil fertilized with toxic chemical commercial fertilizers. Chemicals rob produce of nutrients. The nitrogen in chemical fertilizers can rob food of its protein quality, ascorbic acid and glucose. Pesticides and herbicides bind minerals via chelation, making them unavailable to plants.

Trace-minerals, though labled "trace" are more important than vitamins

Trace minerals can mean the difference between good health and serious disease. They are vital to our health although our daily requirements for them are sometimes thousands of times smaller than for major minerals. They modulate cellular function by stimulating and controlling the rate of cellular reactions.[2] Vitamins have no function in the absence of minerals. Minerals liberate vitamins to do their work. Lacking vitamins, the system can make use of

1) Igram, STN, 287, 63.   2) Whole Life Times, April 1997, page 9.

minerals, but lacking minerals, vitamins are useless. Researchers have discovered trace-mineral deficiencies in the soil of almost every state in the country. Thus, America's food is mineral-deficient even before it is fumigated, bromated, irradiated, refined, or cooked. The vast majority of Americans, living on a diet of commercial foods, are minerally deficient.

60-70% of the foods on your grocery shelves are Gene-Raped Foods. Well-disguised drugfoods.

They have never been a part of the human diet. They are not subjected to pre-market safety testing. **And they are not labled.** Their creators (Albinos, white people) politely call them "genetically engineered food" or "transgenic food." In Europe they are more appropriately called Frankenfood, after the Frankestein monster...for they *are* monsters, whiteman-made freaks. Frankenfood-drugfood is replete with health hazards threatening our bodies, the environment, and future of world-agriculture as Albinos frantically race to replace Nature's safe superior originals with their dangerous inferior re-creations. Thus, "agricultural biotechnology" is **big business**, and another extension of Albinos playing God (really, *Goddess*). And **like all the other "advances" whites make, the effects are destructive.** The altering of genetic codes can now be done in a minute fraction of the time it has taken the process of natural selection to take place. Biotech companies /food manufacturers use genetic meddling to manipulate genes in various produce to "enhance shelf life, size, taste, and resistance to pests." Examples include the "chicken/potato" animal which increases potato immunity; tomatoes with flounder genes to reduce frost damage, ripen on the vine and not easily bruise in shipment; potatoes with silkworm genes to increase disease resistance; and corn with firefly genes to decrease insect damage.[1] Are these freaks plants or animals or what?! One name for them is GEOs ("genetically engineered organisms"). Dr. Afrika enlightens us further:

> "The Caucasian cloned vegetables and fruits have been created with human
> cells, pig cells, insect cells, rat cells, drugs, pus, nuclear mutated cells,
> bacteria, diseased cells and electromagnetically perverted cells that are usually
> grown on petroleum waste without soil. These freak vegetables and fruit are
> causing new mutated spliced genetic diseases of the body, mind, and spirit." [2]

No wonder transgenic food tends to be toxic, allergenic. A transgenic yeast that was engineered for faster fermentation resulted in the accumulation of methyl-glyoxal (a metabolite) at toxic mutagenic levels. Studies suggests that transgenic plants engineered for resistance to diseases and pests have a higher allergenic potential than unmodified (i.e., natural, unmolested) plants. The same cancer-causing potential exists in the "tobacco-tomato" plant as in cooked tobacco.

A Bonus: By choosing *organically* raised produce/meats, you're helping the planet. By choosing *commercially* grown produce/meats, you're supporting Earth's destruction by supporting the "chemical-intensive" anti-Nature habits of "modern" commercial farming. If the demand decreases, they will likely change.

---

1) Pappas, 233.   2) Afrika, N, 191

Dangers of genetically engineered, bastard, mutant, freak-foods

● **Poisonous, Toxic, Lethal:**
Genetic engineering can cause unexpected mutations in an organism, which can create new and higher levels of toxins in foods. In 1989, a genetically engineered form of the food supplement tryptophan produced toxic contaminants. As a result, 37 people died, 1500 others were permanently disabled and 5000 other became very ill. (*The New England Journal of Medicine,* Aug. 9, 1990)

● **Counterfeit Freshness Hiding Nutritional Poverty:** Transgenic foods may mislead consumers with "counterfeit freshness." A luscious-looking, bright red tomato could be several weeks old and of little nutritional worth. Consumers will have no way of accurately judging food quality, if the foods aren't labeled.

● **Increased Pollution:** Scientists estimate that plants genetically engineered to be herbicide-resistant will actually trippple the amount of herbicide use. Farmers, knowing that their crops can tolerate the herbicides, will use them more liberally. Biotech claims that pesticide use will decrease are also misleading. Transgenic corn, altered to contain its own insect-killing toxin, is now registered by the EPA as a pesticide and not a vegetable at all. (*Weed Technology,* June 1994)

● **Allergic (Toxic) Reactions:**
Genetic engineering can produce unforeseen and unknown allergens in foods. Without clear and precise labeling, millions of Americans who suffer from food allergies will have no way of identifying or protecting themselves from offending foods *[unless they know how to use Kinesiology, explained in vol. 3 of this book].*

● **No Long-Term Safety Testing:**
Genetic engineering uses material from organisms that have never been a part of the human food supply. Without long-term testing no one knows if these foods are safe. Time has proven herbicide and pesticide use hazardous to personal and environmental health. Now, genetic engineering is being promoted as the new harmless solution to agricultural problems. But changing the fundamental make-up of food could cause unanticipated problems, just as herbicides and pesticides have.

● **Unknown, Unfathomed, Unpredicted Side Effects:** No one knows the long-range implication of this technology. In one case, a genetically engineered bacterium developed to aid in the production of ethanol, produced residues which rendered the land infertile. Corn crops planted on this soil grew three inches tall and fell over dead. (*The Oregonian,* Aug. 8, 1994) Gene-raped corn has killed 3/4 of the Monarch Butterfly population in some midwestern states.

● **Threatens Our Entire Food Supply:**
Insects, birds and wind can carry genetically altered seeds into neighboring fields and beyond. Once transgenic plants pollinate, genetically original plants and wild relatives can be cross-pollinated. All crops, organic and non-organic, are vulnerable to contamination from gene drift.

● **Irreversible Deadly Harm; Gene Pollution Can't Be Cleaned Up!**
Once genetically engineered organisms, bacteria and viruses are released into the environment it is impossible to contain or recall them. Unlike chemical or nuclear contamination, negative effects are irretrievable and irreversible.

From a pamphlet by *Mothers for Natural Law*

Most commonly detected pesticides on commercial produce

Apples
Diphenylamine	?
Captan	√
Endosulfan	?
Phosmet	√
Azinphos-methyl	√

Bananas
Diazinon	?
Thiabendazole	√
Carbaryl	√

Bell Peppers
Methamidophos	x
Chlorpyrifos	?
Diamethoate	?
Acephate	x
Endosulfan	?

Broccoli
DCPA	?
Methamidophos	x
Demetron	x
Dimethoate	?
Parathion	?

Cabbage
Methamidophos	x
Dimethoate	?
Fenvalerate	?
Permethrin	√
BHC	?

Cantaloupes
Methamidophos	x
Endosulfan	?
Chlorothaonil	√
Dimethoate	√
Methyl Parathion	?

Carrots
DDT	√
Trifluralin	x
Parathion	x
Diazinon	?
Dieldrin	?

Cauliflower
Methamidophos	x
Endosulfan	?
Dimethoate	?
Chlorothalonil	√
Diazinon	?

Celery
Dicloran	√
Chlorothalonil	√
Endosulfan	?
Acephate	x
Methamidophos	x

Cherries
Parathion	?
Malathion	√
Captan	√
Dicloran	√
Diazinon	?

Corn
Sulfallate	?
Carbaryl	√
Chlorpyrifos	?
Dieldrin	?
Lindane	?

Cucumbers
Methamidophos	x
Endosulfan	?
Dieldrin	?
Chlorpyrifos	?
Dimethoate	?

Grapefruit
Thiaboendazole	√
Ethion	√
Methidathion	?
Chlorobenzilate	√
Carbaryl	√

Grapes
Captan	√
Dimethoate	?
Dicloran	√
Carbaryl	√
Iprodione	?

Green Beans
Dimethoate	?
Methamidophos	x
Endosulfan	?
Acephate	x
Chlorothalonil	√

Lettuce
Mevinphos	x
Endosulfan	?
Permethrin	√
Dimethoate	?
Methomyl	

Onions
DCPA	?
DDT	√
Ethion	√
Diazinon	?
Malathion	√

Oranges
Methidathion	?
Chlorpyrifos	?
Ethion	√
Parathion	?
Carbaryl	√

Peaches
Dicloran	√
Captan	√
Parathion	?
Carbaryl	√
Endosulfan	?

Pears
Azinphos-methyl	√
Cyhexatin	?
Phosmet	√
Endosulfan	?
Ethion	√

Potatoes
DDT	√
Chlorpropham	x
Dieldrin	?
Aidicarb	x
Chlordane	?

Spinach
Endosulfan	?
DDT	√
Methomyl	x
Methamidophos	x
Dimethoate	?

Strawberries
Captan	√
Vinclozolin	?
Endosulfan	?
Methamidophos	x
Methyl Parathion	?

Sweet Potatoes
Dicloran	√
DDT	√
Phosmet	√
Dieldrin	?
BHC	?

Tomatoes
Methamidophos	x
Chlorplhyifos	?
Chlorothalonil	√
Permethrin	√
Dimethoate	?

Watermelon
Methamidophos	x
Chlorothalonil	√
Dimethoate	?
Carbaryl	√
Captan	√

√ Residues reduced by washing.
x Residues not reduced by washing.
? Not known if washing reduces pesticides.
Source: FASE (see Bibliography)

Avoid "TTT" –the Top-Toxic Twelve most pesticided produce

Of course, the best way to avoid toxic pesticides is to buy certified organic produce. But less than 4% of America's food is organically grown therefore this option is not available to most Americans. The second best alternative is to **avoid buying the** *most contaminated* **produce. The 12 most contaminated fruits & vegetables present the majority of the health risks from pesticides that cause cancer, neurotoxic, and endocrine effects.** To help consumers minimize their exposure to pesticides in produce, the *Environmental Working Group* analyzed the results of 15,000 food samples tested for pesticides during 1992 and 1993. Compiling FDA and EPA data, they found that more than half of the health risks from pesticides are concentrated in the 12 fruits & vegetables consistently contaminated with the *most* pesticides, plus the most *lethal* pesticides. **By avoiding these 12 fruits & vegetables, eaters can reduce their health risks from pesticides (in/on produce) by half,** and still eat a diet rich in fruits and vegetables. (And remember, most pesticides in America's diet come from eating meat, eggs and dairy). Following is an overview of their findings.

Pesticide Contamination Rankings

The 12 Most Contaminated Fruits & Vegetables

Rank	Crop	Score (200 = most toxic)
1	Strawberries	189
2	Bell Peppers (tie)	155
2	Spinach (tie)	155
4	Cherries (USA)	154
5	Peaches	150
6	Cantaloupe (Mexico)	142
7	Celery	129
8	Apples	124
9	Apricots	123
10	Green Beans	122
11	Grapes (Chile)	118
12	Cucumbers	117

The 12 Least-Pesticided Fruits & Vegetables

Avocados	Corn	Onions	Sweet Potatoes
Cauliflower	Brussels sprouts	U.S. Grapes	Bananas
Plums	Green onions	Watermelon	Broccoli

A closer look at the Top-Toxic Twelve ... plus substitutes

Top Twelve Most Contaminated Produce	Substitutes with far lower pesticide residues
1 **Strawberries** have high levels of fungicides, including carcinogenic captan & iprodione; vinclozolin, that blocks normal functioning of the male hormone androgen; endosulfan, a relative of DDT that interferes with normal hormone function by imitating the hormone estrogen.	**blueberries, raspberries, blackberries, kiwis**
2 **Green & red bell peppers** are more heavily contaminated with neurotoxic insecticides than all other crops analyzed.	**broccoli, romaine lettuce**
3 **Spinach** is high in DDT, permethrin, chlorthalonil and other cancer causing pesticides. Kale, swiss chard, mustard greens, and collard greens equally contaminated.	**broccoli, romaine lettuce, carrots**
4 **U.S. Cherries** are heavily contaminated with 26 different pesticides, more than three times the number found on imported cherries.	**blueberries, other berries, kiwis**
5 **Peaches** deliver a heavy dose of the cancer causing fungicides captan and iprodione, and the neurotoxic pesticide, methyl parathion.	**nectarines, kiwis, oranges, papayas**
6 **Cantaloupes**. To avoid cantaloupes with high pesticide residues, avoid this fruit from January to April, when imports from Mexico are at peak. The rest of the year, enjoy this melon.	**watermelon, cantaloupes after April**
7 **Celery** is a major source of neurotoxic pesticides and carcinogenic chlorthalonil. Celery also had the highest percentage of samples with detectable residues (81%) of all produce vegetables analyzed.	**romaine lettuce, carrots**
8 **Apples** are loaded with pesticides (and toxic wax). More pesticides were detected on apples (36), and more pesticides found on single samples of apples (7) than any other fruit or vegetable analyzed.	**any fruit not on the TTT list.**
9 **Apricots** contain high levels of pesticides, including carcinogenic captan, and the endocrine (hormone) disruptors endosulfan and carbaryl.	**any fruit not on the TTT list**
10 **Green beans** are also a major source of the cancer-causing fungicides chlorthalonil and mancozeb, the neurotoxin methamidophos, and the endocrine disruptor, endosulfan.	**green peas, broccoli, zucchini, etc.**
11 **Grapes** from Chile add a load of cancer-causing and endocrine disrupting fungicides. Eat U.S. grown grapes in season; avoid grapes from January to April, when grapes from Chile dominate the market.	**any fruit not on the TTT list.**
12 **Cucumbers** tend to absorb dieldrin, a banned, potent carcinogen, from the soil. When eaten, dieldrin persists in human body fat for decades. Plus, cukes are heavily waxed.	**any fruit or vegetable not on the TTT list**

Why is commercial produce harmful?

- **Genetically and biologically inferior:** Hybridized, mutated, gene-raped, grafted, picked unripe, shipped long distances refrigerated, unnatural.
- **Genetically engineered food threatens Humanity's future survival.** (see previous section on *Dangers*....)
- **Contaminated with chemicals from poisonous artificial fertilizers:** "American farmers now apply more than 20 million tons of chemical fertilizers to our farmlands every year, more than the combined weight of the entire human population of the country."[1] These poisons are absorbed into plantfood we eat.
- **Contaminated with lethal pesticides:** 35% of U.S. food has detectable pesticide residues. Each year, 1.1 billion pounds of pesticides are used in America. This is 30% of the entire world's use; 5 lbs. for each citizen.[2] Some fruit (peaches, apples, cherries) may be sprayed with insecticides 10 to 15 times a season.
- **Coated with toxic, fungicide-rich wax:** That shiny produce you can see yourself in is shiny because it is coated with wax made from shellac and petrochemicals (like polyethylene).[3] Wax has no nutrition. It's used to make produce look pretty and extend its shelf life. Fungicides are also added to this wax to prevent mold. These fungicides include *ortho-phenylphenol*, which suppresses the immune system and causes cancer;[4] *sodium ortho-phenyl phenate*; and *bemomyl*, which causes cancer, birth defects. Waxed produce includes apples, peppers, cucumbers, tomatoes, eggplant, potatoes and papayas.
- **Deficient in minerals and nutrients:** Grown in abused, mineral-poor soil. Depleted soils and their reduced fertility cause a massive loss of trace minerals. Trace minerals are missing from supermarket produce. Even vitamin C is missing from gas-ripened, supermarket citrus fruits. And bioflavonoid content is deficient.
- **Deranged from nuclear irradiation:** Food irradiation continues, though linked with numerous diseases. Food irradiation destroys food nutrients, disrupts the normal bio-energy field of the food, and creates dangerous new free radicals.
- **Damages our health:**
  - Organophosphates (like malathion) tend to cause memory loss, difficulty concentrating, decreased libido, altered electro-activity of infant's brain, irritability, & potentially longterm brain damage.
  - Environmental chemicals are found in 60-80% of all cancers.
  - An estimated 20% of Americans is being seriously harmed by chemicals. The effect is probably strongest in the young.
  - The use of chemical fertilizers may cause up to 70% of all anemia in the U.S. because these fertilizers do not replace the iron in the soil.
  - Irradiated grains are linked with pituitary, thyroid, heart, and lung problems, plus development of tumors and abnormal chromosomes.[5]

1) Robbins, DNA, 357.   2) Ibid., 334.   3) Steinman, LH, 114..   4) Ibid., 194.   5) Valerian, 0141.

Recommendations for Better Health

Avoid or Reduce Eating:	Healthier Replacements:
• all commercially grown fruit, vegetables, nuts, spices, herbs (in supermarkets & foodstores) • the top toxic 12 (see earlier page) • canned vegetables & fruit • frozen commercial produce • dried fruit/raisins (they're sulfured)	• organically grown, pesticide-free, fruits, vegetables, nuts, spices, herbs (at health stores & "farmers markets") • produce & sprouts you grow yourself! • non-irradiated spices, herbs • least pesticided produce (see earlier page) • non-sulfured dried fruit /raisins

Tips

When organic food is not available, select from the least pesticided supermarket produce (see earlier page), and wash it well. Mostly eat it raw (or lightly cooked /steamed), for cooking makes it more toxic.

Peel all waxed produce before consuming (to remove fungicided, toxic wax)

Be COOL with Celery Juice: Because of its high sodium chloride content, fresh raw celery juice excels at counteracting the effects of extreme heat. Drinking a glass or pint of fresh raw celery juice makes the sizzling summer heat bearable. Simply eating celery is not effective. (Walker FV 12)

Cleansing & Removing Pesticides from Fruit & Vegetables

To effectively cleanse fruit and vegetables of toxic residues and sprays (This takes the load off your liver to do this!):
● **Method I:** Mix 1 ounce of pure <u>hydrochloric acid</u> (sold in drugstores) with 3 quarts of water (use only glass or earthenware utensils). A much weaker solution may also be effective according to some. Place vegetables in solution for 5 minutes, then remove and rinse well with pure water. The solution can be saved and reused many times.
● **Method II:** Add 1 ounce of <u>35%, food-grade hydrogen peroxide</u> (sold in health stores) to 1 gallon of water, then rinse your produce in this water. The oxygen neutralizes toxins on the surface of the produce.
● **If you are not able to do the above,** <u>at least wash your fruits and vegetables</u> carefully with mild <u>organic soap</u> and water. Just rinsing with water does no good. Produce which can't be washed should be peeled.

DRUG # 13

Wannabee Whatever
FakeFoods

They abound in *health-food* stores

They look like and almost taste like the real thang. They are real imitations of the real thang –letting us deliciously indulge and have our real-fake beef, real-fake chicken, real-fake fish, real-fake eggs, real-fake cheese –and eat them too. It is interesting that most of these imitative foods imitate fleshfoods (the more poisonous, hence druglike of foods). Vegetarians will pig out —*oops!*... I mean *carrot* out on eating imitation pig, beef, chicken, hotdogs, burgers, cheese, eggs, and be hardly better off than real-meat flesheaters.

Soy & Gluten are king & queen when it comes to fake fleshfood

Wherever there's fake beef, chicken, duck, pork, fleshfood, etc., there's *Soy*...or *Wheat Gluten*...processed to be anything except themselves. Look on the labels of imitation fleshfoods and you will find Soy and/or Wheat Gluten, at or near the top. Soy is not necessarily healthy, even in its natural state as beans. And by nature, gooey Gluten is a gluey fractionate of wholewheat. Soy is very hard to digest. Research has shown that animals fed on a diet of raw soybeans lose weight and **develop pancreatic problems**, because soybeans are so difficult to digest. It takes more effort on the part of the digestive system to break down the soybeans than the energy provided by the beans. As a result, pancreatic enzymes are overproduced to compensate.[1] *Soy-drugfoods* are a major part of the diet of many *healthfood*-people, preventing them from gaining top, optimum health.

Fakefoods are "something else" !

Fakefoods are heavily processed to get that way, hence are denatured in order to get them to look, feel, and taste like something *entirely different* from what they are. They are frauds and they admit it.

Examples of Fakefoods

● **Fake meats and fake burgers** made mainly from isolated soy protein or wheat gluten. Or *mushrooms*, beware; many "veggie burgers" are really "mushroom burgers." If composed of real grains, lentils and beans (except soy), they are less harmful because they are *real* (that is, made of *real* wholefoods). But if mainly made with mushrooms or isolated protein from soy, gluten, eggwhites, etc., they are highly processed, fractionated, firstclass drugfoods.

● **Fake cheeses** made from anything except real milk. Note that *casein* (a protein from real milk) is a primary ingredient in some artificial "cheeses" at health-food stores. Are such "cheeses" healthy? Not necessarily, but they're usually delicious! –like all prepared drugfoods! So which is worse; *real cheese* from cows' milk or *"rice cheese"* having casein? Probably the rice-cheese because the *rice* had to be *processed* in order to be turned into a big tasty *yellow lie.*

1) Gagne, 236.

- **Fake ice cream, milk,** made from anything except real cream, milk. Plus, they are "enriched" with artificial vitamins and other fractionated nutrients.
- **Fake coffee** or powdered vegetable coffee substitutes.
- **Protein powders.** All are highly concentrated, fractionated products, hence drugfoods. If used at all, only use small amounts; they should not be used in large quantities since they congest the tissues with an excess of amino acids. I'll have more to say about them in the next section on *Fractionated Nutrients.*

Fakefoods are another form of "Franken-foods"

Fakefoods have a lot of nerve proudly displaying themselves as healthfoods. True, many of them are made with "organically grown" ingredients but they still are drugfoods as far as your body is concerned, producing drug-like effects. Fake, artificial, imitative foods are typically made with fractionated nutrients which are drugfoods themselves. Like most prepared foods, they are made with numerous fractioned nutrients in the same food item. Further, these food combinations are usually incompatible.

Recommendations for Better Health

Fakefoods in healthstores are better than fakefoods in regular supermarkets only by virtue of having less toxins and less ingredients. And since many fakefoods taste similar to the food they're imitating, they allow people (especially meat/dairy-loving-but-meat/dairy-abstaining vegetarians) to wonderfully indulge as if they had the real thing. Now if I recommend the real food over the fakefood, we are back where we started, for fakefoods were created to avoid the *ill* effects of eating the *real* but hazardous food.

I am more concerned about you knowing the truth about your food. What you do after that is your choice, your *"true choice,"* for now you are *truly* informed and can *truly* have the *option* of choosing wisely. Whereas before, this was not possible because you have been misled, lied to, or misinformed. When you know the real truth, only then do you have true choice. The truth is withheld from eaters, resulting in their making poor choices while all the time they believe they are making good choices. Then later down the path they wonder why /how they got such-n-such disease.

In general, have your fakefoods and eat'em too, —*sparingly* **though!** Be mindful they are firstclass drugfoods which tax your health in the long run, giving you a different set of health problems from the ones you're avoiding by choosing fakefood. You're still a drugfood addict just the same! Tricked into drugfood-eating only at a slightly higher level. Yes, we all are being fooled but the truth points us to real freedom and closer to *true health.*

DRUG
14
Freaked Fractionated Nutrients

Fractionated nutrients (most "supplements") are drugfoods still

When a single nutrient is totally isolated, fractionated from its "nutritional tribe" (wholefood), hence taken out of its natural state, it loses its status as food and becomes a drug. It becomes potentially harmful or even dangerous because it is now nutritionally incomplete, concentrated, and unbalanced. Drugs and drugfood cause nutritional imbalance and deficiency when eaten. The ingredient-list on the labels of commercial foods, *healthfoods*, and supplements often use words which betray their fractionation, hence true identity as drugs: *extract, isolated, fractioned, "active ingredient, "concentrate, pure, 100%.* Corn oil is an example of an isolated, concentrated, so-called food. Corn oil is a drug, like all extracted, isolated, fractioned foods. It takes about 24 ears of corn to produce a single teaspoon of corn oil. Nature limits the amount of oil a human can safely eat without damaging their biochemical balance and homeostasis. When we regularly cross these biological limits, we tax our body, vitality and thus health.

Fractionated nutrients cause nutritional deficiency /imbalance

When you eat dry or dried out food (like bread, raisins, dried fruit), your body has to put back the missing water before you can assimilate it. Similarly, note that when you buy dehydrated or "instant" food (another form of drugfood) such as powdered mixes, instant soups, you must put the water back into it (usually by boiling) which was earlier removed. The same principle is at work with fractionated nutrients /vitamins, etc. Before your body can use this "incompleted" substance, it tries to make it complete again, –back into a wholefood (almost). It does this by raiding its own reserve of nutrients. Taking an isolated nutrient or vitamin creates a deficiency of other vitamins. Example: taking one or more of the B vitamins increases the need of the other B vitamins not supplied. The oversupply of a particular vitamin or nutrient can cause deficiencies of the unsupplied vitamins which may in turn, produce abnormalities that can do more harm than the vitamins obtained can do good. Fractionated nutrients are standard ingredients in most healthfood /commercial food preparations.

> A drug is any isolated, concentrated substance. Calling a drug a food, spice or condiment does not change its effect upon the body. Drugs cause nutritional imbalances.
>
> *Dr. Llaila Afrika*

In *African Holistic Health,* **Dr. Llaila Afrika further explains:** "Oil and other drugs such as sugars, salt, bleached flour, etc. are partial foods. Because of this, the body tries to make the oil drug a whole food. This is accomplished by taking the necessary nutrients from the eyes, sex organs, heart, kidneys, liver, bones, muscles.... The body tries to duplicate the nutritional value of a whole food before digestion can take place. ...Consequently, the whole body is traumatized and nutritionally shocked by a drug and robs itself (commits nutritional suicide) and then sends its defenses to rid the body of the drug. This is the high feeling that drugs such as sugar or alcohol give. It is also, the defensive reaction of the body sending a rush of nutrients to evict the drug by attempting to make it whole. In due course, the body nutritionally loses this fight and submits to the reactionary alcohol dis-ease of intoxification or...the reactionary sugar drug dis-ease of hyper or hypoglycemia (diabetes) or...the oil drug cholesterol dis-ease of high cholesterol, cellulite, obesity or hardening of the arteries."[1]

At any drug or health store, you'll find neat rows and rows of fractionated, isolated nutrients generally called "supplements"
  – You can buy isolated, fractionated vitamins individually.
  – You can buy isolated, fractionated minerals individually.
  – You can buy isolated amino acids (proteins) individually or mixed with other isolated amino acids in "protein mixes."
  – You can buy isolated "active ingredients" of herbs.
  – You can buy numerous isolated nutrients all individually.

Nature does not work this way! Always, *She* gives us nutrients in wholistic, synergistic clusters; in chords, not single sharp notes. When a nutrient is cut out of its original wholistic cluster, it is unbalanced and fractionated, hence a drug. To the degree that we eat such unbalanced, fractionated stuff, we unbalance and fractionate ourselves from Natural Wholeness we were meant to enjoy and express. When you eat natural whole *living* foods, you get minerals and vitamins in normal proportions. When you take a vitamin pill /supplement, you are getting an incomplete food which your body must handle differently at its own expense. <u>True natural vitamins are metabolized differently from bottled, fractionated so-called vitamins and synthetic vitamins</u>. The only true natural vitamins are those found in natural foods, and extracted by chewing and digestion or juicing /drinking. Vitamins which come in bottles, even if labeled natural, have been extracted by artificial means.

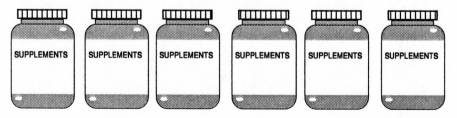

1) Afrika, AHH, 99.

Minerals, Nutrients work only in conjunction with each other.

Scientists keep rediscovering how complex and united Nature is. All the parts are connected and meant to be taken as a whole, not fractionated. Some minerals depend on certain vitamins for maximum absorption by the body. Minerals cannot work to heal when their concentration is increased disproportionately beyond the level of parts per million. Even a dosage of just one tablet of mineral supplementation, can be toxic in effect rather than beneficial, by upsetting the balance of minerals.[1] The nutritional synergy of wholefoods is compromised or damaged by fractionated, isolated nutrients and "enriched" foods.

A year's supply of recommended vitamins would not fill a thimble!

The average person of 160 pounds contains a total of about 7 grams (one fourth of an ounce) of all the various vitamins, including the reserve supplies stored in the tissues and organs! If we took the full quantity of all our vitamin requirements, a whole year's supply –**in pure form**– would not fill a thimble.[2] Vitamin and mineral pills look as big as they do because of fillers and binders. Commercial interests have greatly overblown and misrepresented (lied about) our vitamin situation in order to perpetrate a profitable fraud upon us. *"A reading of the labels of even the most 'natural' of vitamins sold in the market place reveals that they are about 98% of synthetic origin. Even vitamins extracted totally from natural sources are worthless out of context with their food. Synthetic vitamins are totally unusable and, in fact, give _drug effects_."* [3] [–because they _are_ Drugs Masquerading As Foods!]

No supplement can supply all the factors found in raw, LIVING wholefoods.

The human body was not structured for fragmented nutrient intake. Vitamins, minerals, and other nutrients work best in conjunction with other vitamins, minerals, enzymes, etc., as found in whole, living food from Nature. **Thousands of healing, nourishing agents have been identified in natural wholefood that contributes to health:**

- over 20,000 different **bioflavonoids** (like rutin, pycnogenol), regarded as anti-oxidants to slow disease process /chelate heavy metals out the body
- over 800 different **carotenoids** (like beta-carotene), to stimulate immune function and slow aging
- **chlorophyll, phytochemicals** and thousands more **health-giving substances**, including the plant's **lifeforce**

Supplementing with any single, isolated, fractionated nutrient does not work. Nutrients work only by interaction with other nutrients. Get your super-nutrition by juicing organic vegetables and fruit of all kinds and making herbal teas.

---

1) de Langre, 59, 60.   2) Honiball, 104; Nelson, MYN, 50   3) Ibid., 104, 105.

Albinos started & developed "isolated nutrition"...

and they promote it. Vitamin supplements are a 20th-century Albino invention. The first vitamin pill was Vitamin D, synthetically/commercially manufactured in 1927 by Albinos (Mead Johnson & Co.). Humans lived without vitamin supplements for all their existence prior to this time, getting their nutrition from their food. **Isolated Nutrition is disaligned with Nature.** Disconnected from Nature (or rather, apparently *never connected with* Nature, and constantly at War with Nature & anything natur-REAL), the Western-Albino mind fails to see and understand the integrated unity underlying the human body and true nutrition. Nutrition is seen as chemical and mechanistic. Body is seen as a machine with its parts isolated from the whole. Hence, Albinos take B-vitamins for the nervous system, amino acids for the muscle system, calcium for the bones, etc. This is alien to Nature. Melanated people should not live this way; it is harmful. It seems unavoidable, for we live in white people's artificial society and are inundated with white people's glorified, anti-Nature lifestyle. Further, we are trained at their *secular* institutions and proudly display hard-earned degrees they give us, apparently unmindful we are really displaying our ignorance (though we are filled with irrelevant "facts") and disconnection from Nature. De-educating and re-educating ourselves will point us back to the right path that promotes *Balance*, and thereby ensures health, life, and survival.

But why do fractionated nutrients make you feel better?
Fractionated nutrition seems to make you feel better and even healthier. It's counterfeit health! Not *real* health. We may feel and look stronger but really, are weaker. Comparable with the fact that feeding the soil the isolated nutrition of synthetic-chemical-fertilizers produces big, luscious-looking vegetables, etc. But these same veggies are nutritionally deficient, flavor-deficient (compelling eaters to add drugfood-condiments), and are weak. Hence, are very susceptible to disease, insect pests. And they spoil faster. They rapidly become even weaker with each succeeding generation of seeds (if they can reseed at all) and die out completely. Isolated nutrition has a similar effect on its eaters. Like the plants, we too, "spoil" faster *(i.e., get sick more often, succumb to virus-bugs, disease, yeast disorders, immune deficiency)*, and are weaker *(i.e., take longer to heal, die sooner, have less healthy children even weaker than ourselves who are often infertile)*. As detailed later, the apparent energy we feel from taking isolated nutrients is but *stimulation* at the *expense* of our own energy. After the effects ("high") wear off, we need another "hit." *Addiction*, by any other name!

Why do people take fractionated nutritional supplements?
1) There is a massive ongoing campaign (originated and kept going by Albinos) to promote taking supplements.
2) People have been convinced that this unnatural way of (mis)nourishing themselves is necessary in order to be healthy.
3) **People are actually ADDICTED to supplements**, for fractionated supplements are disguised drugs /drugfoods. They stimulate the body, offering a drug-like effect similar to caffeine. This stimulation is misinterpreted as an energy boost. Many health-conscious people consume

many different fractionated (and expensive) supplements. Their kitchen often has a cabinet or drawer literally full of supplements. If they were to abruptly stop taking their supplements for a while (i.e., go "cold turkey" off their supplement-*habit*), they'd soon need a "fix," –just like drug addicts, which they unknowingly are. They would experience "withdrawal symptoms" such as nervousness, irritability, depression, fatigue, "heebie-geebies," etc., which would continue until the body has purged itself of those supplements which are really *Drugs Masquerading As Foods.*

Your nasty noxious nutritional supplements

You'd be horrified at the horrible stuff from which Albinos (drug-chemical corporations) make many so-called natural vitamins and minerals. It's akin to their horrible heartless treatment of diseased, deranged, poison-filled, drugged, steroided "factory farm-animals," –animals which are also key ingredients used in making many of those same commercial supplements. Commercial grade vitamin and mineral concentrates are synthesized by the big deadly, super-rich, truly-*filthy*-rich pharmaceutical-chemical corporations from the same starting material which they make their expensive deadly drugs from: coal tar, petroleum products, animal feces, animal by-products, animal bones, hooves, ground rocks, shells, and metal. They are then wholesaled out to nutrient manufacturers, the "mixing middlemen."

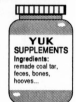

YUK
SUPPLEMENTS
Ingredients:
remade coal tar,
feces, bones,
hooves...

- **All the minerals used in nutrient manufacture are basically DIRT.** The iron, zinc, calcium, etc., are just mined ore, pulverized, powdered to a fine dust. Some calcium is made from ground up oyster shells.
- **Yuk vitamins:** Vitamin A is made from toxic fish-liver juices rich with deadly mercury and PCB's. B-vitamins are made from toxic coal tar and petro-chemicals (*which are respiratory irritants, carcinogens, and nervous-system depressants*). Vitamin B12 is made from fecal matter (it's "natural" and is even high in some vitamins) or ground-up toxic cow livers (*overloaded with drugs, antibiotics, steroids and pesticides consumed by factory-farm cows*).[1] Vitamin C is made from acid blends irritating to the lining of the digestive tract. Vitamin D from irradiated cholesterol.[2] Vitamin E from Eastman Kodak.[1] You get the "picture"? *Ugly,* ain't it?!
- **Yuk capsules:** Unless otherwise stated on the label, the capsule-gelatin is made from the boiled down hooves and bones of factory-farm animals.

No one asks just where these vitamins and minerals come from!
Everyone assumes a vitamin is just a vitamin or a mineral is a mineral. After all, the United States Pharmacopeia (U.S.P.) states that if a substance looks the same under a microscope or in analysis, it *is* the same regardless of what it's made out of. Examples: Glycerin u.s.p. is considered identical whether made from fresh vegetables or toxic minerals or boiled down animal carcasses / cartilage /feet. It considers Salicylic Acid u.s.p. identical whether it comes from wintergreen leaves or by boiling coal in carbolic and sulfuric acids. Which would you rather have?

1) Nutritional pamphlet by *Dr. Richard Schulze.*   2) Igram, STN, 82.

INDUSTRIAL WASTES / by-products sold as healthfood?

Numerous industries have succeeded in getting the public to buy their waste products /by-products as "health food" supplements. They include the following fractionated supplemental foods:

- **Blackstrap molasses** is the "chemicalized, deranged and overcooked waste product" of the sugar industry. Cooked organic minerals become inorganic.
- **Brewer's yeast** is a waste product of the beer industry.
- **Bran** is a waste product of the milling industry. It is used to loosen stools / reduce constipation. Bran is indigestible and high in phytate which impairs calcium/magnesium absorption.
- **Wheat germ** is a waste product of the milling industry.
- **Whey** is a waste product of the dairy industry. **Skim milk** is also a by-product of the dairy industry, once solely fed to hogs.
- **Bone meal** is a by-product of the meat-packing industry. It should be avoided, for it is contaminated with lead and antibiotics.
- **Lecithin** is the by-product of the oil-making industry. As an emulsifier, it prevents and dissolves fat /cholesterol deposits on the walls of the arteries, thus is good in this respect. But most lecithin products are inferior. Avoid: artificial lecithin *(choline chloride)*, liquid lecithin *(gel capsules)*, lecithin having protein or amino acids *(lecithin contains NO protein)*, and most lecithin granules /powder *(they often consist of soy flour & milk solids on which liquid lecithin has been spray-dried)*.
- **Bottled minerals** are often the by-product of the salt industry. In getting fractionated from natural ocean salt, they lose their ionic properties and become inorganic, vastly inassimilable.

The outright poisons in your nutritional & herbal supplements

- **Solvents:** All your *bottled* supplements are solvent-contaminated, unless otherwise noted on the label. The solvents are residues from sterilizing the bottles, and from extracting "active ingredients" from plants. Dr. Hulda Clark wrote: *"Toxic solvents like decane, hexane, carbon tetrachloride and benzene will get more flavor or fat or cholesterol out of things than metabolizable grain alcohol. Of course, the extraction process calls for washing out the solvent later. But it can't all be washed out.."*[1] Dr. Richard Schulze said: *"They use a tremendous amount of solvent and a very small amount of herb and it makes for a much lower quality product. It's not the way it used to be done, at least by the reputable herbalists...The marketing is getting more sophisticated, the process is getting more disgusting."*
- **Heavy Metals & PCBs:** Dr. Clark wrote: *"I have found solvents, heavy metals and lanthanides in 90% or more of the popular vitamin and mineral capsules and tablets I test. ...All the Ester-C™ varieties of vitamin C that I have tested are polluted with thulium!"*[2] Dr. Clark also discovered that some brands of capsules contained PCBs, mercury, ruthenium, thulium, strontium, praseodymium, aluminum, benzalkonium.[3]

1) Clark, CAD, 435, 436.   2) Ibid., 434.   3) Ibid.

- **Pesticides & Irradiation:** How do you know if the herbs you are using were organically grown if the label does not say so? Most herbs on the market today –like commercial produce– are grown with pesticides. Over 90% of the *herbs* sold in the U.S. are grown in countries that have NO regulations on pesticides. Further, these countries are likely using pesticides that have been banned in the U.S. Additionally, many herbs are subjected to fumigation and irradiation when they get to U.S. docks.

- **Hormone disrupters** may be leaching in from the *plastic* container.

- **Alcohol:** Herbs are sometimes in alcohol. *"Alcohol creates an electrical 'black hole' in the body. And any combination with it creates a toxic substance."*[1] Alcohol also causes the body to be more vulnerable to cancers.

- **Calcium Phosphate,** used as a binder. Dicalcium Phosphate (DCP) is usually the main ingredient used to bind tablets. It binds you too. It is also used in capsules. DCP can cause or contribute to hardening of the arteries, arthritis, joint pain /stiffness, osteoporosis, premature aging, excessive wrinkles, digestive problems and memory loss.[3] Other forms are <u>dolomite</u>, <u>lime</u>, <u>monobasic</u> and <u>tri-calcium phosphate</u>. If used as a binder, it does not have to be listed on the label, so beware. Even the dictionary tells us that calcium phosphate is used in glass, ceramics, fertilizers, rubber, baking powders, as a plastic stabilizer, ...and as a <u>food supplement</u>!

- **Electrical Derangement:** Most supplements have no *electrical integrity*, a factor destroyed in most processing such as grinding, steam distilling, and compressing. This is especially true with tablets, which may be made with as much as 14 tons of pressure. As a result, most supplements do not work properly, hence are useless –extra toxins which the body tries to eliminate.

No wonder Dr. Hulda Clark advised:
"Stop Using Supplements ...Stop using your vitamin supplements. They, too, are heavily polluted. ...These substances [pollutants, poisons] will do more harm in the long run than the supplement can make up for in benefits. ...Until all vitamins and minerals and other food supplements have been analyzed for pollutants, <u>after they are encapsulated or tableted</u>, they are not safe. ...No manufactured product is pure." "All supplements must be tested for purity by yourself. If this cannot be done, don't take them. Polluted supplements do much more harm than good."[2]

Thus, instead of getting healthier, we are getting less healthy by ingesting these toxic supplements. They contribute to the waste which our body attempts to eliminate. If our bodies are spending most or all of its time and energy getting rid of wastes, then how can it take the time and energy to repair itself? It can't! That's why we break down...and eventually succumb to degenerative diseases and painful, premature demise.

1) Report by Professional Research Institute; see bibliography.   2) Clark, CAD, 434, 436.
3) according to research by the American Trace Mineral Research Corporation and Nutritional Biologicals, Inc.

A glimpse of frauds and fallacies in nutritional supplements

MINERAL supplements are *inorganic*, thus basically useless.

As noted earlier, all mineral supplements are basically made from dirt...pulverized ores. It matters not that they are powdered to a fine dust; they still are inorganic. *INORGANIC* minerals are *insoluble* (identical with the inorganic minerals composing concrete and nails). Inorganic minerals are essentially inassimilable, hence are useless and even harmful. Inorganic mineral supplements contribute to the toxic materials our body attempts to expel (otherwise deposit them in our tissues /create kidneys stones /harden our arteries, etc.). Modern reseach shows that minerals of this type are 99% inassimilable. So what do manufacturers (white people) do? They add pig digestive enzymes (from factory-farm pigs no doubt), which supposedly pre-digests it or *chelates* it. This "chelation" is an attempt to FORCE the human body to accept the unacceptable, the toxic material. This is a form of biological dictatorship.

To be healthy, our bodies require *ORGANIC* minerals as found in raw plants (herbs, fruit, vegetables); or *ionic* minerals –as found in unheated seawater or undried ocean salt (Celtic salt). *ORGANIC* minerals are *soluble*. Organic and ionic minerals are the most bio-available and electrically alive.

Chemical forms of minerals are not elemental forms of minerals. Example: a 1200 mg. pill of calcium gluconate is only 9% elemental. That is, it contains only 108 mg. of calcium. To get the RDA (Recommended Daily Allowance – another fallacy) for calcium, you have to take 11 of these pills daily. The same goes for every mineral. Magnesium aspartate is only 11% magnesium. Calcium citrate is only 21% calcium. Chromium picolinate is only 12 1/2% chromium. Some forms contain only 1-2% of the mineral element. By law, supplement pills only have to be true to label chemically. That is, if the bottle says the pill contains say 300 mg. of magnesium, that is all it has to do. **But many chemical forms of nutrients are hardly bioavailable. They pass through your intestines without being absorbed.**[1] At best, they are only partially absorbed. Minerals cannot work to heal when their concentration is increased disproportionately beyond the level of parts per million.

VITAMINS: So-called "natural vitamins" are unnatural frauds.

Many companies falsely label their supplements "natural" because the word sells. Most vitamin pill ingredients are synthetic. Manufacturers dodge this issue by using phrases such as "natural source" or "natural grown," but the truth is that most pill ingredients are synthetic and fractionated. They are natural materials (what else is there?) which are so treated with chemical procedures that they are no longer "natural." Example: most vitamin C is made from corn. First the corn is chemically converted to sugar (d-ribose). Next the sugar is chemically converted to pure, ascorbic acid. Not a molecule of corn remains. It

1) Colgan, NN, 105.

Drugs Masquerading As Foods...

is the chemical processing that makes it synthetic, not the raw materials it came from. And what about "natural rose hip" or "acerola" vitamin C? *The best rose hip and acerola powders contain only a few milligrams of vitamin C per gram. A 1000 mg. pill of natural rose hip vitamin C would be about the size of a baseball. All these so-called 'natural' pills are predominantly synthetic ascorbic acid, with a pinch of the natural powder thrown in for marketing.*[1]

Complete with *Fairy Dust.* Deceptively, these nasty "natural" vitamins and minerals might even be in a "base of herbs." More deceptively, some manufacturers will put infinitesimal amounts of one or many herbs in a formula just to have it on the label to make it sell. This is called "**fairy dust**." As noted by Dr. Richard Schulze, *"You'd get just as much out of it if you just yelled the name of the herb at the bottle. There's nothing there."* Even more deceptive, these nasty supplements may have a label on the bottle with a long list of no's like no cellulose, no starch, no soy, no wheat, etc.

SYNTHETIC VITAMINS are not real vitamins but killer chemicals/ drugs.

Synthetic vitamins are even worse than vitamins mislabeled *natural.* Plus they contain preservatives, sugars and other harmful additives. They are produced in laboratories from petroleum, coal tar and isolated chemicals that mirror their counterparts found in Nature.

Synthetic vitamins refract light the opposite of natural vitamin complexes. Synthetic vitamin-producers/sellers claim that synthetic vitamins have the same molecule-structure as natural vitamins, and are therefore the same or at least have the same effect. They never mention that **the polarity of the synthetic is opposite to the natural and has the opposite effect!** Synthetic vitamins always refract light the opposite of natural vitamin complexes. Dr. Royal Lee discovered the light refraction attributes of vitamins in the 1930s. Though synthetic vitamins have the same molecular structure, they are a mirror image of the natural. "Mirror image" suggests they are identical in every detail. But a mirror image is the exact opposite of the real thing, not an exact duplication.

Millions of Americans take synthetic vitamins daily, unknowingly killing themselves while thinking they are helping their health. They have been massively deceived. A Finnish study (published in the *New England Journal of Medicine*) and the Agnes Faye Morgan experiments at University of California, Berkeley in the 1940s proved that taking synthetic vitamins is worse than starvation. The synthetic vitamins killed people quicker. In the Finnish study, there was a "major loss of protection" from lung cancer, stroke, and other degenerative diseases. Apparently, patients died sooner /faster when given synthetic vitamins. Thus, synthetic vitamins do not provide protection; we need to be protected *from* them. They are toxic, reformed, coal-tar chemicals.

1) Colgan, NN, 103.

What about vitamin B12, allegedly deficient in vegetarian diets? Another myth. Studies show that B12 deficiency is rare among healthy vegans and vegetarians.[1] B12-producing bacteria is found throughout the human body. Micro-organisms between the teeth and gums, and around the tonsils, etc., produce an estimated .5 micrograms a day. Only 0.1 micrograms of B12 is needed to get a physiological response in B12-deficient people.[2] While some nutritionists argue that an adequate supply of vitamin B12 cannot be obtained without eating meat, such a viewpoint does not take into account that cooking meat destroys up to 85% of its vitamin B12. Since people do not eat meat raw, meat cannot be a reliable source for this vitamin. The most abundant source of B12 is a healthy intestinal flora.[3] Toxic intestinal tracts can't maintain a high concentration of live lactic-acid and vitamin producing bacteria, even when lactobacteria-rich foods are being eaten. (see later page for plant-sources of B12)

PROTEIN Powder –watch out!

Protein powders are highly concentrated, fractionated, unnatural products, hence firstclass drugfoods which imbalance our metabolism. If used at all, only use small amounts; not large quantities since they congest the tissues with an excess of amino acids. **"Textured vegetable protein"** should not be used at all! It is a totally unnatural form of protein with adherent amino acid chains which are incompatible with the amino needs of the cells. Very high protein intakes as used by many strength athletes and people on high protein diet plans, suck calcium out of your body like a sponge.[4] High-protein meal replacement drinks can seriously deplete your calcium stores if used as the main source of protein in your diet, especially if they contain casein, lactalbumin, and egg white.

Perhaps an artificial diet requires artificial supplementation?

An artificial lifestyle in an artificial environment creates artificial unnatural eating which *apparently* requires artificial supplementation to *simulate* real health. As long as people live on void, empty, "refined", nutrient-deficient, food-deficient drugfood, perhaps then do they need additional "supplements." Those supplements, inferior and unnatural as they are, may be as *good* ("bad" disguised as good) as these people will ever get it on their degenerate, S.A.D. *Western* diet of *Drugs Masquerading As Foods*. It's like bleached-empty-white-bread being supplemented with a few synthetic vitamins and then called "enriched." Stanley Burroughs wrote: *"Just how much [supplementation] and what combination, even with long and complicated tests, will probably never be determined, so this form of unnatural nutrition will always be lacking. Such a plan is a very poor substitute for the right way."*[5]

Only health emergencies justify taking fractionated nutrients & drugs.
Drastic or extreme situations usually call for drastic /extreme measures. Thus, in times of health emergencies, then drugs, fractionated nutrients, and herbs are great tools –even life-saving. However, they are best for short-term use, not long-term usage.

---

1) Cousens, CE, 189.   2) Ibid., 191.   3) Gray, CHH, 20.   4) Colgan, NN, 58.   5) Burroughs, HA, 28.

Energy and Stimulation are not the same. As with drugs, depletion of energy is the secondary effect of supplements.

Fractionated nutrients cause drug-like *Stimulation* because they *are* drugs as far as your body is concerned. *Stimulation* is confused or misinterpreted as being *Energy* (getting energized or an energy boost). Stimulation and Energy are not the same. Stimulation is an *effect* (result, reaction) in the body, and *Energy* is used to produce it. (The word *stimulation* is from the Afrikan root TEM, to pierce, cut, be stung or bitten[1]). We misinterpret this defensive *reaction* of the body as Energy. **The *Stimulation* we feel when we ingest coffee, drugs, tobacco smoke, drugfood, and <u>nutritional supplements</u> is at the <u>*expense*</u> of our <u>*Vital Energy*</u>.** When any stimulating substance is consumed the body defends itself in an effort to maintain its health. It does so by becoming energetic and speedily eliminating the toxic material from its domain. Hence the body is expending energy to rid itself of the toxic substance ingested. As previously noted, the Stimulation this creates is mistaken or misinterpreted for Energy because energy is noticeably expended in the process. However, this Energy is <u>not</u> from the ingested drug or drugfood. This Energy is from the body's Vital Reserve Energy (also called nerve energy). It is <u>not</u> energy being *ADDED* but being *SUBTRACTED*.

As a result of the induced Stimulation, there is a corresponding <u>equal yet opposite secondary effect.</u> It's simply a matter of what goes up must come down. All nervous stimulation ultimately leads to the opposite condition of nervous depression.[2] No wonder people get "hang-overs" from alcohol and other drugs. Another example: when a person smokes, their pulse rate rises within minutes (unknown to them). Smokers experiencing this side effect say the cigarette gives them a lift. What they are experiencing as a "lift" is the *Stimulation* of a toxin causing their heart to beat faster (because the body metabolism speeds up to quickly evict the offending substance).
The more poisonous the substance:
— the more energy your body expends to evict it
— the more addicting it is (the more you crave it)
— the more your body has to adjust itself (at the expense of its vital energy)
In *Maximizing Your Nutrition,* Dennis Nelson informs us that nutritional supplements: "tend to stimulate the body, offering a drug-like effect similar to caffeine ingestion. This stimulation is often misinterpreted as an energy boost. However, neither vitamins nor minerals supply the body with energy. ...What is really happening is an increase in the eliminative activities of the body due to the presence of a foreign, non-usable substance, i.e. the supplement. This is a defensive reaction and energy is used in the process. And, as is true of all stimulants, once the primary effects wear off, secondary effects result which are opposite to the primary effects. In other words, the body must always compensate for any loss of energy as a result of attempting to defend itself from any offensive substance or influence."[3]

1) Suzar, BOTW, 289.   2) Nelson, MYN, 122   3) Ibid., 52, 53.

Excessive abnormal stimulation (from any drugs, medicinal herbs, fractionated nutrients, and toxic nonfoods such as alcohol, coffee, tobacco) may offer a brief illusory respite but they all are ultimately exhausting the body's energy, setting the stage for chronic fatigue. Hard drugfoods (such as donuts, fries, sugar) and fleshfoods also abnormally stimulate the body, but the ultimate result of their consumption, –as with drugs, is depletion of vital nerve energy.[1] Milder drugfoods (such as cooked organic wholefood) only do it more slowly with less problems.

Eating also causes stimulation. Food does not immediately release energy upon ingestion (it has to digest first), yet we feel energy immediately after a meal. This seeming contradiction is explained: "This energy boost is due to the fact that the presence of food within the alimentary canal stimulates digestive activity."[2] For the digestion of food expends energy! The body uses stored energy from its previous meals first, then the new supply later, after hunger signals to again replenish one's energy reserves.

The SOLUTION: Only Mother Nature's way is best.

The best source of assimilable, bio-available, health-producing nutrients are plant-wholefoods from Nature, *organically* grown (ideally from heirloom seeds).

- **Nature offers a superior choice to supplementation in the form of organically grown succulent fruits and vegetables**
These are the richest source of usable vitamins and minerals. **The darker and richer the color, the more minerals and nutrients a fruit or vegetable has.** Fresh fruit contain ample mineral salts. There are more *usable* nutrients in a single piece of organic fruit or vegetable than in a whole bottle of supplements, and in proportions ideal to satisfy the body's needs. When you provide your body with appropriate food, it selects whatever nutrients it requires from the food in the exact proportions necessary to perfectly regulate its own chemistry. No laboratory is capable of duplicating this balanced formula. The RDA's for minerals are several times our actual needs. Even so, all the RDA's added together do not amount to eight grams daily. *"A day's supply of watermelon contains some 24 grams of minerals, about three times our need. Peeled oranges also contain about 24 grams when 2,000 calories are taken. Our RDA of calcium, for instance, is 800 milligrams. Oranges supply over 1,600 milligrams. And so it goes for all the minerals down the line for almost every fruit: Our needs are amply met."[3]*

In addition to eating raw vegetables and fruit, we should also drink them. As fresh juice. There is a vast advantage to consuming **raw vegetable JUICES** as "nutritional supplementation." **When we drink raw vegetable juices, they are digested and assimilated within 10-15 minutes** after drinking them, and are used almost entirely in the nourishment and regeneration of the cells, tissues,

---

1) Nelson MYN, 121.   2) Ibid., 120.   3) Honiball/Fry, 105.

organs. Make sure to include leafy dark greens. Green drinks are powerful, healing, and balancing. Green foods are Nature's protective medicines. They help evict toxins from the body. **Drink as much live juice as you wish. It's best to make your juice right before consuming it.** The longer it stands, the more it loses its *lifeforce* –another form of vital nutrition we need –rarely mentioned in healthbooks. Tip: prewash in advance a lot of veggies /fruit for juicing and store them in the refrigerator in closed containers; when you get ready to make juice, then all you have to do is run them through your juicer.

● **Green, Chlorophyll-rich, "wholefood supplements"**
Spirulina, bluegreen algae, barley-green, wheatgrass, alfalfa... All incredibly endowed with a wide base of nutrients required for optimum human health. High levels of protein, vitamin *complexes*, minerals, enzymes... They can be purchased as powders which can be mixed in drinks /smoothies, or sprinkled over *drugfood* to boost nutrition. Spirulina is *nappy* algae; its cells look just like nappy, kinky, spiraling hair. The same power that spirals the seashells, atoms, and cosmos, also spirals "spirulina" and the "nappy" spiraling, *spiritual* hair of Afrikans.

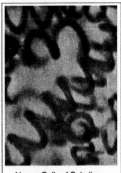
Nappy Cells of Spirulina

Spirulina (a bluegreen algae) has been consumed by Afrikans (Nubians & Egyptians especially) for thousands if not millions of years, particularly in the Afrika's Nile Valley and Chad where it was easily harvested. Even today, Chad, Kenya (& Mexico) have lakes in which Spirulina grows naturally without human assistance. Spirulina and Bluegreen Algae, Earth's most ancient plants, are among the most concentrated of foods, containing some 70% protein, 10% carbohydrates, 9% minerals, plus fats, fiber, enzymes and other nutrients. Spirulina is the world's highest natural source of rare vitamin B12 (containing 225 mcg. per 100 grams as against 27 mcg. in seaweed; 2 mcg. in eggs; 80 mcg. in liver).

Nappy Spirulina's Super-rich Nutrient Composition

*Nutrients are listed according to predominance. (**Bluegreen Algae's composition is similar**)*

Essential Amino Acids:	Carbohydrates:	Lipids:	Minerals:	
Valine	Ramnose	**Fatty Acids:**	Potassium (K)	Cyanocobalamin (B12)
Leucine	Phosphoroled	Linoleic	Phosphorous (P)	Folic Acid
Threonine	cyclitols	Linolenic	Chloride (Cl)	Biotin (H)
Isoleucine	Glucane	Palmitoleic	Magnesium (Mg)	**Carotenoids:**
Lysine	Glucosamine	Oleic	Calcium (Ca)	Carotene
Phenylalanine	acid	Palmitolinoleic	Iron (Fe)	(vitamin A precursor)
Methionine	Muramic acid	Palmitic	Sodium (Na)	Xanthophylis
Tryptophan	Glycogen	Lauric	Zinc (Zn)	Cryptoxanthin
Other Amino Acids:	Sialic acid	Myrstic	Manganese (Mn)	Echinenone
Glutamic Acid	And others	Heptadecanoic	And others	Zeaxanthin
Aspartic Acid	**Nucleic Acids:**	Stearic	**Vitamins:**	Lutein
Arginine	Ribonucleic	And others	Inositol	Euglenanone
Alanine	Acid (RNA)	**Insaponifiable:**	Tocopherol (E)	**Sterols:**
Tyrosine	Deoxyribonucleic	Sterols	Nicotinic Acid (PP)	Cholesterol
Serine	Acid (DNA)	Titerpen alcohols	Thiamine (B1)	Sitosterol
Glycine, Proline		Carotenoids	Riboflavine (B2)	Dihidro 7 Cholesterol
Histidine, Cystine		Chlorophyll a	d-Ca-Pantothenate	Cholesten 7 ol 3
		And others	Pyridoxine (B6)	Stigmasterol
				And others

● **Hemp Seed is a complete food with all the nutrients of mother's milk**
The bond between Hemp and Humanity is ancient. Hemp seed has been
anciently used as food by humans and animals. **Hemp seed** is intensely
nutritious. Yes, it's been *sterilized* (steamed 5 minutes to degerminate it so it
won't grow), thus reduced in nutritional value but it retains, unharmed, enough
of its vast nutrients to still be a worthwhile addition to our diets. It won't make
you "high," it has no intoxicating chemicals or effects (found only in the leaves /
flowers). Hemp seed is a "complete protein" containing all the essential amino
and fatty acids. The globulin *edestin*, found in hemp protein, closely resembles
the globulin found in human blood plasma, and is easily digested and utilized by
the human body. In fact, it is so compatible with humans' digestive tract that a
1955 Czechoslovakian study found Hemp seed to be the only food that can
successfully treat the consumptive disease tuberculosis, in which the nutritive
processes are impaired and the body wastes away.[1] Mothers of the Sotho people
in South Afrika are known to feed their babies with ground hemp seed in pap. [2]
Hemp oil contains a balanced distribution of all the essential fatty acids. The
best oil is green-tinged with hempseed's natural chlorophyll, another bonus.

Hemp is a profound healer. Hemp is of
special importance for People of Color, for it
effectively helps those suffering from Sickle
Cell Anemia. Hemp herb, seeds, and oil
(especially) greatly oxygenates the blood and
decreases blood pressure. Hemp has been used
to treat female disorders: morning sickness,
uterine dysfunctions, menorrhagia (excessive
uterine bleeding), and menstrual cramps.
Queen Victoria herself smoked cannabis to
relieve her menstrual cramps.[3] Hemp has been
used to treat countless dis-eases, including
asthma, respiratory diseases, whooping cough,
muscular dystrophy, multiple sclerosis,
glaucoma, neuralgia, migraines, depression,

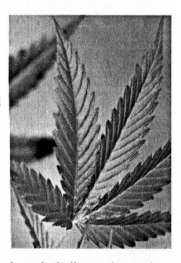

insomnia, malaria, inflammation, digestive disorders, alcoholism and even drug
addiction ...which brings us to another amazing property: *Hemp is not addictive
nor habit forming!* Does this mean it isn't a drug? Smoking marijuana does not
lead to addiction, nor to heroin & cocaine addiction, according to studies.[4]
Cannabis is nontoxic. No deaths from an overdose have ever been verified.

The *holy herb* Hemp has anciently been used for spiritual purposes in cultures
around the world. *Cannabis*-use in Afrika, where it abounds throughout the
continent, predates arrival of the Albinos. The waterpipe was developed in
North Afrika. Known as dagga, hemp is a sacrament and medicine to many
Afrikan peoples including the Twa –humanity's ancestors (derogatorily called
the Pygmies). In ancient times, Ethiopia was known as the "Land of Incense"

1) Robinson, GB, 60.   2) Ibid.   3) Ibid., 54.   4) Ibid., 60.

and is still reknown for its potent *hashish*. **Hemp is even in the Bible.** Some of the references to incense-burning is hemp-burning. The "honeycomb" in Solomon 5:1 and honey "wood" in 1Samuel 14:25-45 is likely hemp. In the latter, Jonathan dipped a rod *"in an honeycomb, and put his hand to his mouth; and his eyes were enlightened" (v27)*. He later declares *"mine eyes have been enlightened, because I tasted a little of this honey" (v29)*.

In addition to feeding, healing, and "enlightening" Humanity, Hemp can help save Earth and solve many of our ecology problems, including deforestation. But the Controllers don't want this! They were responsible for slandering Hemp in the early 1900s, reshaping its image into something bad, relabeling it as "Marijuana" in order to turn the social tide against it to make Hemp illegal. Why? They had their own agenda: pushing petrochemicals, their newfound gold mine.

Hemp used to be America's number one cash crop and 2nd most prescribed medicine from 1840 to 1893 (aspirin was #1). There were no side-effects in all these 53 years! America's first flag was made of Hemp fiber. Hemp is incredibly versatile. It makes the best, most durable, safe "plastic," glue, wood, fiber, paper, nontoxic varnishes & paints, and even bio-fuel. Continuously, it purifies the air, removing detrimental positive ions. If every

---

Very *High* Notes

● The natural chemical in hemp that makes you "high" has great medicinal value. Called THC (tetrahydrocannabinol), it activates when hemp is heated (cooked). For those who smoke hemp, it is safest to smoke it using a waterpipe. When the fumes are drawn through the water, the "bad stuff" (burnt substances) is left behind in the water while the THC escapes. People who smoke both hemp & cigarettes don't get cancer because Hemp cleanses the lungs.

● **THC receptors in the human brain!** *"The discovery of receptors in the human brain specifically designed for cannabinoids should end the debate on their appropriateness for human beings. The receptor site, a protein on the cell surface, activates G-proteins inside the cell and leads to a cascade of other biochemical reactions that generate euphoria."* [1]

● *"In 1992 William Devane identified a cannabinoid-like neurotransmitter produced by the human brain having biological and behavioral effects similar to THC. He named it anandamide, after the Sanskrit word ananda, meaning bliss."* [2]

1) Robinson, GB, 72. 2) Ibid.

Hemp Seed/Oil's Rich Spectrum of Nutrients

Nutrients are listed according to predominance.

Amino Acids in Hemp Seed:	Isoleucine	Oleic, Palmitic	Magnesium	Titanium
Glutamic Acid	Cystine, Cysteine	Stearic	Sulfur	Zirconium
Glutamine	Tryptophan	Gamma Linolenic	Calcium	Iodine
Aspartic Acid	Ethanolamine	Arachidic	Iron	Chromium
Asparagine	**Hemp Oil Analysis**	Palmitoleic	Manganese	Silver
Arginine, Glycine	Moisture	Eicosenoic	Zinc	Lithium, and others
Alanine, Serine	Essential	Behenic	Sodium	**Vitamins:**
Proline, Leucine	Fatty Acids	Lignoceric	Silicon	Carotene (vitamin A)
Tyrosine, Lysine	Vitamin A & E	Heptadecanoic	Copper	Vitamin E
Threonine	Phosphatides	Erucic	Platinum	Niacin (B3)
Phenylalanine	Chlorophyll	Nervonic	Boron, Thorium	Vitamin C
Valine	**Fatty Acids of**	**Minerals**	Strontium	Riboflavin (B2)
Methionine	**Hemp Oil:**	**in Hemp Seed:**	Barium, Nickel	Thiamine (B1)
Histidine	Linoleic	Phosphorous	Germanium	Pyridoxine (B6)
	Linolenic	Potassium	Tin, Tungsten	Vitamin D

one had a hemp plant growing in their backyard, Earth's ozone layer would soon be healed. Being a "weed," it matures fast, thriving in any type of soil. It converts bad soil to good soil. Hemp as an annual rotation crop would eliminate the need for chemical fertilization. For more information: *The Great Book of Hemp*, By R. Robinson; *Hemp, Lifeline of the Future*, by C. Conrad.

● **Bee Pollen, filled with the lifeforce of the entire plant kingdom**
Pollen contains nearly all the elements /nutrients necessary for sustaining human life. Pollen has an estimated more than 5000 different enzymes and co-enzymes, which is more than any other food in existence. Pollen is the richest source of protein in Nature – containing 5-7 times more protein than meat, eggs or cheese, and its protein is predigested –hence easy to assimilate. Pollen contains the richest source of vitamins, minerals, trace minerals, proteins, amino acids, hormones, and fats –including the essential linoleic fatty acid, 15% lecithin, RNA/DNA, nucleic acids, and other goodies. Vitamins in Pollen include A, B, C, D, E, F and even B12. Minerals include potassium, magnesium, calcium, phosphorous, manganese, sulfur, choline, sodium, iron, copper, zinc, – all in organic, highly assimilable form. **The high life force in Pollen** is from the millions of living plant forces it contains. Each pollen granule contains *4 million pollen grains*. One teaspoon contains about *3-10 billion pollen grains*. Each of these grains is the male sperm cells of flowering plants. Each grain has the power to fertilize and create a fruit, a grain, vegetable, flower, or tree. No wonder Pollen is called "the procreative life force of the plant world." The Bible mentions pollen 68 times. Ancient cultures have praised Pollen as a source of rejuvenation, health and longevity. Pollen was believed to hold the secret to eternal youth. It is harvested by female worker bees when they brush up against anthers of flowers. The Pollen sticks to their legs. Upon returning to the hive, they pass through a screen that rubs off some of the Pollen   grains. Like fruit, Pollen does not require killing the plant.

● **Royal Jelly –bee pollen's queen-sista**
Royal Jelly is a thick, milk-like secretion from the head glands of the queen bee's nurse-workers. Royal Jelly is the *only* food eaten by the queen bee, and her lifespan is 35 times longer than that of worker bees. Has every nutrient needed to support life. Loaded with vitamins A, B (complex), C, D, and E. Contains potassium, calcium, iron, silicon, magnesium, manganese, zinc and other minerals. Contains enzyme precursors, sex hormones, and 8 essential amino acids. Is the only natural source of pure *acetylcholine*, a critical neuro-transmitter in the brain (deficient in people with Alzheimer's disease). Stimulates the immune system. Effective for gland and hormone imbalances that reflect in menstruation and prostate problems. Is a natural antibiotic, supplies nutrients for energy and mental alertness. Promotes cell health and longevity (naturally!). Combats stress, fatigue, insomnia. As little as one drop can deliver adequate daily supply. (*Sweet Caution*: It's probably best to avoid Royal Jelly sold mixed with honey –a food which can cause sugar problems.)

● **Wolfberries (Goji berries), richly nutritionally endowed**

People who consumed this fruit in Mongolia typically lived to be over 100 and free of diseases. Wolfberries contain *500* **times more vitamin C** by weight than oranges; **18 amino acids**, **13% protein** by weight –nearly as much protein as bee pollen; **21 trace minerals** including **zinc, potassium, magnesium,** more **beta carotene** than carrots, and **vitamins B1, B2, B6, E.** Its protein displays an insulin-like action. The Chinese use it to replenish vital essences, lower blood pressure and cholesterol, strengthen muscles and bones, protect liver function, treat diabetes, impotence, and much more. **Goji berries regenerate the cells, reverse aging, and stimulates production of HGH** (human growth hormone). One Chinese study found that, when eaten daily, it increases S.O.D. by 48% while decreasing lipid peroxide (a bad thing) by 65%. *(SOD is superoxide dismutase –an antioxidant enzyme which keeps the body young.)* Another study found that it causes the blood of old people to revert to a younger state. Dried raisin-like Goji berries may be found in the "China town" sections of many cities. They are delicious eaten plain or made as tea and eaten afterwards.

● **Organic MSM**

MSM falls on us every time it rains! *Methyl Sulfonyl Methane* is a natural, water-soluble, nutritional form of organic sulfur, one of the five basic elements of life and a major component of your body. MSM is found in rain, dew, all natural foods and all living things; it is especially abundant in trees. Being fragile, it is usually lost in food processing, cooking and storage. It makes our cells permeable and vastly enhances the body's ability to assimilate nutrients and expel wastes. It speeds healing and quickly improves our health in every way. It cleans the blood. It is a free-radical and foreign-protein scavenger. When taking MSM, effects from allergies are quickly reduced or eliminated. MSM works best when taken with vitamin C.

You cannot overdose on MSM. Your body uses what it needs and flushes out the rest within 12 hours. To build and maintain good healthy cells 24 hours a day, take MSM in the morning and evening. The "planetary sulfur cycle" is major way MSM reaches lifeforms. This cycle involves microscopic plants / plankton living in the ocean. These plants "eat" inorganic sulfur in ocean water and then release sulfur as part of their natural life-process. This sulfur escapes from the ocean into the atmosphere and rises to the upper altitudes where it meets ozone and ultraviolet light. These convert the sulfur (dimethylsufide) into MSM and DMSO. MSM is a stable metabolite of DMSO, possessing similar properties; in fact, MSM is chemically DMSO2 (DMSO with an additional oxygen atom). Thus, planetary sulfur recycles from the ocean to the sky and falls in the rain and dew, only to return to the ocean to restart the cycle. Incredible!

● **Apple cider vinegar, a source of assimilable minerals**
Unpasteurized, unfiltered and organic. Two teaspoons in a glass of water. High
in potassium. Also contains organic phosphorus, chlorine, sodium, magnesium,
sulphur, iron, copper, silicon and malic acid. A great regenerating tonic as well.

● **Kelp, Dulse, and Celtic salt**
(or purified seawater) provides assimilable *trace* minerals
Seaweed is a valuable wholefood supplement, rich in assimilable trace minerals
from the ocean. Its roots may reach 30,000 feet below the ocean surface, with its
tentacles floating to the surface where they form nodules and leaves. The leaves
are known as Sea-Lettuce and Dulse. Once dried and ground into granules, it's
known as Kelp. Using Kelp and Dulse in moderation as food supplements
furnishes our system with some of the trace elements so necessary for our well-
being, which are not available in vegetables and fruits. Have a salt shaker filled
with Kelp granules, and a dish of Dulse which you may use freely with your
salads and juices. Replace the use of table salt with Celtic salt. Celtic salt (or
purified seawater) also provides assimilable trace minerals, plus micro-nutrients
necessary for optimum health. Since Celtic Salt has never been heated or dried
out, its minerals are in *ionic*, bio-available form. Celtic salt's 70-plus trace
elements have definite triggering actions on the body's various functions,
feeding the organs with a specific amount –measurable in parts *per million*– of
elements that help to eliminate or prevent disease. (see chart on page 93)

● **What about *herbal* supplements?**
Herbs are generally high in vitamins, minerals, nutrients, and healing
compounds. Thus, herbs are great tools in times of health emergencies (as are
many drugs). Herbs have been used for eons for their healing and other
properties. Most herbal supplements are whole, dehydrated plants sold as tea, in
loose form, or powdered and encapsulated. When herbs /plants are dehydrated,
as done in modern processing, 98% of the oils are evaporated out of the
plant. This oil is the agent /catalyst that delivers the herb's nutrients to
the cells. Effects: 10% absorption at best, of the herb. When the oils
are put back in (as done with companies like *Young Living
Essential Oils,* and *Perankh*) the absorption rate goes up to 89%.
Since herbs are dehydrated, they are more concentrated,
however (as far as your body is concerned) herbs are more
acceptable as supplements, both in bulk and capsules, but not as
extracts, concentrates, or concoctions. As with true natural
whole nutrients, WHOLE-herbs (not fractionated or extracted),
are metabolized differently from artificially produced drugs, even
if the drugs are made from "natural ingredients."

Herbs are sometimes referred to as "natural drugs." Indeed many outright
drugs are essentially the extracted (fractionated) "active ingredient" of herbs. I
do not call herbs drugs though many herbs are undeniably drug-like in their
effects. Drugs have been artificially mucked with to become that way; herbs are
the way they are from Nature, not through artificial means.

Homeostasis. The drug-like property of most herbs is evident with the phenomena of *homeostasis*, clearly described by Robert Gray: *"Homeostasis is the tendency of the body to maintain an equilibrium condition wherein all bodily functions are stabilized at normal levels. The body will gradually neutralize the effect of almost any substance that is repeatedly put into it over a long enough period of time. Most herbs lose all effectiveness when taken over a period of eight to nine months. ...When an herb subject to homeostasis (and almost all are) is taken regularly, sensitivity to it decreases linearly until all of the herb's effectiveness has been lost. Once full homeostatic resistance has been reached, it takes five to seven years of abstinence from the substance in question before maximum sensitivity is regained. In order to prevent homeostatic resistance from reaching the point where an herb is no longer useful, one should not take the herb more than one third of the time."[1]*

Herbal Notes: Herbs lose strength with age and should be discarded after 12-15 months, depending on the herb. **To prepare an herb as tea**, place the herb in a ceramic or glass container, pour on boiling water and allow to steep. To better draw out the herb's medicinal properties, **use *distilled water* for making herbal teas.** Generally, teas are made with a ratio of 1 teaspoon herb to 1 cup boiling water. **Do not boil the herb** (unless recipe instructs otherwise), as that can destroy the herb's beneficial characteristics. Boiled herbs are more or less a drugfood depending on length of boiling (cooking) time. Since many teas contain toxic alkaloids, they should be used in moderation (see next chapter).

The Human Body can make protein, minerals, vitamins and other nutrients from sunlight & air

Contrary to popular belief, the human body can make minerals and vitamins not supplied in the diet, and even make protein from the nitrogen in the air. The human body can especially do all these things and more when the body is pure and healthy and the owner is living in harmony with Mother Nature. In his book, *The Secret Life*, Dr. George Lakhovsky, discusses an experiment where he relates cosmic radiation to nutrition. His thesis is that *"body growth and maintenance depends not on food, but on cosmic rays; the body itself being a condensation of these rays"* which are said to be *"streams of substance of ultrasonic form which condense into minerals"* as they contact the Earth's atmosphere. He deducted this by measuring the amount of iron in unicellular organisms kept in sealed tubes. After a period of time he found that, as the cells multiplied, the iron content of the organism increased.[2] As verified by L. Kervan in his book, *Biological Transmutations*, colored women on a natural, wholefood diet can make vitamin C in their bodies.[3] Kervan's experiments showed that matter is being created from solar radiation through the condensing effect of cell geometry. Example: *"the nitrogen diet is lowered below the level*

1) Gray, *The Colon Health Handbook*, 70. 2) Kulvinskas, STC, 120. 3) Afrika, AHH, 58.

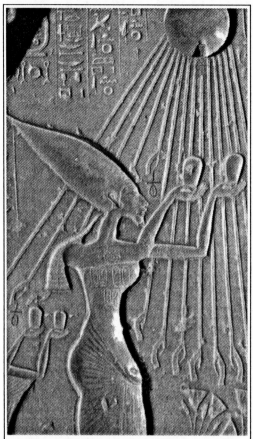

As in this relief of the Sun blessing Akhenaten, Nile Valley Afrikans often showed "hands" of the Sunrays holding "ankhs," –symbol of Life & Joining

of normal excretion by the intestine. The excreted quantity remains higher than the total ingested quantity. Since nutrition could not supply nitrogen, endogenic production must be responsible." [1]

Dr. Norman Walker wrote: "...the air we breathe is taken into our lungs as a combination of approximately 20% Oxygen and 80% Nitrogen. The air we expel from our lungs, is mainly carbonic acid and carbon dioxide. What happens to the Nitrogen? ...This is what happens when we breathe. Two main classes of enzymes in our lungs come into action the moment air reaches the tiny bunch-of-grapes-like interior of our lungs, known as alveoli. One set of enzymes, known as Oxidase, separates the Oxygen while the other set of enzymes, known as Nitrase, separate the Nitrogen from the air. The Oxygen is collected, by enzyme action, by the blood and circulates it through the body, while the Nitrogen, by the action of 'transportation' enzymes, passes into the body for protein generation." [2]

Stanley Burroughs, author of "The Master Cleanser" wrote:
"Many elements needed by the body are absorbed from the air through the lungs. It is recognized that oxygen and hydrogen are taken from the air, but few realize that nitrogen is also taken from the air and used as a protein builder. Breathing fresh air and eating of fresh fruits and vegetables eliminates completely any possible need for any of the animal forms of food." [3]

People who smoke can't pick up the nitrogen from the air so easily, but can still get enough from proper food without the use of animal flesh. Dr. Mikhail Valsky's experiments showed that even animals can assimilate nitrogen from the air to make protein in their bodies in his experiments with egg-embryos in incubators containing nitrogen-tagged atoms. [4]

1) Kulvinskas, STC, 120.   2) Walker, FV, 13.   3) Burroughs, 113.   4) Kulvinskas, STC, 120.

Why are fractionated vitamins /nutrients harmful?

- **The human body was not designed to handle fractionated nutrients.** Supplementing our diet with any isolated, fractionated vitamin /mineral /nutrient does not work. Instead, it imbalances us and creates a deficiency of other vitamins and nutrients. Examples: *Taking one or more of the B-vitamins increases the need of the other B vitamins not supplied. Though zinc deficiency is common, excess zinc disrupts copper metabolism, which disrupts iron metabolism, which disrupts... and so on.* Vitamins, minerals and other nutrients work only in conjunction with other vitamins, minerals, etc., as found in raw, wholefood (fruit, plants, herbs) from Nature.
- **People become addicted** to fractionated nutrients, for such are drugs.
- **They are** *Drugs* as far as your body is concerned. **Hence, they are** *Stimulants,* substances speeding body metabolism They stimulate the body with a drug-like effect similar to caffeine. The *Stimulation* we feel when we consume nutritional supplements is at the *expense* of our vital *Energy.* As with taking drugs, **depletion of energy is the secondary effect of taking fractionated nutrients /supplements. They may make you feel better in the short run, but they do this by over-stimulating your system.** Over a long period, most supplements cause you to fall into degenerative disease faster.
- **Most supplements do not have** *electrical integrity,* a quality usually destroyed in processing. This is especially true with hard tablets (14 tons of pressure may be used). As a result, they do not work properly, hence are useless, hence are toxins the body tries to eliminate.
- **Synthetic, lab-made vitamins** /supplements are harmful chemicals, not food. Their polarity and light refraction is the opposite of natural vitamin complexes. They also contain preservatives/sugar/additives.
- **Synthetic, commercial grade vitamin /mineral** concentrates are synthesized from the same horrible starting material of commercial drugs: coal tar, petroleum products, animal feces, animal by-products, animal bones, hooves, ground rocks, shells and metal.
- **Nearly all nutritional supplements are polluted.** Solvents, heavy metals and lanthanides are found in 90% or more of the popular vitamin and mineral capsules. Herbal supplements often contain pesticides and sometimes alcohol. Dicalcium phosphate, a common binder used in tablets, can cause artery-hardening, arthritis, and other health problems. Polluted supplements do much more harm than good.

Continued >>

Continued: **Why are fractionated nutrients harmful?**

- **Mega-vitamin/mineral therapy** (taking massive quantities of isolated nutrients) imparts little benefit as it depletes one's cash while enriching one's urine. Because once the body receives what it needs, any additional must be excreted by the body's eliminative organs. Megadoses can also result in disease symptoms.
- **Chelated nutrients:** "Chelation" is an attempt to FORCE the human body to accept the unacceptable (toxic, *fractionated* material).
- **Most synthetic vitamins (including yeast) are acid-forming**, especially vitamin C, which is even called "ascorbic *acid*" (synthetic vitamin C). When taken too much, they can cause acidosis. Vitamins from natural food do not usually cause acidosis. According to NIH researchers, "Taking 1000 or more milligrams can cause nausea and kidney stones and will not prevent colds."
- **All the minerals used in nutrient manufacture are basically DIRT** (pulverized mined ore). And they are *inorganic,* therefore are 99% inassimilable. Hence, they contribute to the toxic materials our body attempts to expel (otherwise deposit them in our tissues /create kidneys stones /harden our arteries, etc.).
- **Calcium** supplements don't work at all.[1] Some calcium supplements are made from oyster shells. Bone meal (used as a calcium source) is contaminated with lead and antibiotics.
- **Iodine** supplements in inorganic form (iodized table salt or tablets) is responsible for many vague "borderline" glandular symptoms without actual pathology.[2]
- Long-term use of **iron** tablets can result in decreased absorption of copper, zinc, and selenium. Since **iron** never leaves our bodies except through bleeding, excess iron in the brain can cause Alzheimer's disease; excess iron in the cardiovascular system can cause artherosclerosis and heart attacks.[3] (Low iron levels in the body are seldom due to iron shortage; it is mainly due to a lack of the nutrients required to mobilize iron stores in the liver, etc.)
- **Protein powders**, especially when eaten in high amounts, suck calcium out your body like a sponge. High-protein meal replacement drinks can seriously deplete your calcium stores if used as the main source of protein in your diet.
- **"Textured vegetable protein"** is a totally unnatural form of protein with adherent amino acid chains which are incompatible with the amino needs of the cells.
- Because it's high in phytates, **plant protein**, especially from soy, causes zinc deficiency if eaten in large amounts. Vegetarians who eat primarily soy as a protein source often develop zinc deficiency.
- **Bran** is indigestible and high in phytate which impairs calcium and magnesium absorption.

1) Colgan, NN, 62.   2) de Langre, 45.   3) Healthiatry Course V, 23.

Recommendations for Better Health

Avoid /Reduce Eating:	Healthier Replacements:
• fractionated nutrients • isolated nutrients • isolated vitamins (vitamin "complexes" are better) • vitamin supplements • so-called "natural vitamins" • ascorbic acid (vitamin C) • mineral supplements • vast majority of nutritional supplements • synthetic lab-made nutrients (in drugstores, supermarkets) • "textured vegetable protein" • chelated nutrients • protein powders • protein bars • "energy" bars • "breakfast" bars • most lecithin products including granules and liquid form (they are made with artificial lecithin and contain soy flour, milk solids, etc.) • "enriched" breads, cereals, foods	**Best:** • **fresh JUICE of living fruit & vegetables** (best form of high-level, assimilable, true-natural vitamins, organic minerals, enzymes, nutrients, plus the lifeforce of the plant; see chart on next pages) **Very Good to Excellent:** • **spirulina, bluegreen algae** (has nearly all nutrients needed by humans including vit. B12) • *wholefood nonfractionated* **supplements** such as spirulina, barley-green or alfalfa powder • **hemp seed** (has nearly all nutrients needed by humans) • **wolfberries** (loaded with vit. C, 18 amino acids, 21 minerals, beta-carotene, B-vitamins, E...) • **bee pollen** (highest source of nearly all nutrients required by humans; has 5-7 times more protein than meat. Rich in vitamins A, B, B12, C, D, E, minerals, fats, linoleic acid, lecithin, RNA/DNA...) • **royal jelly** (has every nutrient needed to support life) • **organic MSM** • **steeped herbal teas** • **pure whole herbs** /herb supplements (use moderately, preferably with supervision. be careful here too, for they are drug-like) • **dehydrated vegetable juice capsules** • **digestive enzymes** (especially w/ fleshfood meals) • **raw apple cider vinegar** (2 T. in water) • **"true lecithin"** (as found in 15% of pollen or lecithin by *Lewis Labs* which has 95% phosphatides) **Improvement:** • *buffered* **vitamin C** (not as *ascorbic* acid but in *ascorbate form*, like calcium or sodium ascorbate, which is alkalinizing instead of acidifying) • *electrically whole* nutrients • **colloidal** liquid form of minerals • **homeopathic** cell salts (all 12)

Tips

– If using an herb regularly, use for no more than a few months, then stop for a few months, then use again –in order to prevent **homeostatic neutralization** (see p173)

– If you take supplements, it's better to do it in moderation, perhaps every other day(s) rather than daily. Unless otherwise specified, best to take supplements with meals, not on an empty stomach.

– A way to accurately know what to take and how much /often is through **kinesiology** (discussed in *Don't Worry, Be Healthy!* –vol 3 of this book)

Top Sources of Organic Minerals in Raw Plantfood

Only raw *wholefoods* are listed here. (Problematic veggies, omitted). They may all be eaten RAW, or juiced (ideally), or made as herbal tea –or in some cases, sprinkled on/in *drugfood*. **Best to take your "supplements" as fresh vegetable /fruit JUICES.** The best way to get high-level nutrients from fresh organic vegetables is to run them through a juicer. Experiment with different combinations like spinach /parsley /cucumber, or carrot /celery /beet. Recommended: Norman Walker's juice-therapy book: *Fresh Vegetable and Fruit Juices.* Nutrient-tables in healthbooks do not take into account that cooking destroys 70%-100% of the nutrients they list (vitamins & enzymes), plus, cooking turns organic minerals inorganic.

Mineral	Fruit		Nuts & Seeds	Raw & Juiced Vegetables	Herbs	Wholefood Supplements
Organic **Potassium**	Watermelon Papaya Bananas Plantains Nectarines Peaches Lemons Oranges	Grape,Date Persimmon Cantaloupe Berries, Fig Pear, Plum Cherimoyas Avocado Cherries	Hemp seed Filberts Cashews Coconut Sunflower Walnuts Almonds Pecans	Dark leafy greens Kale Watercress Corn Beets Leaf lettuce Romaine lettuce Cucumbers	Alfalfa Parsley Peppermint Dandelion Eyebright Fennel Yellow Dock Aloe Vera	Spirulina Bluegreen Algae Apple cider vinegar Wolfberries Pollen, Royal Jelly Celtic Salt Seaweed, Kelp
Organic **Calcium**	All fruits Cranberries Avocado Cherimoyas Apples Citrus	Watermelon Cherries Peaches Prunes Dates, Figs Grapes	Sesame Filberts Coconut Carob Walnuts Flaxseed	Dark leafy greens Broccoli, Carrots Leaf/Rm. Lettuce Parsley, Sprouts Watercress	Alfalfa Irish Moss Chamomile Bittersweet Oat straw Aloe Vera	Spirulina Bluegreen Algae Pollen, Royal Jelly Celtic Salt Seaweed Kelp, Dulse
Organic **Magnesium**	Apples Avocados Dates Papaya Peaches Cucumbers	Oranges Cherimoyas Bananas Lemons Figs	Brazil nuts Sesame Hemp seed Almonds Walnuts Flaxseed	Dark leafy greens Spinach Leaf Lettuce Romaine lettuce Celery, Carrots Corn	Alfalfa Parsley Dandelion Watercress Aloe Vera Nettle	Spirulina Bluegreen Algae Wolfberries Pollen, Royal Jelly Apple cider vinegar Celtic salt, Kelp
Organic **Phosphorus**	Elderberries Avocados Prunes, Dates Papaya Cherries	Lemons Raspberries Figs, Grapes Apricots Peaches	Sesame Hemp, Carob Sunflower Pumpkin Almonds	Spinach, Peas Leaf/Rm. Lettuce Cucumbers Cabbage, Corn Broccoli	Alfalfa Rosehips Rosemary Licorice Caraway	Spirulina, Pollen Bluegreen Algae Apple cider vinegar Seaweed Kelp, Dulse
Organic **Iron**	Avocado Black currant Blackberries Watermelon	Plum, Prune Cherries Apricot, Fig Strawberry	Hemp seed Sesame Sunflower Walnut,Seeds	Dark leafy greens Spinach Leaf lettuce Sprouts	Alfalfa Yerbamate Watercress Burdock	Spirulina, BG Algae Pollen, Royal Jelly Apple cider vinegar Celtic Salt
Organic **Sodium**	Strawberries Pomegranate Figs	Lemons Peaches Cherries	Hemp seed	Celery, Beets Spinach, Kale Romaine lettuce Cucumbers	Alfalfa Dandelion Irish Moss Aloe Vera	Celtic Salt, Kelp Spirulina, Pollen Bluegreen Algae Apple cider vinegar
Organic **Zinc**	Apples		Hemp, Pecan Sunflower Pumpkin	Dark leafy greens Sprouts, Beets Broccoli	Dandelion Chickweed Rosehips Marshmallow	Spirulina, BG Algae Wolfberries, Pollen Kelp, Celtic Salt
Organic **Sulphur**	Avocado Pumpkin Red currant	Raspberries Cranberries Cherimoya	Hemp seed Coconut Nuts	Celery, Cabbage Spinach, Kale Broccoli, Peas Cauliflower, Corn	Alfalfa Horsetail Irish Moss Eyebright	Aloe Vera (has MSM) Organic MSM (is 30% sulfur) Fresh Rain or Dew (has much MSM) Pollen, Celtic Salt
Organic **Chromium**	Apple peels		Hemp seed	Broccoli, Corn Sprouted Grains Raw Sugar Cane	Alfalfa	Royal Jelly, Kelp Spirulina,Celtic Salt
Organic **Manganese**	Avocado Cucumber Squash Pineapple	Apricots Oranges Blueberries Cherries	Nuts, Seeds Filberts Pecans Walnuts	Dark leafy greens Carrots, Beet, Peas Dandelion	Ginger, Parsley Wintergreen Primrose Yellow Dock	Bee Pollen Royal Jelly Kelp, Seaweed Celtic Salt

Top Sources of Vitamins /Nutrients in Raw Plantfood

Nutrient	Fruit		Nuts & Seeds	Raw & Juiced Vegetables	Herbs	Wholefood Supplements
Vitamin A Or Carotene	Apricots Yellow squash Persimmons Muskmelon Cantaloupe	Papaya Melons Prunes Peaches Avocado	Hemp, Pecan Cashews Black walnuts Pistachio Pumpkin	Dark leafy greens Carrots, Corn Kale, Spinach Parsley, Sprouts Leaf Lettuce	Wheatgrass Alfalfa, Suma Rosehips Lemon grass Dandelion	Spirulina Bluegreen Algae Wolfberries Pollen, oyal Jelly Kelp, ulse
B Complex B12 content shown by "(B12)"	Prunes, Figs Avocados Cherimoyas Bananas (B12) Concord Grapes (B12)	Cherries Cantaloupe Oranges Rosehips	Hemp seed Sunfl'wr (B12) Walnuts Pecans Carob Coconut	Dark leafy greens Carrots Kale, Spinach Leaf Lettuce Peas, Corn Cabbage	Wheatgrass (B12 Alfalfa (B12) Dandelion (B12) Suma Aloe Vera Comfrey (B12)	Spirulina (B12 high) Bluegreen Algae (B12) Wolfberries Bee Pollen (B12) Kelp, Dulse (B12) Ginseng (B12) Royal Jelly
Vitamin C	All fruits Acerolas Papaya Oranges Strawberry Black currants	Guavas Star fruit Citrus fruit Persimmons Pineapple	Hemp seed Brazil nuts Fresh coconut	Sprouts, Broccoli Corn, Watercress Leaf Lettuce Kale, Spinach Cauliflower	Rosehips Wheatgrass Alfalfa, Suma Yerbamate Hibiscus	Wolfberries Bee Pollen oyal Jelly Bluegreen Algae Kelp
Vitamin E	Avocados Mangoes Apples	Cucumbers Bananas	Hemp seed Flaxseed Nuts, Seeds	Dark leafy greens Parsley, Celery Sprouted seeds	Wheatgrass Alfalfa, Suma Watercress	Spirulina, BG Algae Wolfberries Pollen, oyal Jelly
F **Fatty Acids**	Avocados Apricots Cherries Rosehips Berries	Apple peels /pits Orange peels Prunes Watermelon Grapes	Hemp, Flax Sesame Pine nuts Sunflower Pecans	Corn Dark leafy greens	Alfalfa Dandelion Uva Ursi Suma Huckleberries	Bee Pollen Spirulina
Protein Amino Acids	Avocado, Fig Elderberries Watermelon Cherimoyas	Bananas Apricots Cherries Squash	Hemp seed All Nuts All Seeds	Dark leafy greens Spinach Kale Parsley	Alfalfa Aloe Vera Irish Moss	Spirulina Bluegreen Algae Wolfberries Pollen, Royal Jelly
Vitamin D a hormone	Vitamin D isn't a vitamin but a hormone. 1/2 hour of **Sunshine** per day may fulfill one's vitamin D needs. Sunlight touching the skin provokes synthesis of D. Body makes D from cholesterol abundant in skin's oil glands. Sources: **Pollen, Royal Jelly, Spinach, Apricots, Alfalfa, Lemon juice/grass, Wheatgrass juice, sprouted seeds.**				
Vitamin O **Oxygen**	Our most important nutrient. 80% of oxygen intake goes to the Brain. All <u>raw</u> plantfood & Fruit is rich in **Oxygen**. Cooking drives out the oxygen. _Sunlit_ **AIR** is additionally loaded with "**Prana**," a vital life-energy from the Sun. Wholeplant **Hyssop-extract**, organic **MSM, Hemp herb-seed-oil** (especially) intensely oxygenate the blood.				
Enzymes	Enzymes are vital to life. Without enzymes, no life! Cooking destroys enzymes 100%. • All **RAW food, especially Sprouts,** are rich with many types of Enzymes. • Dried barley juice ("**Green Magma**") has 1000s of enzymes plus **SOD** (Superoxide Dismutase). • Raw **Pineapple** is loaded with **Bromelain**; raw **Papaya** (especially unripe/green) is loaded with **Papain**, both protein-digesting enzymes with many other benefits. • **Wheatgrass juice** and **Aloe Vera,** both super-healers, are super rich in enzymes. • **Bee Pollen** has some 5000 different enzymes. **Royal Jelly** is also enzyme-rich.				
LifeForce **"Light"** Color	**All living plantfoods** have the LifeForce of the plant, seed. Some super-healing herbs, like **Hyssop** and **Wheatgrass** seem to link the body to great amounts of light & vitality, measurable with Kirlian photography, and usually felt as increased strength. • Right after taking properly made, wholeplant **Hyssop-extract** (as made by _Hyssop Enterprises_; see _Southall_ in Bibliography), your aura (bio-electric field) blazes with intense light, raising your vibrations. Dis-ease is usually gone in 12 days with daily use (2-4oz./day). • The trace-minerals **Rhodium & Iridium** are super-conductors of spiritual light; they enhance our LifeForce & vitality. Foods containing both are **Hyssop, Concord Grape Juice, Essiac Tea, Aloe Vera, Watercress, fresh Carrot Juice,** and **St. John's Wort.** • **Bluegreen Algae** is one of the most concentrated sources of "stored light." • **Bee Pollen** contains the most concentrated essence of LifeForce. • **Color** (light) is nutrition; Color is the active principle of all vitamins. For instructions on color therapy, read _Healing for the Age of Enlightenment,_ by Stanley Burroughs.				

DRUG

15

Vitality-Sapping Cooked Food

Sadly, less than 5% of America's daily calorie intake is from fresh, raw foods.

Why is all cooked food harmful?

—OVERVIEW —

1) All cooked foods are drugs!
   And cooked food is the foundation of all drug addiction.
2) All cooked food is poison.
   Cooking itself creates additional toxins in the food.
3) Whenever you eat cooked foods, your
   white blood cell count GOES UP immediately.
4) Cooking destroys almost all the food's nutrients.
5) In cooked food, 100% of the enzymes are destroyed,
   thus cooked food robs your body of precious enzymes.
6) Cooking turns the food's *organic*
   minerals into <u>*inorganic*</u> minerals (as in concrete).
7) In cooked food, animal proteins coagulate,
   becoming almost digestion-proof.
8) Cooked starches & sugars ferment quickly,
   turning your body into an alcohol factory.
9) Cooked food turns your body into a smorgasbord
   and free-hotel for germs, fungus, flukes, and parasites.
10) Cooked food MAL-nourishes you while making you fat.
11) Cooked food is the foundation of dis-ease and ill-being.
12) Cooked food COOKS YOU!
13) Cooked food is dead food; dead food saps your
    Vitality (Lifeforce) and dims your *Light.*

**Now let's look at
the *Overview*
in steaming
DETAIL...**

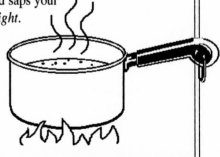

—DETAIL—

1) All cooked foods are drugs! And cooked food is the foundation of all drug addiction.

Cooking automatically turns all food into drugs. Drugfood. The mo it's cooked, the mo it's a drug. Note that high temperatures are used in manufacturing drugs and processed food. Any wonder that most addicting substances are *cooked*: tobacco, coffee, alcohol, sugar, cocaine. Since all cooked foods are drugs, then **all cooked foods are addictive.** The desire and craving for cooked food is a symptom of addiction. **In fact, cooked food is the foundation of all drug addiction.** Thus, all drug-addicts are cooked-foodarians. They all live on (die on) cooked food. And all people that eat any cooked food are cooked-food addicts. Drugfood addicts. This includes health-conscious people that eat tofu, sprouts and buy organic food from the healthfood store, food which they *cook* and eat (get a fix). It follows then, that the most effective way of destroying a drug habit is to eat RAW food and avoid eating cooked food.

"A herb in its natural state is raw and fresh. Once the herb is cooked (as in tea) it becomes a drug. Heat causes the nutritional tribe to segregate and concentrate. This isolation of the internal nutritional tribes creates a drug reaction in the plant. Consequently, the plant becomes a drug. All heated herbs are drugs. Technically, all cooked or fired (heated by fire) foods are drugs. In this respect, most of the addicting substances are cooked, such as tobacco, cocaine...coffee, sugar, heroin, cola drinks... pastries... alcohol."

Dr. Llaila Afrika: *Afrikan Holistic Health*, p99-100

"...we discovered that all refined (dead) food acts as a drug on the system. When a particular food is consumed it acts as a stimulant to the nervous system....The process of bodily purification releases the body from the above cravings and enables it to be [out] of this harmful cycle."

Drs. Gael & Patrick Flanagan: *Elixir of Life*, p58

2) All cooked food is slow poison.
Cooking itself creates additional toxins in the food.

Whenever raw food is cooked, it is corrupted at the molecular level and no longer qualifies as health-giving food. The higher the heat or longer it's cooked, the more toxic the food becomes. Worse yet, if the food is cooked over direct flameheat or charcoal fire, benzopyrene (a powerful carcinogen) is produced; a pound of charcoal-broiled steak (or any charcoal-broiled food?) is estimated to have as much benzopyrene as in the smoke of 300 cigarettes. When foods are cooked, the preservatives, dyes, and the thousands of other chemicals added to commercial drugfood become even worse. Pesticides and fungicides break down to form even more toxic compounds, and so on. The results are scrumptious delicious toxins. Which slowly compromising our health, slowly killing us little by little, meal by meal, bite by bite. Gradually accelerating, then rapidly accelerating and sometimes suddenly shifting (or catapulting) us into another dimension, permanently. With the cooking of any food, <u>free radical</u> production greatly increases. Cooked oils and fats break down into toxins which proliferate free radicals. Free radicals are highly reactive, incomplete, electrically unbalanced molecules. They rebalance themselves by robbing molecules and electrons from other molecules. This unbalances the next molecule in a chain reaction fashion. Free radicals can destroy enzymes, lipids, and proteins and cause cells to die. They cause cross-linkage among tissue proteins. They disrupt the function of the cell membranes, DNA/RNA structure, protein synthesis, and cell metabolism. *(Some foods are actually <u>less</u> toxic only when cooked [or sprouted], therefore must be cooked before eating to reduce their toxicity. These foods include cassava and most beans. They taste disagreeable raw anyway –a hint that we should not eat them in the first place. In general, if a food has to be cooked in order to make it edible, that food is not meant for humans to eat.)*

Worse and more harmful than cooking is *microwaving* **food. This is cooking the cooking!** Microwaves vibrate the food molecules up to 2.5 billion times per second. Thus, microwaved food is freak-mucked molecularly; the actual structure of the molecules are changed, deranged. Microwaved food is much more harmful than conventionally cooked food. Microwaved food causes pathological changes in the blood and body cells. The body responds to microwaved food as if it were an infectious agent. (see page 61)

Carcinogens (cancer-causing agents) is produced by cooking

Regarding this subject, Dr. William Havender wrote: "The burned and browned matter produced when meats are char broiled, smoked or fried is highly mutagenic. Some of this matter comes from the smoke of burned material deposited on the meat by the cooking process, but much of it originates from the breakdown of the meat protein itself. This charred material has been analyzed, and several of its chemicals have been identified as both mutagenic and carcinogenic. One important class of such chemicals are the heterocyclic amines, formed when certain amino acids (the building blocks of proteins) in foods are heated.... These compounds have been shown in some bacterial tests to be highly mutagenic [gene damaging], rivaling or exceeding some of the most potent mutagens known, such as aflatoxin B1... All are carcinogenic in animal tests. Heterocyclic amines can be found in such burnt foods as broiled beef and fish, toast, bread crusts, coffee, fried potatoes and a variety of other foods, and the amounts of them in the foods appear to be related to cooking temperatures. More heterocyclic amines are formed when meat is broiled than when it is cooked at lower temperatures... Another class of compounds formed in cooked foods are the polycyclic aromatic hydrocarbons, of which benzo(a)pyrene is a notable representative. Not only is this substance carcinogenic in its own right, but under laboratory conditions it can 'promote' (i.e., enhance) the carcinogenic action of other chemicals."[1]

3) Whenever you eat cooked foods, your white blood cell count GOES UP immediately.

This abnormality was called "digestive leukocytosis" and doctors thought it was normal, since it seemed to happen to everyone. Then in 1930, Dr. Paul Kouchakoff discovered that eating raw food did not produce leukocytosis –*only* cooked foods produced it![2] White blood cells are the defense organisms that prevent infection and intoxication of the blood. Any pathological condition, including the intoxication of the digestive system with cooked foods or other toxic materials, causes these white cells to increase. Interestingly, when raw food is eaten with cooked food of the same type, in a 50/50 ration, leukocytosis does not happen.[3]

4) Cooking destroys almost all of the food's nutrients.

70-90% of the vitamins are destroyed. 100% of the enzymes are destroyed (at 130°F). The nutritive value of fats and oils are mostly destroyed. The protein coagulates. The starches and sugars readily spoil and ferment quickly in the body. The *organic* bio-assimilable minerals become *inorganic* and inassimilable. The RNA and DNA structure is disrupted.[4] The oxygen ("Vitamin O"), is lost. And the *Lifeforce* (another vital but unrecognized or unacknowledged nutrient) is dissipated, driven out.

---

1) Havender, DNKB report. 2) Cousens, SN, 101; Kulvinskas, STC, 45.
3) Cousens, SN, 101. 4) Cousens, CE, 364.

5) In cooked food, 100% of the enzymes are destroyed, thus cooked food robs your body of precious enzymes.

...and this results in early aging and health disorders. All our life processes depend on enzyme function. When enzymes are depleted, so is our vital lifeforce and health. Dr. Edward Howell, pioneer in the enzyme field stated: "When we eat cooked, enzyme-free food, the body is forced to produce enzymes needed for digestion. This depletes the body's limited enzyme capacity. This 'stealing' of enzymes from other parts of the body sets up a competition for enzymes among the various organ system and tissues of the body. The resulting metabolic dislocations may be the direct cause of cancer, coronary heart disease, diabetes, and many other chronic incurable diseases."

The human body and digestive system were not designed to consume cooked food. Enzymes are vital catalysts essential for the proper functioning of your body and assimilation of food. Enzymes occurring in raw food assist digestion so that your body's enzymes do not have to do all the work of digestion. When enzymes are missing from your food, the full burden of digestion falls on your digestive system. Over time, this depletes your body's enzyme reserve and causes early degeneration and aging. While health experts agree that a 100% raw food diet is ideal, they recognize that such a diet is difficult for most people to follow (because they are all drugfood addicts!). They generally recommend that a ratio of 80% raw to 20% cooked as adequate for supporting general health, with a little less raw foods in a colder climate.

Really, enzymes are a *vibration*, a "Cosmic Energy Principle"

In his book, *Fresh Vegetable and Fruit Juices*, Dr. Norman Walker enlightens us about the true, non-physical nature of enzymes:

"...enzymes are not 'substances.' Enzymes are an intangible magnetic Cosmic Energy of Life **Principle** (not a substance) which is intimately involved in the action and activity of every atom in the human body, in vegetation, and in every form of life. ...Once we get this clearly into our consciousness, we will know definitely why our food should be intelligently and properly selected, and why it should be raw, uncooked and unprocessed. ...We cannot have life and death at the same time, either in connection with our body, or with vegetables, fruits, nuts and seeds. Where there is life, there are enzymes. ...Life as LIFE cannot be explained, so we describe enzymes as a Cosmic Energy Principle or vibration which promotes a chemical action or change in atoms and molecules, causing a reaction, without changing, destroying or using up the enzymes themselves in the process. In other words, enzymes are catalysts and as such they **promote** action or change without altering or changing their own status."

Take <u>digestive enzymes</u> with your cooked food / flesh

Most people are enzyme-deficient, plus are not fully digesting food. Papayas (papain enzyme) and pineapples (bromelain enzyme) are especially enzyme-rich and helps digest protein. Always take digestive enzymes about 10 minutes before mealtime, then eat proteins first.

Drinking Willard Water boosts your enzymes

Among other marvels, it makes the body's enzymes work 10 times more effectively, thus producing a 10-fold increase in body's own natural healing power. It is also called "liquid crystal water" and "catalyst altered water." To make, add 1 ounce of "Willard Water Concentrate" to 1 gallon *distilled* water.

6) Cooking turns the food's *organic* minerals into *inorganic* minerals (as in concrete).

Cooking converts *organic* minerals in plants into *inorganic* minerals.[1] As such, they are not soluble in water. Since inorganic minerals are insoluble, they enter the bloodstream in inassimilable form and tend to deposit out in areas of slow blood velocity (highly congested tissues). Inorganic substances clog up our circulation if not eliminated. They combine with body fluids, oils, and waste materials to form plaques or stones which saturate our vascular system, or are abnormally deposited within our joints, muscles, lymphatic system, and various organs, especially the gallbladder and kidneys. The results include gall & kidney stones, arthritis, diabetes, heart problems, varicose veins, and hemorrhoids.

7) In cooked food, animal proteins coagulate, becoming almost digestion-proof.

When animal flesh /protein is cooked, the protein *coagulates* or changes from a hydro**phile** (water-loving) to a hydro**phobe** (water-hating) colloid. This is why a raw egg will mix in water but a cooked one will not. One half of assimilable protein is destroyed by cooking. Coagulated protein is 50% less assimilable (or 50% bio-available). You only need half the amount of protein if it's eaten raw. Hydrophile colloids absorb water, secretions and enzymes, thus they are easily broken down, hydrolyzed, and used by the body. But once cooked, they become hydrophobe colloids that will not absorb water, secretions, or enzymes, thus cannot be hydrolyzed and properly broken down by digestion. Hence it feeds the Escherichia Coli bacteria in your colon. This bacteria produces large amounts of toxic, harmful waste products as it literally rots the cooked protein.[2] This applies to pasteurized milk/cheese/yogurt and cooked eggs. Better to have raw milk/cheese, etc. This is very important for babies. Cooked milk formulas cause them much acid and foul smelling stool. Babies on raw milk (and raw fruit juices) don't have these problems.

1) Walker, FV, 47.   2) Preston, 110

8) Cooked starches & sugars ferment quickly, turning your body into an alcohol factory.

In your body, cooked starches and sugars ferment quickly in the presence of heat /moisture, producing alcohol, vinegar, carbonic acid gas and other poisons, especially when eaten with proteins. Alcohol is made from fermenting grains. People who eat a lot of starches (bread, cereal, pasta...) –hence nearly the entire American population– have made their bodies into a distillery constantly producing alcohol. As a result, most people are semi-alcoholics unknowingly! Hence "are always in an auto-intoxicated state, to which their bodies have become so completely adjusted, that when the toxic effects begin to fade, an uncomfortable feeling appears in the sensations of hunger, weakness, nervousness, headache, etc."[1]

9) Cooked food turns your body into a smorgasbord and free-hotel for germs, fungus, flukes, and parasites.

Cooked dead food is food and fertile soil for bacteria, which ferments and decomposes it. Germs (bacteria) are everywhere. They are attracted to and proliferate in dead matter, dead cooked food, and dis-eased tissues. Their job is to decompose dead matter. Example: when a plant dies, bacteria come in and eat the plant and it eventually becomes soil. Germs/bacteria does not eat a live, healthy plant. Same thing is true in people -- germs /bacteria are attracted to dead matter. Therefore, if you have dead matter in your body (whether dead cells or dead-cooked-food), bacteria will come in and get to work decomposing the dead matter so that it may eventually become soil.

The average American has about 2 pounds of bacteria in their intestinal tract, whereas healthy raw-foodarians have only a few ounces. Why? Those who live exclusively on a raw food diet have very little fermentation and very little –if any, putrefaction. To understand this take two apples –one raw, one cooked. The cooked apple ferments within 24-36 hours while the raw apple keeps fresh at least 24-36 days! Cooked food spoils readily whether inside or outside our body. Of course, it spoils faster in our warm, 96 degrees-plus, intestinal tract, where it putrefies, depending on the type of food.

1) Hotema, MHC, lesson 13 /page 21.

Living healthy cells are not soil or food for bacteria, but decomposing substances are. **Germs and bacteria are scavengers that only feed on dead food and mucus. Virulent bacteria thrives in cooked food but cannot live on raw living food. Cancer cells also thrive in a cooked food medium but die in a raw food medium!** Cooked animal protein (flesh, eggs, milk, cheese, yogurt) especially feeds the Escherichia Coli bacteria in your colon. **Germs, viruses, fungi, parasites,** and **flukes** can only thrive in a foul, polluted, congested body. **Everyone has billions of bacteria, germs, fungi,** viruses, in their body, even when healthy. **Each day, millions of cancer cells occur in the body,** and billions or trillions of bacteria and fungi are absorbed from the intestinal tract into the portal blood. These are effectively "taken care of" by the body's defense mechanism, especially in a detoxified bloodstream (made possible through a diet high in raw plantfood). Thus, scarcely any bacteria or fungi ever enter the circulating blood. So long as our body is relatively pure, waste materials do not accumulate and the scavenging assistance of bacterial germs are not called upon

.

10)   Cooked food MAL-nourishes you while making you fat.

Cooked food causes malnutrition and obesity at the same time. And no wonder, for its nutrients are 70-100% destroyed so it is mostly empty *calories*. It does not truly nourish you though it fills your stomach. As a result, cooked food, especially hard drugfood, stimulates craving for food because the organs are not getting the nutrients they would normally get in raw food. The body's craving for more nutrients may turn into an uncontrollable appetite and lack of will-power. Over half the American population is overweight –overfed yet undernourished. *Ever* eating because they are *ever* hungry because their bodies are *ever* craving the nourishment it can *never* get on a diet of toxic, foodless drugfoods. Farmers know if they feed raw potatoes to hogs they will *not* gain weight, but if fed cooked potatoes they gain weight. People lose weight easily on a rawfood diet. Often this is all that is needed to help people lose weight. When you are mainly eating living food, you are satisfied on *less* food.

11) Cooked food is the foundation of dis-ease and ill-being.

All degenerative diseases are toxic reactions to living on cooked foods, drugfoods...because they are toxic. **When the load of toxins in your body becomes too great, your body produces an emergency state of *rapid toxic discharge*. This state is called "dis-ease"!** Mind you, germs and bacteria do NOT cause disease; they indicate that you were already unbalanced to begin with. Only internal filth (which the body has not been able to expel because you kept putting it in faster than your eliminative organs could evict it) causes disease by giving the germs food to thrive on. Blaming disease on germs is like blaming garbage on flies. Clear the garbage and the flies go away. Further, germs are *pleomorphic*; they change form (like a caterpillar into a butterfly), becoming bad or good, or back to good or bad, depending on their pH environment. Only when the body's balance is off do these organisms change form and become nasty. Progressive slow degeneration of the physical body is the result of a continuous diet of cooked food.

12) Cooked food COOKS YOU!

What's done to the food you eat is done to you biologically!

We read on page 39 of The Essene Gospel of Peace: *"And Jesus continued: 'God commanded your forefathers: Thou shalt not kill.' I say to you: Kill neither men, nor beasts, nor yet the food which goes into your mouth. For if you eat living food, the same will quicken you, but if you kill your food, the dead food will kill you also. For life comes only from life, and from death comes always death. For everything which kills your foods, kills your bodies also. And everything which kills your bodies kills your souls also. And your bodies become what your foods are, even as your spirits, likewise, become what your thoughts are. Therefore, eat not anything which fire, or frost, or water has destroyed. For burned, frozen and rotted foods will burn, freeze and rot your body also."*

This applies to **microwaving** and **irradiation** as well; eating irradiated sugar can produce the same results as irradiation directly applied to the living cell!

Cooked food has the vibration of burning fire, –the fire that cooked /killed it. Microwaved food is worse. Therefore, cooked or microwaved food "burns" and "microwaves" and inflames our cells, organs, tissues. This produces internal irritation which causes short tempers, persistent anger and stress. Living on cooked foods keep our body temperature cooked. The body temperature of cooked-food eaters is 98.6. The temperature of raw-food eaters is 96.8. The temperature of fruitarians is likely even less. The average Afrikan and American is *well-cooked* plus very highly *seasoned* (loaded with poisons / chemicals).

13) Cooked food is dead food; dead food saps your Vitality (*Lifeforce*) and dims your *Light*.

As previously documented, when a fractionated nutrient is eaten, the body tries to turn it into a wholefood –by robbing its own reserves– before it can use it. The *same thing* happens with *deadfood:*

> **When you eat DEADFOOD, your body tries to RESURRECT the deadfood at the expense of your own lifeforce.** Before the body can use deadfood, it must put *LIFE* back into it...life it takes from itself. Thus, deadfood slowly robs the body of its lifeforce, *your* Lifeforce. Eating cooked dead food slowly depletes your lifeforce and lowers your vitality because dead things have the vibration of Death. *(This is why it is best for sick, diseased, or cancerous people to avoid eating dead cooked foods until they are well.)*

Although dead cooked foods sustain life, they are not life-giving or regenerating. Only life begats life. Only living, raw, wholefoods begat life. Anything less than this is slow death. Living food imparts its vitality and Lifeforce directly to your body when eaten.

We are designed to be creatures of Light. We radiate light as our aura (bioelectric field), which is visible to clairvoyants and through Kirlian photography, which shows that *living* food has life-energy around it, while *dead* cooked food has darkness (no light) around it. Cooked food is full of darkness and has no aura of light. **Raw living food radiates light /lifeforce energy because it is** *alive*. When you cook it you kill it, driving out all its light, turning it into toxic drugfood. No wonder it looks so dull and drab. And limp. When you eat such, it steals Light, Life, Vitality from your body –just like it steals your vitamins, nutrients. Your body robs from its own Light and nutrients in order to make this drugfood assimilable to any degree at all. If you live mainly on cooked foods, you are eating darkness and thus diminish your Light, Lifeforce.

Thus, a diet high in cooked food and animal flesh clogs our system, slows or obstructs our flow of life-energy, and steals our Light –literally dimming our aura. Hence, we are in darkness relative to the obstruction. And feel separated from the light, joy, peace, harmony, divinity (God/Goddess) which should be our birthright. We feel empty. We try to fill this void with the wrong things.

> **Cooked Food is *Denied Food*.** Denied Food denies us. Denied Food holds *Denied Light* (darkness). If our cells are made of Denied food then our body is largely a Denied Body, thus is always in subhealth and has less energy (light) than what it's suppose to. This leads to slow physical degeneration and premature demise.

Raw plant foods increase the micro-electric tension in the cell tissue.
Increased micro-electric tension in the cell tissue improves cell oxygenation, stimulates cell metabolism, increases the cell's resistances to aging, speeds the process of cell renewal –in short, improves the cell's metabolism and prevents biochemical suffocation.[1]

In *Survival Into the 21st Century,* Viktoras Kulvinskas wrote:
"Under a microscope the etheric body of a living cell scintillates with sunlight. Dead cells do not polarize light and the color display is extinguished. The minerals of live food act as magnets, holding the suns's energy, filling our bodies with sunlight. Technically, the electron orbit of a mineral takes a quantum orbit jump because of the absorption of sun energy. An inorganic mineral becomes an organic mineral through the action of sunlight on a plant. Live food elements make it possible to charge the body with an enormous amount of energy from natural breathing which provides optimal power for the mental and spiritual faculties. On a cooked food diet, to generate the same power requires forced breathing exercises."[2]

Again, in *The Essene Gospel of Peace*:
"For I tell you truly, live only by the fire of life, and prepare not your foods with the fire of death... 'Master, where is the fire of life?'...In you, in your blood, and in your bodies. ...And the fire of death? asked others. ...It is the fire which blazes outside your body, which is hotter than your blood. With that fire of death you cook your foods in your homes and in your fields. I tell you truly, it is the same fire which destroys your foods and your bodies, even as the fire of malice, which ravages your thoughts, ravages your spirits. For your body is that which you eat, and your spirit is that which you think. Eat nothing therefore, which a stronger fire than the fire of life has killed."[3]

1) Airola, AYC, 48, 49.   2) Kulvinska, STC, 48.   3)Szekely, 40.

It's not the food in your life but the life in your food!
Live food promotes Life. Dead food promotes Death.
The vast majority of people eat dead food
the vast majority of the time.
Therefore, they are dying more than they are living.
Only **LIVING** *foods*
build the **HEALTHIEST** *bodies!*

Advantages & benefits of a Rawfood diet

- Truly radiant health and abundant vitality.
- The absence of sickness and dis-ease, hence no more medical bills.
- Rejuvenation and longevity. You grow younger, more beautiful, more handsome. Your hair stops falling out –might even grow back. Raw plantfood rebuilds the vital regenerative force of the total organism.
- Greatly increased strength, endurance, and muscle tone without exercising.
- You feel better, lighter, more energized, happier, and youthful.
- You sleep better, wake up alert and energetic, and need much less sleep.
- A purified body, free of offensive body odors. A rawfood diet is a cleansing diet.
- Your body will be very well nourished on small amounts of foods. Most raw foods are easier to digest than cooked foods (especially fruits, veggies).
- Your food bill cut at least in half, saving you money.
- You will no longer be a "kitchen slave" –bound to your stove.
- Raw foods are easier to prepare. They are also much easier to clean up after: no greasy dirty skillets, pots, pans, dishes, etc.
- You achieve the normal weight Nature intended for you. Obesity disappears steadily, painlessly and effortlessly.
- You needn't worry about putting on weight unnaturally; live foods are not fattening, not even bananas and avocados.
- No swings from *high* to *low* –as experienced on a drugfood diet of stimulants (sugar, coffee, coke) and depressants (heavy rich foods, overeating).
- Menstruation and menopausal problems disappear.
- Bloody menstruation decreases; menstrual flow becomes clear and bloodless, and takes less time (decreasing from days to hours or minutes).
- Your body can become pregnant –when you had given up.
- Your spermcount increases or doubles (unless you're a smoker)
- Increased mental clarity, inner peace. Your sight, hearing, senses sharpen.
- Great improvement spiritually. You feel closer to Goddess /God.

You sick? Gotta health problem? Want to heal FAST? Then "go raw."

Eat only raw living food (fruit & vegetables) and the juices of such. A 100% rawfood diet is a 100% healing diet. For the treatment of illness, Alvenia Fulton, Dick Gregory, Queen Afua, Aris LaTham, Dr. Yuki Kudo, "Doctah B," Dr. Paul Goss, Dr. Llaila Afrika, Tarik ibn Freeman, Dr. Sebi, Dr. Nathan Rabb, Asara Tsehai and innumerable other health leaders /educators, including our ancient Afrikan ancestors, recommend a regenerative or raw food diet. Raw plantfood rebuilds the vital regenerative force of the total organism. As a result, sickness and even so-called incurable diseases disappear.

Societies having many centenarians eat mainly living food.

All the societies in the world which have produced large numbers of people living to be 100 and beyond in excellent health, are societies that live primarily on LIVING food. The largest amount of the food they eat is raw, organic food. Such food is rich in electro potential. The minerals are in an ionic state; that is, they are electrically charged. The enzymes and vitamins are also electrically charged. When such ionic substances enter our body, they are ready to assume their proper role within the cells.

Plants connect us to the cosmic forces of Life.

The closer food is to sun energy, the higher it is in all levels of nutrition for humans. Plant food (especially fruit) is at the top of the nutritional scale. Animal food is at the bottom. Nothing clouds the nervous system when nourishment comes from the plant realm. By the nourishment of plants, humanity can enter cosmic relationships which take us beyond mundane worldly limitations. This was common practice by our Afrikan ancestors. The "Real People" of Australia have not lost this gift.

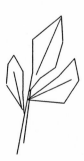

Recommendations for Better Health

Avoid or Reduce Eating:	Healthier Replacements:
• all microwaved food 　(*restaurant* food is often microwaved) • grilled food, toasted food • smoked food • fried food • pre-cooked and canned food • burned food	**Best:** • raw, uncooked plant food • "sun-baked" (sun-heated) food **Improvement:** • undercooked or lightly cooked food • low-temperature cooked food • steamed food • baked food

Tips

● **Avoid?** No, *gradually REDUCE* eating cooked foods, while increasingly eating raw living produce (organic as much as possible) because the ideal diet may make you uncomfortable in this less-than-ideal environment!
A *gradual* change to more wholesome eating is better than changing suddenly. For as a "recovering drugfood addict" you need *time* to adjust, both metabolically and psychologically. So take your time. Your present destructive eating habits and present body state were years or decades in the making. It will take some time to regenerate, rebuild and reprogram.

● **At least 50%** of the food you eat should be raw, living, water-rich food (fruit & veggies) in order to maintain *fair* health and comfortable vitality.

● **About 90-100% of your food** needs to be raw living food for vibrant radiant outstanding health and vitality.

● **Meals:** One or two large salads daily, featuring leafy greens is a big plus for health. All fruits and most vegetables can be eaten raw. You can make a delicious *drugfood* sauce /dressing and use it over diced raw veggies. A "mono diet" (just eating one natural food item per meal) is ideal.

● **Begin each meal with a raw food,** like a fruit, salad, or fresh vegetable juice. This results in the most effective digestion. Cooked foods eaten with raw foods are more acceptable, more healthy and less harmful.

● **Take digestive enzymes** with your meals of cooked food, especially flesh.

● **If you cook:**
  – Cook your food in glass or enameled pots. Totally avoid aluminum.
  – Use low heat. If vegetables are cut into small pieces, less heat is required for cooking. Low-temperature cooking also keeps food crispy /tasty.
  – Use *steaming* rather than boiling (the broth should also be used).
  – Use *baking* or broiling rather than frying.
  – Cook with fewer ingredients; the less ingredients, the better.
  – Consume the water/broth you cook in; it has nutrients cooked out of the food.
  – Do not grill or toast food (or eat such), to avoid carcinogenic benzopyrenes.
  – Do not use microwave ovens at all or eat any nuked (microwaved) foods; microwaves are deadly, both for your food and environment.

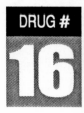

DRUG #

Personal Allergy Food

Allergic? Then that food is your *poison*.

Even if it's organic and "healthy." Let's address **genetic nutrition**. There are genetic and biochemical differences from one race or ethnic group to another. The bodies of your ancestors adapted to the foods of their environment. Your ethnic background gives you special nutritional needs. When you eat foods that your body is not genetically adapted to handle, this food is POISON to your body, more or less. Thus you are "allergic" to that food.

Many common dis-eases are food allergies (toxic food reactions)

arthritis	asthma	skin eruptions
headaches	migraines	post nasal drip
depression	dizziness	mental /emotional disorders
edema	indigestion	chronic fatigue
eczema	diabetes	heart palpitations
weakness	epilepsy	heart disease

These and other health problems will disappear once you stop eating the offending food. Foods you are allergic to raise your blood pressure, speed your heartbeat, and act as a stimulant, a poison. Allergies to otherwise healthful foods make them into poisons (drugfoods!) as far as your body is concerned, and thus into addictive substances, resulting in countless variations of pathology, not just rashes or runny noses. Individuals can be allergic to, and thus addicted to just about anything. Common allergens include wheat, corn, eggs, soy, cow's milk, beans, white potatoes, oranges, shellfish, beef, sugar and yeast –plus thousands of chemicals added to foods. Then there's "transgenic" food (genetically-altered produce) providing more allergenic health hazards.

A toxic food reaction (allergy) may appear minutes, hours or even several days later after you eat the offending food

...hence go totally unrecognized or linked with the culprit-food that produced it. Worse yet, the reaction is misdiagnosed and the true cause is never suspected by the physician, who inappropriately treats the patient with symptom-suppressing toxic drugs, hence, compounding the problem.

Often, allergy responses are occurring on top of previous allergy responses before they have worn off. Thus, if you are constantly eating foods/chemicals you are unknowingly allergic to, **you have battles and wars going on constantly in your body (!)** making your body a biological war zone. And you are the victim ...deliciously unknowingly killing yourself. In fact, most degenerative diseases (heart disease, cancer, diabetes, etc.) are toxic food reactions (allergies). Nearly 90% of the population has a toxic food reaction to some food(s) they eat.

A glimpse at the allergy mechanism

We genetically lack the code to digest certain foods. When such foods are only partially digestible, this is a *food intolerance*. Partially digested foods increase the amount and variety of harmful intestinal bacteria and fungus. Harmful intestinal bacteria and fungus create toxic by-products as a result of rotting and fermenting the partially digested food. These toxic chemical by-products frequently cause intestinal gas, bloating, pain, inflammation, and diarrhea or constipation. Toxic chemical by-products are absorbed into the bloodstream and go to the liver. The liver detoxifies most of these toxic chemicals, but when the load is too much, some leak past the liver into general circulation. Toxic chemical by-products of harmful intestinal bacteria and fungus in the general circulation poison the cells, tissues, organs and create many health problems. Harmful intestinal bacteria, fungus, and toxic chemical-by-products make microscopic holes in the walls of the intestines. Partially digested starch, fat, and protein molecules pass through these holes into the bloodstream. Once in the bloodstream, these partially digested molecules are interpreted by your immune system as bacterial, fungal, or viral invaders. Your immune system then launches a war against these molecules every time the offending food is eaten, often creating symptoms of illness. This toxic food reaction is called an "allergy."

Dietary *lectins* are *antigens* that can trigger toxic reactions from the immune system

They (are used to) agglutinate blood according to blood type. They are high in grains, common in beans and present in other foods. Those who eat foods high in lectin content *specific for their blood type* are at an increased risk. Strong stomach acid, pancreatic enzymes, and thorough cooking tend to degrade lectins, thus destroying their antigen capability (but cooking creates other problems).

Dietary *lectins* can affect the body in three ways:

1) **Blood Agglutination**: clumping of blood cells leading to reduced blood flow in capillaries /tissues. As the effect builds up in larger vessels, this leads to plaque formation, clots, loss of oxygen, arterial closure, blockage of blood flow to organs.

2) **Immune Response**: immune stimulating antigens promoting several toxic reactions at the same time, causing headaches, aches, diarrhea, vomiting, fatigue, irritability, hemolytic anemia, asthma, hay fever, eczema, hives, hyperactivity in children, migraine, joint/muscle pain, bladder inflammation... **Virtually any non-infective health problem involving inflammation, congestion, and swelling is the result of the "slow anaphylactic response"** of the immune system to some type of food molecule (*anaphylactic* =overprotective).

3) **Digestive Distress**: many dietary lectins attach to cells of the small intestines' mucosal wall, causing inflammation, reduction of carbohydrate absorption as much as 50%, Coeliac & Chron's disease, multiple sclerosis and other dis-eases. Entering the blood, they block insulin-sugar intake, hence elevate blood sugar levels.

Recommendations for Better Health

Avoid or Reduce Eating:	Healthier Replacements:
• foods you are allergic to	• foods you are *not* allergic to • foods you are mildly allergic to

Find out what your food allergies are

This is a worthwhile investment for your health. By primarily eating foods you are not allergic to, your physical /mental /emotional health, vitality, and well being greatly improves. Diseases even disappear. Don't just eat "healthy" food, eat food your body can handle. Complete instructions for accurately and easily determining your allergies (to *anything*, including foods) are presented in the third volume of this book, entitled: ***Don't Worry, Be Healthy!*** Several options are given, including *kinesiology* (muscle testing), which lets you determine allergies almost instantly, plus, it's free.

Vegetables & Grains are Unnatural and Contain Poisons

Most vegetables are not natural!
Plus they contain natural poisons!

Healthfood books apparently avoid this topic; they almost *never* address the *unnaturalness* of vegetables or the natural poisons which vegetables contain. If they did, it might become obvious that vegetables and grains are not Humanity's natural food! The unnatural cultivated vegetables and grains of today are lesser, unrecognized drugfoods. While not as lethal as hard drugfoods, they are harmful enough to slowly damage our health over time.

Few people know that most vegetables we eat are not natural

Most vegetables and grains are not found growing wild in Nature. Many of them did not even exist in Nature just a hundred years ago. Vegetables and grains are the product of careful artificial cultivation. They are difficult to produce and contain many natural poisons. The fields in which they grow are artificial. Annual crops are artificial. Their cultivation is artificial. All these cultivated things would die and disappear without the pampering hands and *machines* of humans.

- **Grains and cereals** have been developed from grass seeds now unknown to botany. All cereal-grains belong to the grass family. Grains are both the *fruit* and *seed* of grasses. By long ages of seed selection, careful breeding, intensive cultivation and constant fertilization, small grass seeds were developed by this artificial process into the modern grains and cereals.
- **Beans, peas, lentils, cabbage, lettuce, celery**, etc., were developed in the same way from the grass family.
- **Tubers, which include potatoes, onions, carrots, turnips, beets, radishes**, etc., are nothing more than wild weed roots developed by the artificial process described earlier.
- In addition to having suffered cultivation, the vegetables and grains of today have been **hybred and genetically mucked with**, including the organically grown produce in healthfood stores.

Humans were never intended to eat vegetables and grains as food!

Vegetables are not natural, nor are they the natural food of humans. Hue-mans (the original Black people, humanity's parents) adopted this habit because they migrated from their natural home in tropical and subtropical regions. Humans discovered the therapeutic value of vegetables after becoming sick from unnatural foods in an unnatural environment.[1] The human diet has changed drastically in the last few thousand years. Most humans are eating many recently introduced plants that our ancestors did not eat, such as corn, tomatoes, potatoes, avocados, olives, tea, coffee and cocoa.

Pesticide-defenders make an apparent good argument that...

...vegetables contain many natural toxins that are greatly higher in quantity than the "residues" of pesticides on /in the plant. I contend there is a significant difference! The plant-toxins are <u>organic and part of a living system</u>. But the whiteman-made toxins are NOT organic, NOR living. (Consider the vast difference between organic minerals and inorganic minerals.). Therefore the Human Body handles them much differently, than if they were organic and living --just like the Body handles synthetic vitamins or man-altered nutrients differently than true-natural, unmolested, wholefood vitamins /nutrients.

Cultivation. All forms of artificialization disturbs the balance of Nature and produce disastrous results.

Cultivation is the name of the unnatural, quick crop growing method. Cultivation exposes the land to excessive sunlight, wind and water which nutritionally drains the soil of its vital elements. Fields are sun-baked in dry weather and muddy and eroded in the rainy season. In time, cultivation destroys the land, regardless of how shallow the land is plowed. It creates disharmony in the Earth's soil and alters the ecological balance of plants, insects, air, water, animals and people. A more natural form of plant farming is **non-cultivation farming**. In this form of farming, the trees, waters, animals and land resources are left as they are and farming is done around them. The plants are allowed to live free and wild. Afrikan people originated and practiced both types of farming. These non-cultivated crops were not domesticated. Subsequently, they produced a more wholistic higher nutritional food value. This non-cultivation farming did not have a higher crop production, but it did require the humans to be in tune with the rhythm and cycles of the Earth's and the cosmic's atmosphere.[2]

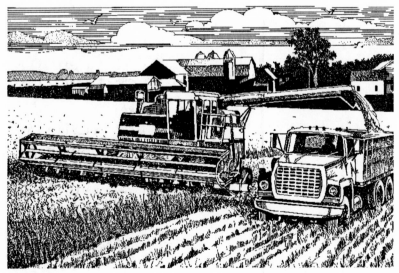

1) Kulvinskas, STC, 88.   2) Afrika, AHH, 97.

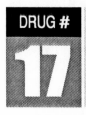

DRUG
17
Cultivated:
Gravity Grains

Grains are the most harmful of plant foods

Vegetarians and Flesharians both overeat starches (grains, cereals, breads, pasta). Our bodies have not evolved on grains. All grains are detrimental to humans. Grains (wheat, barley, oats, rye, etc.) are no more a part of humanity's true food than oranges the food of cows. **Grain is a *recent* entry to human diet in the overall length of human history.**

The unnaturalness and harmfulness of grains
as fuel for humans is evident in a number of ways:

– **Grains have to be <u>cooked</u> just to make them edible.** Cooking is unnatural, plus it corrupts the food. **If we have to cook a food to make it edible, that food is not meant for us to eat!** Grains contains large amounts of minerals –which become *inorganic* when cooked.

– **Of all plant foods**, grains are most often associated with food allergies, especially *wheat* and corn. **There are over 30,000 varieties of wheat!** –hence 30,000 allergenic wheaty ways of harming ourselves.

– **Humans have only one starch-splitting enzyme, *ptyalin*,** whereas true starch eaters (graminivores) have several starch-splitting enzymes.

– **Gluten**, a protein component in wheat /rye /barley is opium-like and indigestible to humans. As we shall later see, gluten causes many diseases and health problems.

– **Bran** (tough coating of grains) is also indigestible to humans. Barley has such a thick bran that only pearled barley, having some of its bran polished away, is sold for human consumption.

– **All grains /starches are mucus-producing** (except millet). Because Americans eat so much wheat and other starches, they suffer from sinus congestion, headaches, asthma, excess mucus in the respiratory and digestive tracts, arthritis, constipation, and many other problems.

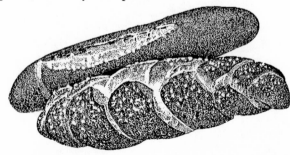

DRUG # 18

Cultivated:
Vice Veggies

A vegetarian diet causes diseases (like flesh-eating diets)

Vegetarians are hardly better off than flesh-eaters. Vegetarians do not live much longer than *flesharians* (meat eaters). A vegetarian diet causes calciferous degeneration, atheroma, arteriosclerosis, hardening of the blood-vessels, ossification of the tissues and joints, and premature decrepitude or aging.

Vegetables are biological *fractionates*, hence drugfoods

A fraction (trait) of their original wholeness has been overdeveloped or "selected." The word *selected* itself betrays fractionation. I would call vegetables *natural drugfoods* except they are *unnatural*; they **appear natural** and the world is fooled. Thus, the vegetables and grains which currently compose Humanity's predominant diet, are unbalanced. They win *first place* as the best disguised drugfoods! Your body knows the difference! As with drugs, the body will adapt to the drugfood that is constantly forced upon it. The body adjusts itself to the point where it craves these stimulating substances. This adaptation is at the expense (decrease) of the body's vitality.

Vegetables are mild narcotics

Health advocate Hilton Hotema lived to be about 95. As far as he was concerned, these unnatural vegetables are mild narcotics to the body. In *Man's Higher Consciousness,* one of the few books addressing natural poisons in vegetables, he wrote:

"The vegetarian's [and flesh-eater's] body is stimulated and saturated with poisons of the substances he eats; and the vegetables [or drugfood] one craves most are those that poison one most. The vegetable poisons are usually mild in character and slow in action, but their damaging effects are cumulative, increasing with the years, and are responsible for many disorders, the basic causes of which are never suspected.

"The flesh-eating man is in a steady state of mild irritation, or auto-intoxication, rising from the excessive stimulation caused by the decaying flesh food in his stomach, bowels and blood. ...Just as in the case of the flesh-eater, the vegetarian has eaten his diet from childhood, and the condition of auto-intoxication is deep-seated and chronic. The victim's body and organs are adjusted to it.[1]

"The vegetarian goes through life in that weakened condition with his vitality much below par, but he knows it not because he never knew anything else. He has no reason to believe his vitality and health are not what they should be. He cannot miss what he never had. He is dying by inches all the day of his life, while believing that he is following a high standard of living."[2]

1) Hotema, MHC, lesson 13, page 21.   2) Ibid., lesson 15, page 30-31

The Natural Poisons in Vegetables!

No wonder children naturally tend to dislike eating vegetables. Why are natural poisons in vegetables at all? Plants have evolved natural toxic chemicals in order to defend themselves from insects and other predators. Also, to protect themselves from diseases such as viruses and molds. Other plant chemicals have therapeutic, medicinal, stimulatory, hallucinatory, or narcotic effects. From earliest times people have been aware that some plants are poisonous and should be avoided as food. Humans' sensory perception of bitter, acrid, astringent, and pungent tasting plants is a defense which warn us against a wide range of natural toxins in foods. We often ignore these warnings...and indulge anyway, in eating mustard, pepper, garlic, and other plants having these attributes. Today's unnatural cultivated vegetables are unsuspected, unrecognized, seemingly innocent, lesser drugfoods. True, they are not as harmful as *hard* drugfoods (sugar, coffee...) but they are harmful enough to damage our health over time –they just do it even more *s l o w l y*. So let's find out about these poisons:

1. **Potatoes, tomatoes, eggplants, bell peppers** and **tobacco** (!) are all narcotics. They all belong to the toxic Nightshade or Solanaceae family. The term *nightshade* is from *nihtscada*, meaning the shade or shadow of night, a name referring to the narcotic qualities of the various flowering nightshade plants. All nightshades have an above average *nitrogen* content. They all contain *nicotine*; **tobacco** has the highest concentration, **eggplant** is next. They all have a common *"allergen"* that produces joint pain. In fact, the nightshades cause or aggravate rheumatoid arthritis and osteo-arthritis (pain, swelling, creaking in the joints).[1] The toxicity of tobacco is well established. Natural toxins abundantly found in nightshades include *solanine, glycoalkaloids* and *alkamines.* *Glycoalkaloids* have been shown to cause red blood cells to self-destruct in vitro (test tubes). *Alkamines*, which are absorbed by the intestines, have been shown to contribute to nervous disorders in humans and animals. *"Altogether, these substances have been linked with kidney stones, calcium depletion, nausea, abdominal pain and swelling, loss of red blood cells, ulcers, jaundice, rashes, muscle wasting, breathing difficulties, trembling, drowsiness and paralysis."* [2]

1) Clark, CD, 83; Murray, EN, 449; Gagne, 207.   2) Gagne, 207.

2. The common **white potato** contains two *narcotic alkaloids* called *chaconine* and *solanine* which cause potato poisoning. Buildups of solanine is visible as *green spots* on the potato. They are poisonous even when cooked. *Solanine* poisoning from green potatoes will produce throat burning, weakness, rashes, diarrhea or constipation, stomach pains, ulceration, intestinal irritation, hemorrhage and even convulsions with collapse and coma, requiring hospital care. Few animals will eat potato vines because of their poisonous properties. Fowls won't eat potato bugs because they're so poisonous. Because of its toxicity, the **Lenape potato** was withdrawn from the market. Red potatoes are recommended over white varieties since they do not have this poison, due to their different chemistry. Avoid eating green potatoes, and store potatoes in the dark to avoid the greening effect of light. White potatoes also contain *gamma-amino butyric acid* (GABA), that may have sedative activity.[1] **Potatoes** are true salt-suckers, and can be very helpful for reducing the sodium in tissues of people who have consumed far too much salt.[2] **Sweet potatoes** contain *phytoalexins* that can cause lung edema and are liver-toxic to mice. Sweet potatoes are not the same as **yams**, though similar. Most so-called yams sold in America are really varieties of sweet potatoes. Many species of (real) **yams**, eaten in other parts of the world, contain toxic *alkaloid compounds*, including *dioscorine*. They may weigh a hundred pounds, and are put through a laborious washing/cutting process to reduce their toxins enough to make them safely edible.

3. The enzyme, cholinesterase, plays an important role in nerve impulses. The toxins *chaconine* and *solanine,* found in **potatoes, tomatoes** and **eggplant,** are *cholinesterase inhibitors* (like malathion), that is, they affect nerve transmission much like the most toxic chemical-warfare agents. They block nerve transmission. Solanine and chaconine are present in potatoes at 15 mg per 200 g (75 ppm). Bruised potatoes and potatoes that have begun to sprout have substantially higher levels and can be lethal. *Solanine* and *chaconine* are also *teratogens*, substances that cause fetal malformations. Both compounds are found in the tissues of potato eaters.

4. Toxic *cholinesterase inhibitors* are also found in **eggplant** and the roots and leaves of **tomatoes**. Small amounts are found in **asparagus, turnips, radishes, celery, valencia oranges,** and **carrots**.

1) Quillin, 127.   2) Gagne, 210.

5. *Methyl glyoxal*, a potent mutagenic substance which causes cancer in rats, is found in **tomatoes** and **potatoes** (plus coffee and alcoholic beverages). **Fermented potatoes** is the source of *vodka*, one of the scourges of Russian society.

6. **Tomatoes** have *"the uncanny ability to deplete the body of minerals."* [1]   Blood crystallization studies done in Germany show that cancerous blood and the juice of fresh tomato reveal a striking structural similarity.[2] **Tomato vines** are as poisonous as **potato vines.** Few animals will eat them. Tomatoes (especially unripe and green) also contain *tomatine*, a toxic *glycoalkaloid*. Adverse and allergic reactions to **tomatoes** and **peppers** are common.

7. **Eggplant** has been linked with cancer in that its slightly mutagenic qualities have caused genetic damage to cells in vitro (test tube).[3] It was once regarded as a contraceptive by Nigerians. According to Chinese medicine theory, **eggplant** and **tomatoes** slow the healing process, plus contribute to wound infections /complications.[4] (Is this the real reason hospitals often serve tomato products to patients after surgery?!)

8. **Lettuce** is a narcotic. Lettuce got its name from its milky juice, *lactis*, milk. Wild lettuce grows 6 feet high. The whole plant is rich in a milky, bitter juice that flows freely from any wound. When dry, it hardens, turns reddish brown, and is known as *lactucarium*, a *narcotic alkaloid* which is sometimes used as a substitute for *opium,*[5] and was smoked by Native North Americans. It tastes and smells just like opium and used to be called "Poor man's opium." In early Mesopotamia, **wild lettuce** (or bitter lettuce) was popularly used as a sedative. All varieties of lettuce possess some of this *narcotic juice*. The wild varieties called **Lactuca Virosa** (virosa means poisonous) and **Lettuce Sacriola** have the most. The latter is believed to be the progenitor of the cultivated varieties. Cultivation has lessened the narcotic properties of **Garden Lettuce. Bibb Lettuce** contains *morphine*. **Iceberg Lettuce** contains *strychnine* and *ammonia*. Iceburg lettuce has *no* nutritional value; it's all water, roughage and toxins.

9. Dr. Hilton Hotema wrote: *"Potatoes, lettuce and practically all so-called vegetables dull the brain and produce enervation. One may speak of solanin psychosis or potato psychosis or lettuce psychosis as a mental disorder caused by eating these substances as one speaks of alcoholic and opium psychosis. ...Beets, eggplant, spinach, Swiss chard, rhubarb, all contain certain poisons."* [6]

1) Gagne, 211. 2) Ibid., 211. 3) Ibid., 212. 4) Tien, 70. 5) Hotema, MH, lesson 15 /pg 29, 30. 6) Ibid. 30.

10. **Garlic**, especially **raw garlic**, is harmful to the body when consumed regularly. Though endowed with many beneficial attributes, garlic also causes extensive edema, bleeding and ulceration of the stomach mucosa, reduction of red-blood cell count, increase in reticulocytes (immature blood cells), and it knocks sugar out of balance – *'being very hypoglycemic.'*[1]

11. **Garlic, onions, leeks, shallots, chives, cress, radishes,** and **mustard** all contain toxic, non-metabolizable *mustard oil*, a very irritating and indigestible substance which contains *allyl isothiocyanate*, a mucous membrane irritant which causes cancer in rats. The soporific oil irritates the kidneys and bladder. It makes the eyes water and the genital mucus membrane do the same. Some people assert that it acts as a powerful aphrodisiac. Cooking evaporates this oil to a degree. *Allyl isothiocyanate* gives pungent flavor to **mustard** and **horse-radish**, etc., where it is present at about 50–100 ppm. Much lower levels are present in **broccoli**, **cabbage** and **arugula**.

12. Many **beans**, even when sprouted, have *trypsin inhibitors* which block trypsin (a pancreatic digestive enzyme), causing poor digestion of the protein within the beans, which results in putrefaction and gas. These include **lentils, black-eyed peas, partridge peas, mung beans, kidney, peanuts, lima** and **soybeans**. Bean allergies are as common as wheat allergies.

13. Many species of **legumes** and **beans**, especially **red kidney beans** and **castor beans**, have *lectin proteins* (phytohemagglutinins) that can agglutinate red blood cells. Poisoning can occur if those beans are eaten raw or not completely cooked. The *hemagluttins* found in many **beans** suppress growth in rats, and are believed to line the intestines and block fat and protein uptake. Hence, unless thoroughly cooked to degrade or destroy the hemagluttins, beans are poorly absorbed.

14. **Coffee beans** contain *caffeine*, a neurotoxin, and many other toxins. Caffeine's adverse effects are undisputed. **Cocoa** and **vanilla beans** contain *methylxanthines,* nervous system stimulants from the same chemical family as the caffeine.

1) Health Freedom News, 3/92, p29.

15. **Celery, tomatoes, spinach** and **beets** are loaded with beneficial organic sodium which, when _cooked_, becomes *inorganic sodium* which causes fluid-retention, just like table salt (sodium-chloride). Likewise, the abundant organic acid in **tomatoes** and **tomato juice** becomes detrimental *inorganic acid* when cooked /canned, and causes kidney and bladder stones if eaten with starches and sugars.[1] Examples of such food are pizza, spaghetti /pasta with tomato sauces.

16. Many consider **rhubarb** to be a tasty, tangy vegetable. But only the stalks of the leaves are relatively safe to eat. The leaves, being large, may be tempting as a source of greens, but they contain very high amounts of *oxalic acid*, which enters the bloodstream. There it clots the blood, crystallizes in the kidneys, and eventually leads to death. During WWI, the English government, in an effort to conserve food, mistakenly encouraged people to eat the leaf blades of rhubarb and many people died as a result.

17. **Mustard greens, collard greens, turnip greens, spinach, rhubarb, Swiss chard, kale, beet greens** and **sorrel** contain a high percentage of *oxalic acid (oxalates)*. *"They should therefore never be eaten when cooked,"* advises Dr. Norman Walker. When these are cooked, the organic oxalic acid becomes inorganic and *'results in causing inorganic oxalic acid crystals to form in the kidneys, with the consequent pain and kidney trouble.'*[2] In its raw, organic state, oxalic acid is beneficial to the body. **Mustard** and **collard greens** are "soul food" to many Blacks. Now we see that they are definitely drugfood when cooked. Also the high content of calcium in spinach is bound by its oxalates (cooked or raw?) so that not even a milligram can be absorbed![3]

18. **Peanuts** and **almonds** contribute to forming kidney stones. Kidney stones are most commonly formed of *calcium oxalate*. Though peanuts and almonds contain only moderate amounts of oxalate, its bio-availability is very high and therefore peanuts and almonds *"pose more of a risk than [foods /vegetables] with more oxalate."*[4]

1) Walker, FV, 75, 76.   2) Ibid., 75, 73.   3) Colgan NN, 59.   4) Williams, DW, 35

19. **Asparagus, celery, cabbage** and **turnips** contain *arsenic*. According to Dr. Carey Reams: *"The arsenic in vegetables is in the phosphate form and is not poisonous. In fact it is vital for a strong heart! Our hearts contain a large amount of arsenic compared with the other organs and this is what really makes the heart different from all the other organs."* [1] But you can bet that <u>cooking</u> alters this arsenic, making it inorganic and probably toxic.

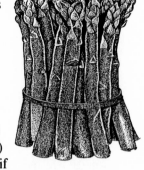

20. *Nitrates* are natural components of plants. They occur in small amounts in fruits but are high in certain vegetables. **Beets, radishes, rhubarb, celery, spinach** and **lettuce** contain the highest levels of nitrates. They all contain about 200 mg (2,000 ppm or parts per million) of nitrate per 100 gram portion. (100 g is about a quarter of a pound) This level could increase to more than 3,500 ppm if *nitrate fertilizers* are used. Nitrates are also high in **eggplant, collards, mustard, kale, turnip, potatoes, carrots** and **cabbage**; and present in **asparagus** and **onions**. The two most important factors responsible for large accumulations of nitrates in vegetables are the <u>high levels of fertilization with *nitrate fertilizers*</u> and the tendency of the species to accumulate nitrate.[2] Nitrates combine with natural stomach and food chemicals to create carcinogenic *nitrosamines*. The FDA allows 200 ppm in processed meats even though sodium nitrate /nitrite is a potential cancer hazard at levels higher than 10 parts per *billion*. The nitrate limit in drinking water, established by the government, is 10 ppm. Tap water accounts for 5-10% of nitrates consumed. In the U.S., the average dietary intake of nitrate is about 75-100 mg per day. Most of this is from vegetables. Vegetarians may ingest about twice this amount daily.

21. *Canavanine* in **alfalfa seeds** and **sprouts** may a cause hypersensitivity illness. Alfalfa sprouts, eaten in excess and harvested before maturity (7 days) contain toxic *canavanine*, an amino acid which worsens lupus and rheumatoid arthritis.[3] The concentration (1.5 percent by weight, or 15,000 ppm) is highest on the 3rd day. Feeding alfalfa sprouts to monkeys causes a severe toxic syndrome resembling the human disease lupus erythematosus.

22. Naturally occurring *estrogens* are present in **carrots, alfalfa, soybeans, potatoes, garlic, sage** and **parsley.** Usually, they don't seem to be a problem, although **ginseng** has caused breast enlargement in men (gynecomastia), due to the presence of an estrogen-like substance.

1) Kirban, 127.   2) Winter, FA 281.   3) Cousens, CE, 372.

23. Many vegetables and plants contain *cyanide-producing compounds* called *cyanogenetic glycosides*, which give them protection from insects, disease, and grazing animals. Most cyanogenetic compounds are poisonous; cattle and other range animals have died from eating plants containing them. And cases of human poisoning from the cyanide released from certain varieties of **lima beans, bitter almonds** and **cassava** have been reported. When broken down in the body, these compounds liberate *cyanide*, one of the most toxic substances known to humans and animals. Its lethal dose is only 1 mg/kg body weight. Fortunately for us, the concentration in these plants is usually far below the toxic dose. And the breakdown of the compounds is often not complete. Your body produces PIT, a food chemical which detoxifies cyanide-containing foods. It can take the liver a week to detoxify a meal full of cyanides.[1] *Cyanide compounds* are found in **cabbage, peas, chickpeas, alfalfa, yams, corn, sprouts, bamboo sprouts** and especially **fruit pits** and **cassava.**

24. **Cassava (manioc)** is inherently toxic. It is poisonous when raw or improperly prepared. It contains high levels of *cyanide-producing compounds* (cyanogenetic glycosides) such as *linamarin* which converts to hydrocyanic acid. Cassava, unfortunately, is widely consumed by People of Color. **Cassava** is a major food crop in Afrika, Southeast Asia and South America. A crossbred plant made in Europe, cassava was brought to Afrika by the Europeans. It is extremely insect-resistant because it contains so much natural *cyanide*, therefore it does not require pesticides. But it does require extensive processing. Cassava root is put through a laborious process of soaking, washing, grinding, boiling, drying and fermenting to reduce its toxic cyanide effects and make it safe to eat. Barely though. For neurological disorders and thyroid enlargement occur in Afrikans and other peoples who eat large amounts of inadequately processed cassava. And ataxia (loss of muscular coordination) due to chronic cyanide poisoning is endemic and prevalent in many of the cassava-eating areas of Afrika.[2]

25. **Lima** and **kidney beans** are toxic when raw. Both contain *cyanide-producing compounds*, including *linamarin*, which can be largely destroyed by adequate cooking. Cyanide is also found in **bean sprouts, butter beans, broad beans, soybeans** and **lentils.**

1) Clark, CAD, 84.   2) Cooke, R. & Cock, J. (1989) New Scientist 17, 63-68.

26. All **nuts** and many **fruit-pits** are high in both <u>beneficial</u> and <u>toxic</u> *cyanide compounds*. For example, **almonds** and **apricot pits** are very rich in anti-cancer *Laetrile,* also called *vitamin B17* and *amygdalin*. Apricot pits have the highest content of Laetrile on Earth. Laetrile is a diglucoside with a cyanide radical that is highly "bio-accessible." This cyanide radical once made the vitamin controversial, but B17 has been proven to be completely non-toxic.

A special explanation is needed here: <u>*Laetrile destroys*</u> <u>*cancer cells without harming normal tissue.*</u> *No wonder the FDA has declared it illegal. Chemically, Laetrile is a cyanide molecule safely sandwiched between two other molecules. Don't cringe at the thought of cyanide. This was the FDA's way of scaring most of the public away from the use of Laetrile. Cyanide is always present in the body, since it is a normal product of metabolism just like ammonia and carbon dioxide (these, too, are poisons). Our body cells produce an enzyme (rhodanese) which neutralizes metabolic cyanide before it can harm our tissues. Trophoblast cells (such as cancer), however, do <u>not</u> produce this protective enzyme. Instead they manufacture another enzyme (beta-glucuronidase) <u>which</u>* <u>*releases from the Laetrile that deadly cyanide (deadly to the trophoblasts/*</u> <u>*cancer cells only) right at the site of the cancer. In brief, the cancer cell*</u> <u>*contains the perfect trap for its own destruction but no defense, while the*</u> <u>*normal cell contains the perfect defense against the cyanide but no trap.*</u>

Nuts containing *laetrile* include: **almonds** (especially), **cashews, filberts, pistachios, pecans, brazil nuts, chestnuts** and **bitter nuts.** The greatest concentration of laetrile is found in the **pits /seeds** of rosaceous fruits: **apple & pear seeds, cherry & plum pits, peach & nectarine pits**, and also **papaya seeds** and **alfalfa seeds.** It is wise to follow the simple rule that one should not eat at one time more seeds of any kind than they likely could consume if they were also eating a reasonable quantity of the whole fruit. This is a common sense rule with a large safety margin that can be followed with confidence. For many seeds also contain other toxic substances which can be harmful. (*Kinesiology* can be used to determine whether something is safe for you personally, and in what amount.)

27. **Black pepper** is considered more harmful to the liver than alcohol.[1] Extracts of black pepper have caused cancer in mice. Black pepper contains toxic *alkaloids* called *chavicine, piperettine* and about 10% *piperine* by weight. *Piperine* is found in the **pepper family** (black & white pepper but not cayenne).

1) Nelson, MY, 88.

28. Found in **cayenne pepper,** the poisons *piperidin* and *capsaicin* irritate the body so severely that circulation is increased in order to promptly eliminate it. Its use can damage the liver and kidneys. The body outpours mucus when such hot peppers are used in order to protect itself from irritating *alkaloids* in peppers. This defense response is misinterpreted as aiding the healing process.

29. **Carrots** (a crossbred), **parsley, celery, dill** and **black pepper** contain a little *myristicin*, a psychotropic, hallucinogenic toxin which in large doses (such as an ounce) may cause shock, stupor, acidosis, or other intoxicating symptoms with euphoria for up to 24 hours after ingestion. **Nutmeg** has high concentrations of this toxin, including other toxic compounds such as **eugenol, isoeugenol, elemicin, limolene** and **safrole** (a liver carcinogen to mice). Depending on the dose, some of these substances are toxic or therapeutic.

30. *Goitrogens* interfere with thyroid functions, prevent iodine utilization and promote thyroid enlargement (goitre). Besides being gas-producing, the Brassica family of vegetables contain high levels of *goitrogenic* (anti-thyroid) *chemicals*. **Cabbage, brussel sprouts,** and **kohlrabi** contain *progoitrin* (in the range of 65-140 mg per 100 gram of fresh vegetable). *Goitrogens* are found in **cauliflower, broccoli, spinach, beets, kale, turnips, radishes, mustard, rutabaga, cassava root, legumes, beans, soybeans, peanuts, pine nuts, rapeseed, millet,** and **carrots**. Cooking reduces the goitre effect of these vegetables (but creates other problems). *Goitrogens* are further liberated by juicing. The daily consumption of **raw carrot juice** may induce a mild hypothyroid state.[1] On the positive side, there is evidence that eating Brassicas regularly helps prevent bowel cancer.

31. Health books praise "cruciferous vegetables" for their *"anti-cancer indoles."* An abstract on the internet stated: "Although crucifers may provide some protection from cancer when taken prior to a carcinogen, when taken after a carcinogen they act as promoters of carcinogenesis."[2] What that sounds like is that cruciferous vegetables may promote cancer if carcinogens are present in the body. (And carcinogens seem unavoidable in western society.) So it looks as if eating crucifers do not necessarily protect against cancer. Crucifers such as **cabbage, broccoli, kale, cauliflower,** and **mustard** were used in ancient times "primarily for medicinal purposes" (another way of saying they are drugfoods!) and were spread as foods across Europe only in the middle ages.

1) Igram 249. 2) "Beier RC..Reviews of Environmental Contamination and Toxicology, 1990, 113:47-137."

32. **Canola** and **Soy** are health hazards. Re-read about them on page 87. The *rape* plant (of the mustard family) is appropriately named, and the genetically re-engineered version of this plant is the source of "**canola oil**." Rape is the most toxic of all food-oil plants. Rape and soy are weeds. Their toxic oils form *latex-like substances* that agglutinate the red blood corpuscles, congesting bloodflow. Rape (canola) oil contains *isothiocyanates* (cyanide compounds) and causes respiratory distress, emphysema, anemia, constipation, irritability and blindness.

33. The **soybean plant** is a weed. Soybeans are very hard to digest and have a high *toxin content*. Soybeans contain *indigestible carbohydrates* and *inhibitors* of digestive enzymes (soybean trypsin inhibitor) which also cause excessive gas and occasional abdominal pain and diarrhea. Research has shown that animals fed a diet of raw soybeans lose weight and develop pancreatic problems, because soybeans are so difficult to digest. It takes more effort on the part of the digestive system to break down the soybeans than the energy provided by the beans. As a result, pancreatic enzymes are overproduced to compensate.[1]

34. **Soybeans** are high in *copper,* a zinc antagonist, hence, vegetarians who eat primarily soy as a protein source frequently develop zinc deficiency. Zinc is a crucial component of a wide range of human enzyme systems.

35. *Psoralens* (furano coumarins) are present in umbelliferous plants (**celery, parsnips, parsley**). The level is so low they are not normally harmful. But plant-breeders have made new strains with high amounts. Psoralens are *mutagenic* and *phototoxic* (photo means light); they cause toxic reactions when the person is exposed to sunlight. Photodermatitis often occurs with people who frequently handles celery, such as grocery employees and celery field workers. Many psoralens are carcinogenic, especially to rats (in high doses). Psoralens are sensitizing agents that increase erythematous (skin-reddening /inflammation) effects of UV radiation from sunlight or fluorescent tubes. Absorption of such light in the presence of psoralens temporarily inhibits DNA synthesis and alters immune system reactions. *"When a major grower introduced a new variety of highly insect-resistant celery into commerce, a flurry of complaints were made to the Centers for Disease Control from all over the country because people who handled the celery developed rashes and burns when they were subsequently exposed to sunlight. ...[It was] found that the pest-resistant celery contained 6,200 ppb of ...psoralens instead of the 800 ppb present in normal celery...The celery is still on the market."* [3]

1) Gagne, 236.   2) Report by Bruce Ames, *"Nature's Chemicals...Toxicology,"* UC Berkeley, 8/15/90.

36. Due to **mold** (which produces **mycotoxins,** some of the most toxic chemicals known), **soybeans** and **peanuts** (hence peanut butter) have **aflatoxin,** which kills portions of the liver on contact. Soy products include *tofu, soy cheese, soy milk, soy fake-fleshfoods, soy sauce, tamari, miso, and most commercial "bean" products.*

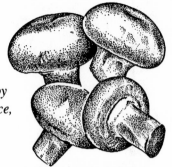

37. While some **mushrooms** are therapeutic, some species are outright lethal. It's probably wisest to use mushrooms as **medicine,** not as food. Mushrooms grow in the dark, thriving on decaying matter. Like you, they are what they eat. They are a form of **fungus** which is very putrefactive in your gut. Raymond Rife discovered mushrooms were a natural cause of cancer and that cancer cells thrived in a mushroom medium.[1] The common **white mushrooms** in grocery stores are one of the most highly **chemicalized** plant foods available.[2] The common cultivated mushroom contains the carcinogen, **para-hydrazinobenzoic acid**, at a level of 10 ppm.

38. **Hydrazines** are abundant in edible mushrooms. Many hydrazine compounds are carcinogens. Cooking reduces the amount hydrazines in mushrooms. The three most commonly eaten mushrooms are the **False Morel**, the common **Cultivated Mushroom** (Agaricus bisporus) and the **Shiitake Mushroom**. All contain large amounts of hydrazines. The False Morel mushroom is edible in some areas; deadly in other areas. It contains **gyromitrin**, which the body breaks down into **monomethylhydrazine**, a compound similar to what is used in rocket fuel. The **shiitake mushroom** and **common cultivated mushroom** both contain **agaritine**, another hydrazine, at a level of 300 mg/ 100 g portion (3,000 ppm). A metabolic product of agaritine has been shown to be mutagenic to bacteria and highly carcinogenic.

39. Many **herbs** are toxic if ingested in too large dosages. Many herbs are **natural poisons** which are beneficial when properly used. Medicinal herbs are drug-containing plants which should not be used everyday. Like other drugs, medicinal herbs have side effects, toxic effects, allergenic effects, as well as therapeutic effects. Many medicines are **extracts** of "active ingredients" of herbs and plants. Examples of harmful substances in herbs: **Comfrey** (a hybrid plant) has **aloin** and **pyrrolizidine**, both known to help cause hepatitis. Heavy use of **Ginseng** can cause elevated blood pressure, skin eruptions and adverse hormonal effects.[3] **Sassafras** contains **safrole**, which causes liver cancer in rodents, and makes up 75% of oil of sassafras.

1) Lynes, 51, 52.   2) Gagne, 205.   3) Canning, ES, 22.

40. *Pyrrolizidine alkaloids* are present in many **herbal teas** and traditional **herbal remedies**. These natural chemicals are often carcinogenic, mutagenic, teratogenic (capable of causing birth defects) and chronically toxic. Pyrrolizidine alkaloids form irreversible "cross-links" with DNA, thereby preventing cell division. Human diseases such as liver cirrhosis (scarring of the liver) and liver cancer are linked to consumption of plants containing these alkaloids. *Pyrrolizidine alkaloids* are present in hundreds of **plant species,** and at very high levels—as much as 5 percent of the plant's dry weight. But don't dismay; you can still have your herbal tea and drink it too. For the most part, herb teas are relatively safe; if they were not, there would be many poisoning cases reported. Reports of adverse reactions to herbs are few. *Moderation* generally ensures safety. Almost any substance can be toxic in large enough doses.

41. Liver toxicity has been linked with a number of **herbal teas.** *Tannins* in tea, including ordinary tea and peppermint tea, are surface irritants to the gastrointestinal tract and have been linked to cancer of the esophagus and stomach. Adding milk (preferably, raw milk) to the tea binds the *plant tannins* and may protect the digestive tract from irritant effects. Paradoxically, some tannins are anti-carcinogenic and also beneficial.

42. **Comfrey** is a popular herb because of its supposed universal healing properties. It is sold in both, healthfood stores and supermarkets. Its leaves and roots are used to make teas and compress pastes to treat a variety of external and internal diseases. Numerous vegetarian recipes call for comfrey leaves to make soufflés, salads and breads. Unfortunately, comfrey is potentially liver-toxic because it contain as many as nine *pyrrolizidine alkaloids*, known to cause liver diseases in humans and cancer /bladder tumors in rats. Comfrey leaves and roots contain up to 0.29 percent pyrrolizidine alkaloids such as *intermedine, lycopsamine, symphytine* and others. Comfrey's well-demonstrated reported toxicity and carcinogenicity is such a major cause for concern that the governments of four European countries (Australia, Canada, Britain, Germany) either restrict comfrey's availability or have banned its sale entirely.

43. *And what about* **fruit** *–do they contain natural toxins?* Hardly. The amount of natural toxins in fruit is far less than found in vegetables. Fruit are vastly safer than vegetables or any other plantfood.

Despite their natural poisons, vegetables have many benefits

While vegetables are very poor in our primary need, *glucose*, they are very rich in our other major nutritional needs: proteins, carbohydrates, fiber, minerals and vitamins. They also contain many anti-oxidants, anti-carcinogens, nucleic acids, live enzymes, paciferans (plant antibiotics), fatty acids, chlorophyll, carotenoids, and other goodies. Apparently for the most part, **it is the *COOKING* of vegetables (organic or not) that *really* makes them toxic** (beyond their natural toxicity), hence rendering them even more of a drugfood.

Most of the cultivated plant foods we eat have less natural toxins than their progenitor wild counterparts. For example, the wild potato *Solanum Acaule*, progenitor of cultivated potatoes, has a toxic glycoalkaloid content about 3 times that of cultivated strains. The leaves of the wild cabbage *Brassica oleracea* (progenitor of cabbage, broccoli, cauliflower) contain twice as many toxic glucosinolates as cultivated cabbage. The wild bean *Phaseolus lunatus* contains 3 times as many toxic cyanogenic glucosides as the cultivated bean. Similar reduced toxicity through agriculture has been reported in lettuce, lima bean, mango, and cassava. **People that eat abundantly of fresh fruit and vegetables rarely, if ever, get cancer. This is true even though the very vegetables they eat contain many natural chemicals that are carcinogenic to rats (in high doses).** But we don't eat "high doses" of vegetables (though we do eat "high doses" of starches –and yes, this causes its own set of problems, later addressed). The "most striking carcinogen" ever discovered through "rodent carcinogenicity studies" is excesssive calorie intake or over-eating. In other words, overfed rats get cancer more often than normally fed rats.

Usually, a healthy body is able to detoxify the natural poisons in vegetables if not eaten in excess; "excess" is for you to determine. In *Fresh Vegetable and Fruit Juices*, Dr. Norman Walker shows that the freshly squeezed JUICE of RAW vegetables (and fruits) have great healing powers. They regenerate the physical body. He tells you how to use specific combinations (formulas) of different vegetable/fruit juices to heal many diseases and restore the body's impaired functions back to normal. He was a health advocate who apparently lived what he preached, for he lived to be over 110 years old.

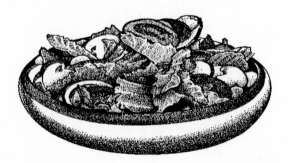

Natural toxins in Grains

1. **Grains** have to be <u>cooked</u> to make them edible. Raw grains contain large amounts of organic calcium and other minerals, which become *inorganic,* hence *insoluble* and toxic when <u>cooked</u>, These *inorganic minerals* of **cooked grains** slowly turn us to stone, ossifying our tissues, depositing out in our muscles, arteries and organs if we eat grains /starches often. Results include painful joints /muscles, arthritis, gallstones, kidney stones, varicose veins, and hemorrhoids.

2. *Alcohol* is made from fermenting **grains**. **Cooked grains** (starch) ferment quickly in the body, producing *alcohol*, *carbonic acid*, and other toxins. People who eat lots of starches (almost everyone) make their body into a distillery, producing alcohol. *"These vegetarians* [or starcharians] *are always in an auto-intoxicated state, to which their bodies have become so completely adjusted, that when the toxic effects begin to fade, an uncomfortable feeling appears in the sensations of hunger, weakness, nervousness, headache, etc."*[1]

3. Grains are *mold*-prone. *Mold* produces *mycotoxins*, some of the most toxic chemicals known. These include *ergot*, a fungus on grains such as **rye**, producing the most potent hallucinogen known, *LSD*.[2] Ergoted bread caused epidemics of madness and "Saint Anthony's Fire" in Europe.[3] *Gluten*, a component of wheat and rye, is a feast for yeasts, mold. All packaged breads, pasta contains mold, even if you can't see or smell it.

4. **Corn** is often contaminated with *fumonisins*, which are produced by the fungi in the genus Fusaria. Fumonisins are carcinogenic in animals and are thought to be a cause of human liver cancer in some parts of the world.

5. *Zearalenone* is an almost universal contaminant in corn. Other big sources are commercial **cereal grains, brown rice, popcorn** and **corn chips**. Also in **wheat, barley, oats, sorghum** and **soybeans**, particularly if these have been improperly stored. A toxin produced by Fusarium molds, **"zear"** has immune-lowering effects and it prevents you from detoxing deadly benzene. It is also carcinogenic to mice and has estrogenic activity; it causes over-estrogenization. Zear looks like *extra estrogen* to the body. In women, the effects include breast sensitivity, especially during menstruation (this is also conducive to breast lumps and breast cancer). Over-estrogenized women are over-emotional and often develop a high pitched, almost squeaky voice. In exposed female animals, zearalenone causes vaginal prolapse, swollen vulva and mammae and enlargement of the uterus. Men and boys are affected too; it affects the male maturing process. It also causes signs of feminization, such as shrunken testicles and enlarged nipples.

1) Hotema, MHC, lesson 13/page 21. 2) Cummings, 23. 3) Ibid. 4) Murray, 223. 5) Nelson, MYN, 66.

6. **Wheat, rice, oats, barley** and most **cereal grains** have naturally occurring *estrogen* (female hormone) which, when concentrated and cooked into bread and such, can cause problems with male sexuality.

7. Traces of natural *cyanide compounds*, mostly *beneficial vitamin B17 (laetrile)* are found in **millet, corn** and **sorghum.**

8. *Gluten* is a protein component in **wheat, rye** and **barley**. Gluten is a toxin causing many problems including schizophrenia and coeliac disease (intestinal malabsorption). Gluten has been linked to thyroid abnormalities, psychiatric disturbances, diabetes, hives and increased cancer risk.[4] Gluten components have *opioid* (opium-like) activity.[4] *Gluten* and *bran* are indigestible to humans and mucus-forming. GLUten makes an effective *glue*, which glues us too. Other problems include excess mucus clogging the respiratory and digestive tracts, sinus congestion, asthma, headaches and constipation. **Buckwheat** and **millet** also contain *antigenic elements* similar to wheat gluten. *(Papain, the papaya's protein-digesting enzyme, digests gluten, allowing some people to tolerate gluten, plus renders gluten harmless in coeliac disease).*

9. Americans eat too much **starch**! Regularly eating a lot of starch (**bread, cereals, grains, pasta, pastry, gravy**, etc.) can create mineral deficiency because starches bind certain minerals in the body, making them unavailable.

10. *Phytate (phytic acid)* is found in **wholegrains (wheat, rye, oats, rice,** etc.) and **beans**. Phytate inhibits and impairs absorption of calcium, iron and zinc. Phytate binds calcium and magnesium in the diet, making them unavailable for absorption. It combines with calcium, forming an *insoluble salt*, preventing calcium absorption.[5] Healthy intestines allegedly produces an enzyme which neutralizes this, but *healthy* intestines are rare in a population of drugfood eaters! *Phytate* is mainly in the **bran portion** of grains. **Wheat bran** has over 80% of the phytate present in the whole grain. Although **wheat bran** lowers mucus in the stools, it does so at the expense of creating more mucus in other parts of the body.[1] The phytate in wholemeal flour has been related to the negative calcium balance that develops in people living largely on wholemeal bread.

11. **Grains** are high in *lectins*, key culprits in allergies. In susceptible individuals with a high grain intake, lectins create intestinal degeneration which can result in Coeliac or Chron's disease, Inflammatory Bowel disease, multiple sclerosis, systemic lupus erythmatus, and other diseases.

1) Gray, CH, 41.

Why are all grains harmful?

- **Grains have to be <u>cooked</u> just to make them <u>edible</u>.** If we have to cook a food to make it edible, that food is not for us to eat! Grains have large amounts of minerals which become inorganic /toxic when cooked.
- **Regular consumption <u>hardens the tissues and joints</u>, plus results in**:[1]
arthritis	gallstones	kidney stones	heart problems
tumors	diabetes	hemorrhoids	varicose veins
- **The reason for the above:** When any starch is cooked, its calcium becomes insoluble inorganic calcium (like that in cement) which your body cannot use. This clogs your system, and if your body is not able to excrete it, it dumps it wherever convenient, such as the gallbladder (resulting in gallstones); kidneys (hence kidney stones); dead-ends of blood vessels in the abdomen /anus (resulting in tumors /hemorrhoids).
- **Are <u>mucus forming</u> and <u>acidic</u> in the body** (except for millet). This results in sinus congestion, excess mucus in the respiratory & digestive tracts, asthma, headaches, and constipation (promoting colon cancer).
- **Cooked cereals causes nervous afflictions** due to its high content of inorganic sulfur and phosphorous.[2]
- **Grains are high in dietary lectins**, which can trigger toxic food reactions (allergies) from the immune system. Lectins are responsible for numerous health disorders and diseases, depending on your blood type.
- **When we eat starch**, our body must convert it to glucose before it can absorb it. **We have only one starch-splitting enzyme, *ptyalin*,** whereas true starch eaters have many starch-splitting enzymes.
- **Of all plant foods, grains are most often associated with food allergies,** especially wheat and corn.
- **Promotes calcium deficiency and tooth decay.**
- **Are the most constipating of foods.**
- **Gluten**, a protein component in wheat /rye /barley is indigestible to humans. It makes an effective glue. It will glue you too.
- **Bran** (tough coating of grains) is also indigestible to humans.
- **Wholegrains (especially bran portion) are high in phytate**. Phytate blocks or impairs absorption of calcium, magnesium, iron and zinc.
- **Mold is common in grains, producing** mycotoxins (mold poisons), some of the most toxic chemicals known. All <u>packaged</u> starches (bread, cold cereals, pasta, brown rice, etc.) contain mycotoxins.
- **Cooked starches quickly ferment in your body** in the presence of heat and moisture, producing harmful alcohol, carbonic acid gas and other poisons, especially if eaten with sugars or proteins. People who eat lots of starches (almost everyone) have made their body into a distillery, constantly producing alcohol.

1) Walker, FV, 33-34, 47.   2) Ibid., 60.

Why are vegetables harmful?

- **Most vegetables contain natural poisons** (see earlier pages).
- **Like grains, vegetables are not the natural food of Humanity.**
- **The majority of vegetables are unnatural.** They are cultivated and not found naturally growing in the wild (see earlier pages). Additionally, **they are hybrid and genetically altered,** even the organic ones in healthstores. **Many species did not exist a hundred years ago.** Very few of the plants which humans eat would have been present in an Afrikan hunter-gatherer's diet. Our diet, as humans, has drastically changed in the last few thousand years. Most humans are eating many recently introduced plants that our ancestors did not eat (potatoes, tomatoes, corn, cassava, coffee, cocoa, tea, mangoes, olives, kiwi, cabbage, broccoli, kale, cauliflower, mustard...).
- **Since most of the foods humans eat are** *new* **to our diet** –relative to our evolution on this planet– we have not had enough time to biologically adapt to them and evolve biological defenses for the natural toxins they contain. Natural selection works far too slowly for humans to have evolved specific resistance to the toxins in these newly introduced plants.
- **On top of all this, we COOK these foods, rendering them more toxic.** When cooked, the vast majority of vegetables become even more harmful; their organic minerals, compounds and other substances become perverted and inorganic, thus toxic. Therefore, reaching optimum health is a fantasy for the majority of us, while subhealth is normal and standard.

Recommendations for Better Health

- **DRINK your vegetables too!** Get a juicer (*Champion* brand is an excellent choice) and make /drink a large glass of fresh raw vegetable juice at least a few times a week. This is especially important if you mainly eat cooked food. Meat-eaters and vegetarians both need to do this! Marvel at how much better you WILL feel only after a short time.
- **Avoid or drastically cut back on eating the most toxic vegetables**
  – nightshade veggies: white potatoes, eggplant, tomatoes, bell peppers
  – the top-toxic twelve of commercially-grown veggies on pages149-150
  – cassava and mushrooms
- **Cut back drastically on eating grains /starches.** Yes, this might be a challenge! But try this anyway: for 7-10 days, completely abstain from eating any grain/starch food (breads, cereals, pastry, pasta, potatoes, gravies, etc.). At the end of this period, note the distinct difference in how you feel.
- **See the end of the next chapter for complete Recommendations.**

So What is Humanity's Proper Food?

Raw FRUIT, Humanity's perfect food and diet?

The highest food for Humanity to eat, and the food to which humans are best biologically adapted, is *Fruit*. Fruit is the most perfect food. It takes the least amount of energy to digest and gives your body the most in return. **Anatomically and physiologically, the Human is a fruit-eater (fruitarian, frugivore). The digestive system and the teeth of humans correspond in almost every detail with the teeth of gorillas and other fruit-eating animals** (monkeys, apes, lemurs, chimpanzees, orangutans, gibbons). Like other frugivores, humans have *alkaline* saliva which promotes carbohydrate digestion of fruit and starts the neutralization of the acids of fruits. However, the saliva of meat-eating animals (carnivores) is extremely acidic in order to digest concentrated protein and dissolve flesh with almost no chewing. **Anthropological findings indicate that humans were *exclusively* fruit eaters for millions of years.** Although we have become Veget-arians, Grain-arians, Flesh-arians, and Drugfood-arians, **we have biologically remained Fruit-arians**! No wonder we're in such a health mess! For most of the food we eat is unsuited to humans' biological adaptation. Though flesh and grains have been a diet of humans for a long time, this period is short compared to the millions of years of human existence.

- **We are not herbivores,**
  animals that feed mainly on grass and vegetation (cattle, horses, zebras, deer, goats, rabbits). We don't have the four stomachs herbivores usually have, nor the teeth and very long intestines. This rules out most herbiage as our diet.

- **We are not graminivores,**
  animals that feed mainly on grains (most birds). We have only one starch-splitting enzyme versus the numerous starch-splitting enzymes possessed by starch-eating animals. This rules out grains and grasses.

- **We are not carnivores,**
  animals that feed on flesh, blood, bones (tigers, lions, dogs, wolves, jackals). It is not our nature to kill and eat an animal while it is yet warm and bloody, to eat its heart, brains, organs, and blood as true carnivores do. True carnivores do not chew meat. For their hydrochloric acid is hundreds of times stronger and more concentrated than ours; and it would digest our hands quickly if swallowed whole. It also digests feathers, fur, cartilage, bone. Their rasping tongues also serve to tear flesh from bone, as compared to the smooth tongue of humans.

> **We do not require vegetables and grains in our diet. For if we eat sufficiently of (organically grown) fruit to meet our *caloric* needs, we will simultaneously meet all our needs for vitamins, minerals, proteins (amino acids), essential fatty acids, and other nutrients.**

The foods that are "naturally right" for humans to eat have great appeal –in their <u>natural state</u>– to *all* of our senses!

They look beautiful, smell good, feel good, and taste delicious. And they require little or no preparation. The foods humans are *not* supposed to eat do *not* have natural appeal to our senses; they have a repelling, bitter, or disagreeable taste, odor, appearance, etc., that would prevent people from eating them in their natural state. This is The Great Mother's way of protecting us –Her children, keeping harmful things out of our precious bodies so we may stay healthy. Unfortunately, we disregard this...and pay a penalty as the adverse effects catch up with us. If we have to put a food through extensive preparation, drastically altering its natural state, just to make it edible, then that food is not our natural food! –is not meant for us to eat! Examples: grains and beans (have to be cooked, seasoned); animals (have to be killed, skinned, de-feathered, dismembered, cooked, seasoned). But Fruit need only be picked off the tree and perhaps rinsed, then relished. Fruit, the food to which humans are biologically adapted, is relished in its natural raw ripe state like no other food in Nature.

Dr. Hibbs wrote:

"Grains are responsible for nearly all of man's disease, for wheat, barley, oats and rye are no more a part of his food than oranges the food of the cow, or grains the food of dogs and cats. Man's food consists of the fruit and nuts of the tree. They are beautifully wrapped and hung on trees where the common herd cannot get to them. Man is given hands with which to remove this food and its wrappings, and eat to his content and perfect health. ...The [Albino] medical profession dare not take a group of children and feed them according to Nature's law for a period of six months, and then truly publish the results."[1]

Dr. Abramowski wrote:

"Raw fruit diet supplies every want of the human body, and it is not only as nourishing and sustaining as the most expensive mixed diet, but it produces more energy and endurance, and is more easily assimilated, and is absolutely free from any dangerous matter." [2]

1) Hotema, MHC   2) Abramowski, 16..

Fruit is the BEST and RICHEST part of the Tree /plant

Now you know the true source of your "sweet tooth"!

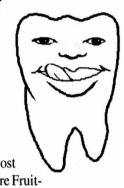

...and BEAUTIFUL and colorful like the *flowers* they developed from. Fruit has the highest concentration of nutrition that the plant produces. There are more varieties of Fruit than any other form of food. Over 300 edible varieties are known. Fruit is the natural gift of the plant, just for eating. Fruit (and milk) are the only foods that are *karma-free*. All other food involves killing, whether it be of animals, plants, or seed. The closer food is to Sun Energy, the higher it is in all levels of nutrition for humans. Plantfood, especially Fruit, is at the top of the nutritional scale. And Fruit grows in the *higher* atmosphere, literally closer to the Sun, on Trees. Animal food is at the bottom. Most animals are plant-eaters. The highest developed plant-eaters are Fruit-eaters and the highest developed Fruit-eater is the Human.

The craving for "sweets" is a craving for Love. Fruit is Love.

Food is really condensed SunLight. Light is our food. True Light is our true food. True Light is *Loving Light* or simply, *Love* –the original and perfect food, Humanity's truest food, which nourishes us like nothing else. The highest manifestation of Loving Light as food is *Fruit*, the edible form of Love. The highest and most perfect food for humans, *Hue*-mans. The most nourishing part of the Tree. The Tree itself expresses the essence of Heart, the *Connection and Balance Point.* Opposites connect and unify in the Tree, reaching deep down into Mother's dark Earth, and equally high up into Father's bright Heaven, connecting Heaven and Earth in a planetary Balance that sustains Nature and all life on Earth. Most Fruit grow on Trees. Fruit even comes in all the *Hues* or colors of the *Rainbow* ...which is *Light!* **The pure essence of Love is SWEETNESS.** No wonder Fruit is sweet! Sweetness is the primary quality of Fruit...and Love. The root of the word **FRU**it (fer/fru/fre as in <u>fri</u>end) means Love! Sweet *glucose* is the brain's only food. You see, we are supposed to be living off Sweetness. And we do, except it's the wrong sweetness: White Sugar. The #1 drug to which the whole world is addicted. Sweet sugar. Deadly sugar. **Thus, the desire and craving for Sugar ("sweets") is a craving for LOVE! White Sugar is false love! Counterfeit love.** See how the addiction to Sugar is pointing to Humanity's need and craving for one basic thing: LOVE? The foremost nutrient we need the most but get the LEAST! No wonder the world is the way it is. We settle for counterfeit love. False love. Sugar. The Drug. Lie. Deception. Death. Humanity's *Return To Fruit* as our main nourishment is our return to our Long Lost Love.

"Then God [Goddess] said, 'I give you every seed-bearing plant on the face of the whole earth and **every tree that has fruit with seed in it. They will be yours for food**. And to all the beasts of the earth and all the birds of the air and all the creatures that move on the ground –everything that has the breath of life in it —I give every green plant for food." (Gen. 1:29, 30 NI translation) "Now the Lord God had **planted a garden in the east,** in Eden; and there he **put the man he had formed**. And the Lord God made all kinds of trees grow out of the ground —**trees that were pleasing to the eye and good for food**. (Gen. 2:8, 9 NI translation)

Sweet Properties of Raw Fruit (organically grown)

- **Fruit, Humanity's natural diet, has great appeal to the senses:** it is beautiful to the eye, pleasant to smell, and sweet to taste.
- **Fruit is the easiest food to digest.** It takes the least amount of energy to digest while giving your body the most in return.
- **When ripe, fruit is in a predigested state.** Thus fruit digests in 10 to 30 minutes –in the small intestines, *not* the stomach, from which it passes within minutes of ingestion. Contrast this with meat and fat which takes 3-5 hours just to pass out the stomach.
- **Fruit is the only food which does not introduce toxins into the body,** nor produces such while passing through.
- **Fruit is clean, pure, hygienic in its natural peel.**
- **Fruit is food and drink at the same time; it satisfies hunger and also thirst.** It is most often 90-95% water. Therefore, it cleanses as it nourishes.
- **The only food your brain can work on is glucose.** Fruit is primarily fructose, which is easily converted into glucose.
- **Fruit contains bioflavonoids** (also known as vitamin P), which keep the blood from thickening and plugging up the arteries. It also strengthens the capillaries, and weak capillaries often lead to internal bleeding and heart attacks.
- **Citrus fruit is essentially a total anti-cancer package** because it possess every class of natural substances (carotenoids, flavonoids, terpenes, limonoids, coumarins) that neutralize chemical carcinogens. One analysis found that citrus fruit possess 58 known anti-cancer compounds, more than any other food!
- **The citrus peels** are also one of the highest sources of pectin which has been proven to remove heavy metals (lead, mercury, cadmium, etc.) from the body. It even removes radioactive contamination like strontium-90.

Advantages & Benefits of a Rawfood, Fruitarian diet

- **True, radiant health and abundant vitality and energy**, even in "old age."
- **The absence of sickness and disease,** hence no more medical bills and buying medicines, drugs. Rawfood is therapeutic and prevents disease.
- **You rejuvenate,** grow younger, more beautiful, live much longer. Your hair stops falling out –might even grow back and stop graying.
- **Rawfood rebuilds the regenerative force** of the total organism. The higher the percentage of fruit /rawfood we eat, the slower the rate of tissue degeneration.
- **Euphoria.** Feeling good. Being "high" becomes your natural state, like children.
- **Superior nutrition.** Raw, living foods contain all the nutritive elements in the right proportion and balance, and is easier to digest than the same food cooked.
- **Drinking water is not necessary** on a fruitarian diet. You won't feel thirsty, even after strenuous exercises.
- **Greatly increased strength,** endurance, and muscle tone without exercising.
- **No fatigue,** even with strenuous activity. Said one fruitarian: *"I surprised myself...when I swam hundreds of meters...a high speed – after not having swum for years – without even being short of breath at the end of the race."*
- **You feel better, lighter,** more energized, happier, and youthful.
- **You need much less sleep,** and you sleep better, wake up alert and energetic.
- **You will stay clean on the inside,** for fruit /raw plantfood is a cleansing diet.
- **A purified body;** offensive body odor and bad breath disappears. On a *fruit* diet, even your feces smell sweet, and you won't even need toilet paper! You become "sweet" and clean as the fruit you eat.
- **Your food bill cut** at least in half, saving you money.
- **You'll no longer be a "kitchen slave"** –bound to your stove.
- **Raw foods are easier to prepare and** much easier to clean up after: no greasy dirty skillets, pots, pans, dishes, etc.
- **You achieve the normal weight** Nature intended for you; if overweight you lose, if underweight you gain. Obesity vanishes steadily, painlessly, effortlessly.
- **You needn't worry** about putting on weight unnaturally; live foods are not fattening, not even bananas & avocados.
- **No swings from "high" to "low"** –as experienced on a drugfood diet of stimulants (sugar, coffee, coke...) & depressants (heavy rich foods, overeating).
- **Your menstrual flow becomes clear, bloodless,** decreasing in length, taking minutes instead of days. Menstruation and menopausal problems disappear.
- **You can become pregnant** –when you had given up.
- **Painless, easy childbirth.**
- **You will be able to safely suckle your young,** producing abundant milk rich in all necessary nutrients and free of toxins.
- **Your spermcount doubles** (unless you smoke).

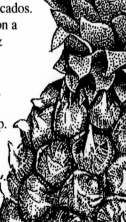

- **Increased mental clarity and inner peace.**
- **Your sight, hearing and senses sharpen.**
- **More LOVE in your home. Great improvement spiritually.**
- **You feel closer to Goddess /God.**
- **You become a Super Being. Your body *TRANSFORMS*,** becoming more alive, sensitive, and cosmically/spiritually *connected* (described later).

Nuts are part of the fruitarian diet

Nuts are single-seeded *fruits* with hard, inedible coatings, according to botanists. Nuts grow on trees. The only true nuts are acorns, sweet chestnuts, hazelnuts and beechnuts, –all belonging to the Fagales family of trees. The other things we call nuts (almonds, walnuts, filberts, pecans...) are seeds or relatives of various fruit trees. Nuts and seeds provide concentrated nutrition. They are very high in protein and polyunsaturated oil. They have a wide variety of vitamins and minerals, plus starches, sugars, etc. Like other protein foods, nuts are acid-forming (except for coconuts). Nuts supply everything we can get from fleshfood, in much better form, better condition, cleaner, more easily used, and without risk of eating diseased flesh. Nut protein is easily assimilated and does not form uric acid. Eat all nuts raw. They are tastier, healthier, and easier to digest in their raw state, than when roasted and salted. Nuts can take up to 3 hours to digest. When *soaked* and *sprouted*, many of their nutrients are increased and the nuts, seeds, (and grains) become easier to digest. Their naturally occurring inhibitors of digestive enzymes – are washed away, and their proteins, fats, complex carbohydrates become predigested into free amino / fatty acids, and simpler carbohydrates.

It's best to eat nuts (and seeds) in *moderation*, *–small* quantities. To ensure freshness and flavor, buy nuts in their shells and do your own cracking. The best seeds are hemp, sunflower, pumpkin, sesame, and flax. A problem with nuts is mold. (Instructions for demolding shelled nuts are later in this chapter) **And all nuts are high in anti-cancer compounds.** For example, almonds contain laetrile, an effective cancer-killer. Kernels of many stoneseed fruit contain laetrile, especially apricot pits. In eating such, one must be judicious and not consume more than what one consumed if they ate the whole fruit (for many seeds also contain natural toxic compounds). One herbalist recommended taking 4 or so apricot kernels and 2 pieces of dried apricots.

Is an all-fruit diet unhealthy?
The charges against fruits are baseless

In *"I Live On Fruit,"* the fruitarian authors Essie Honiball and T.C. Fry show that the charges made against the fruitarian diet are baseless. I recommend their book if you are considering changing to a fruitarian diet. It will quell your fears about the safety and sufficiency of an all-fruit diet. It presents *"proof that the fruitarian diet is not only nutritionally adequate in every respect to sustain life, but is actually superior to any and all other foods for humans!"* Following is a summary of selected charges made against fruits and fruit-eaters, and rebuttals to these charges:

Charge 1: Fruits are protein poor:

Only when unfairly compared with high protein food. Protein content in food is relevant only to our protein need. Fruit amply supplies our need for protein; almost every fruit has more amino acids (protein) than we actually need.[1] Many fruit have the same percentage of "complete protein" as mother's milk.[2] And, as any **fruitarian GORILLA proves, fruit protein builds big strong bodies!** When ripe, fruit is in a predigested state. Its "protein" is ready-to-absorb amino acids. Its fats are simple fatty acids – monoglycerides and glycerol. Remember, the body recycles 90% of its protein from its own protein wastes. Thus the much touted requirement of 70-100 grams of protein a day is a meat-and-dairy-industry-fostered myth. Our actual protein needs are only 20-30 grams per day (one ounce = 28.35 grams). "When we've eaten some 2,250 calories worth of almost any fruit except apples, we've also ingested some 25 to 40 grams of protein."[3] Relatively speaking, a human adult does <u>not</u> need more protein than a human baby, yet human milk is only 1.1% protein (about 7.5% by dry weight) for a fast-growing baby. Watermelon contains 7% protein by dry weight! Protein only needs to be about 5% of a food's dry weight to meet our needs. Most fruit adequately meet this need.[4]

Charge 2: Fruit eaters cannot maintain weight and are too thin.

<u>Gorillas are fruitarians</u>. They grow much larger and heavier than humans! Earth's biggest animals are plant eaters. Initially, on a fruitarian diet or even a vegetarian diet, one loses weight as the body cleanses and adjusts. Then one begins to gain weight again. When you eat living foods you don't have to worry about putting on weight unnaturally. Live foods are not fattening. If you are overweight, you lose weight automatically; if underweight, you gain –to the norm Nature intended for you.

1) Honiball, 103.   2) Cousens, CE, 177.   3) Honiball, 92. 4) Ibid., 104.

Charge 3:
An all-fruit diet causes nutritional deficiencies /imbalances:

False! Eaten judiciously, fruits amply supply us with all the nutrients we need, known and unknown.

● **Fruit amply supplies all the vitamins we need**
–in their best form– many times beyond our need when we have met our caloric requirements. "If we took all our vitamin requirements quantitatively for a whole year, all of them together in their pure form would not fill a thimble. Commercial interests have vastly overblown and misrepresented our vitamin situation in order to perpetrate a profitable fraud upon us." [1]

More fallacies:
– Fruit is said to be deficient in calcium. This is false, for calcium composes every gram of fruit food.
– Fruit are charged as being too poor in iron and causing anemia. This is false, for the body recycles 95% of its iron and needs very little iron from outside. Most anemic people are meat eaters!
– Fruit are charged as being poor in vitamin B12. Review the B12 section under *Fractionated Nutrients*. Like all other plant-eating animals, we get ample B12 from bacterial production in our intestines and other places.

● **Fruit amply supplies the organic minerals we need.**
"Fruits contain ample mineral salts. The RDA's for minerals are several times our actual needs. Even so, all the RDA's added together do not amount to eight grams daily. A day's supply of watermelon contains some 24 grams of minerals, about three times our need. Peeled oranges also contain about 24 grams when 2,000 calories are taken."

● **Fruit supplies our fatty acid needs**.
Nutritional science teaches we must get three fatty acids from our diet (linolenic, linoleic, and arachidonic). Today, only linoleic is said to be essential. They are contained amply in fruit! Our total fat need from our diet is less than 1%.[2] Fruit adequately supplies this. For example, watermelon contains about 16 grams of fat when eaten to the extent of our caloric needs for a day. That amounts to some 3-4% of intake.

Charge 4:
Fruit, especially dried fruit, have too much sugar.

90% of our nutrient requirements are for monosaccharides or simple sugars for energy. Until this need is met, it's ridiculous to cry "too much sugar." Sugar in fruits comes to us predigested, hence cannot be beyond our digestive capacity no matter how much fruit you eat. Starch (grain food), a "complex carbohydrate," must be cooked before eating; heating dextrinizes starches. Our body converts dextrinized starches to the simple sugar of glucose, hence we're back where we started. **Only dextrinized starches ferment in the digestive tract, intoxicating us. Raw, uncooked sugars are not fermentable until they have been oxidized**.[3] The body has ample opportunity to absorb them long before oxidation will have occurred in normal digestion.

1) Honiball/Fry, 104.   2) Ibid., 105..   3) Ibid., 97

Charge 5:
Those who live on fruit become neurotics.

This has never been substantiated. To the contrary, all neurotic psychotic people eat typical drugfood diets like most people; none are fruitarians! If they became fruitarians, they would undoubtedly heal and become sane! European psychologists do not recognize the physical bases of neuroses; they give credence almost completely to emotional, social, economic and mental factors. The ancient Afrikans did not separate the mind, body, spirit and soul, but understood that all are intimately and inseparably connected. A toxic body adversely affects its mind. Purified bodies however, suffer neither mental nor physical disturbances. The people of fruit-eating societies had the most peaceable, congenial and harmonious dispositions of any peoples on Earth.

Charge 6:
Fruits have too many free acids.

Fruits (lemons, grapefruit, sour grapes, plums...) have no "free" acids, only organic acids. Vinegar, cheese and fermented milks have free acids (acetic, lactic acids). Humans metabolize most fruit acids very well (main ones: citric, tartaric, malic acid). The acids which give us metabolic problems (benzoic, tannic, oxalic, prussic), none of which are free acids, are rarely found in fruit. Eating acid fruits incompatibly with other foods or even with sweet fruit (bananas, dates, persimmons) can cause discomfort. Also, acid fruits excel at stirring up stored toxins to be eliminated; this too may cause discomfort. Acids which are the *end product of metabolism* can be eliminated ONLY after they are changed to neutral salts, then they are no longer harmful to the kidneys and intestine walls.[1]

Charge 7:
Fruit eaters become over-alkaline and suffer alkalosis.

This is baseless. Humans readily, harmlessly excrete excess alkaline substances, but have great difficulty handling acid end-products. Acid products must first be neutralized by alkaline minerals before excretion, otherwise our eliminatory organs (especially kidneys, liver) will be damaged. With an abundance of acid in our diet (from flesh/protein foods, grains), the body robs from its bones, teeth and other alkaline structures for the alkalis, mostly calcium, necessary to neutralize the acids from acid-forming foods. Fresh fruits are alkaline-forming in every case. (The acid-forming exceptions are *cooked* or *unripened* fruit, *dried /sulphured* fruit, and prunes/plums.)

Our natural foods need to be predominantly alkaline in metabolic reaction for our acid-generating metabolism. Fruit accomplishes this. Acid and alkaline elements are present in all foods. Body balance (homeostasis) in humans requires an alkaline pH for our acidic metabolic end products.

1) Aihara, 10.

Shivapuri Baba
A 112 Year Old Fruitarian

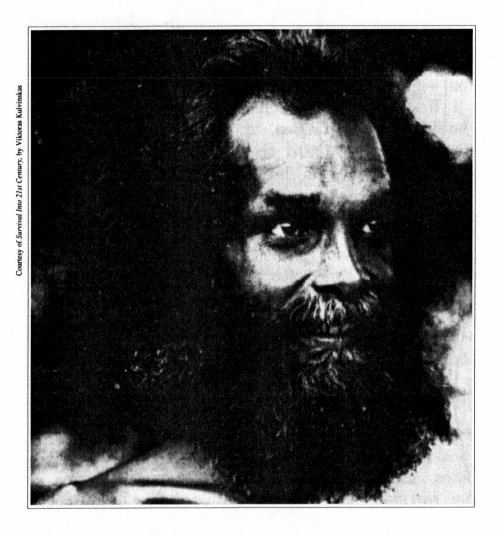

Courtesy of Survival Into 21st Century, by Viktoras Kulvinskas

Shivapuri Baba at the age of 112 years.
A fruitarian for at least 20 years, in India,
he died at age 135.*

* Kulvinskas, STC, 123.

"Changes" and *Transformations* you may go through when you "go raw" or Fruitarian

When toxic people go on a rawfood or fruitarian diet, at first they will likely experience "cleansing reactions" as their body evicts years of accumulated filth, waste, mucus, pus, toxins, pesticides, additives, etc. In a toxic body, the organic fluid of fruit dissolves old waste

> **"But eating fruit gives me diarrhea! Why?"**
> It's cleaning you out! –stirring up the cleansing process of your body.

deposits and stored chemicals, dumping them into the bloodstream (and colon) for elimination. As a result, you feel cleansing reactions. While toxins are being eliminated, one might suffer cleansing reactions of tiredness, weakness, irritableness, dizziness, headaches, nausea, vomiting, pimples, rashes, itching, puffy eyes, mucus-coated tongue, stankness, discharge of foul fluids, symptoms of sickness, and other discomforts. Rejoice! Don't give up because of these symptoms. They signify a massive housecleansing. Your body is detoxifying, going into a catabolic stage (thus causing drastic weight loss), **repairing and rebuilding itself.** *If things get too uncomfortable, you can slow down the detoxifying process –by eating cooked foods– in order to reduce discomforts and escape some of the more intense crisis that can occur.* The *gradual* approach is definitely best and recommended, the older you are. Weight gain comes after detoxification is more or less complete. Gradually, any symptoms or cleansing reactions clear up as the body purges on this purifying diet.

Will one be able to keep up strength on rawfood or fruitarian diets?

Initially, a fruitarian or rawfood diet may seem inadequate to supply strength (unless you move into this diet *gradually,* since you are a *recovering* drugfood addict!) ...because digesting this light food does not form **uric acid** and other toxins to saturate the body and act as **stimulants**. As you clean out, you become increasingly stronger, much stronger than you ever were.

At the beginning why does one feel hungry/weak a lot on a rawfood diet?

Some people think it's because the body has been starved for so long for living foods, thus just can't get enough. They call this a **hangover** or "hangover deficiency disease" from having lived on dead foods for so long. While this is largely true, I think it's also equally due to another reason: The body has been used to functioning on a low vibration several octaves down. With the introduction of raw vegetables and fruit, the body gradually begins to "vibe up." At first, the body is not used to operating on finer /higher vibratory food; it's used to coarse toxic vibrations. Plus, the body is still literally composed of substances from inferior toxic drugfoods. Further, it is loaded with toxins. So as the body's existing molecules are replaced with molecules from the finer, more superior (i.e., raw, live, organic, pure, natural) food, correspondingly, its vibrations are raised. This compares with being used to loud deafening noises for a long time then suddenly having very soft harmonious musical sounds. At first you almost can't hear them. Then as your ears adapt, you begin to hear these soft sounds in all their subtle richness. Another comparison: it's like being at a movie theater and getting used to the dark, then suddenly exiting the theater directly into the bright sun light. You squint, becoming temporarily near-blind until your eyes adjust.

Likewise, the drugfood-nourished body is adapting, going from low-vibe-dead-drugfood to high-vibration-living-rawfood. Literally more light (lifeforce energy of live food) is entering the body. Literally, vibrations of real musical harmony are entering too, for the *molecule* vibrations of livefood are beautiful complex symphonies. (in contrast to the cacophonous, discordant *noise* of cooked food molecules).

Thus, a GRADUAL change to a rawfood diet is best for most people. (If you prefer to speed things up, add fasting to your regime). Most meat-eaters need about 1 or 2 years to transition to a vegetarian diet (containing cooked food). Transitioning to a rawfood diet may take slightly longer. A gradual changeover gives the body (and mind and soul) time to adjust and adapt to the higher, healthier, *(w)holier* way. **Gradually replace cooked dead food with raw live food,** with the ultimate goal of becoming largely a Fruitarian. As you achieve this, you will increasingly have abundant strength, far more than you had before, and it will astound you. Case examples include Dick Gregory, Mahatma Ghandi, Arnold Ehret and numerous others.

> **Fruit for Thought**
> There is a relationship between the fact that eating food produces stimulation (see page 166), and that fruit (a naturally predigested food) digests in the small intestines –not in the stomach where everything else digests, breaks down. Eating fruit, especially with a purified body and colon, produces very little stimulation compared with eating any other food. Humans have become used to the unnatural stimulation from their unnatural diet in a world increasingly being made unnatural.

The Great Purge Happens

As a person continues their rawfood diet, especially if they also do periodic fasting, their body detoxifies at increasingly deeper and deeper levels. And at some point (perhaps after 1-3 years) they will experience a special Great Purging, though they think that by now they are clean. The Purge may happen more than once. When the Great Purge happens, huge amounts of mucus and other nasty stuff are quickly expelled from the body, often making the person feel very sick just prior to the purge. Afterwards, the person feels a vast, unbelievable surge in energy and vitality. When it happened to Arnold Ehret (who had been on a rawfood diet for a while, before vomiting –after generously eating of grapes /grapejuice), he did 326 knee-bending /arm-stretching exercises consecutively. He relates this in his books: *Mucusless Healing Diet System* and *Rational Fasting*.

Your body *TRANSFORMS*, becoming more alive, sensitive, literally *RADIANT*, and cosmically *connected*.

As your rawfood /fruitarian diet continues, (along with periodic fasting and colon cleansing) your body's organs began to work differently –the way they were intended! – not the compromised way they presently have to work under their toxic heavy load of degenerate drugfood. Your body is repatterning itself. In time, your body's deeper faculties and unused organs slowly awaken; like infants learning to walk for the first time. Your body goes through a *Transformation*, a *Rebirth*. You begin functioning at a higher octave(s). Thus, your body slowly begins responding differently to the physical laws. For example, in cold weather you may remain warm even if you're wearing no coat. In hot weather, you may remain cool and comfortable though people around you are sweating. Gravity does not "pull" on you as hard, hence you feel so *light*. You'll be able to do strenuous physical activity and not get tired. You won't even need to "exercise" in order to stay fit. Your aura gets brighter and brighter. In fact, you may sometimes literally glow a radiance that can be physically seen by others. Afrikan and Indian "holy people" have done this. White-but-well-tanned Arnold Ehret did it too. (Remember, the Human Body is electrical and has a mild electric current covering it.) You become conscious of your connection with the Cosmos (Universe) and cosmic rays. The cleaner your body becomes (internally), the higher the cosmic energy vibrations available to your brain. You may sometimes even hear the beautiful, exquisite, legendary "music of the spheres." The genius within you awakens. You effortlessly have insights into the nature of Life, your Self, and the Cosmos –easily "tuning in" to higher knowledge, awareness, answers. You become one with Mother Nature, living constantly in a natural "high." You become more conscious of your connection to God/dess. The Temple of your precious Body becomes a true *joy* to live in, as was meant to be by our Divine Parents (Goddess, God).

Encouragement

Nothing worth striving for is free of frustration, including the rawfood or fruitarian diet. The process of Rebuilding and Rebirth is joyful, but not necessarily easy. So do not be discouraged if things do not immediately get right; or if changes in health are not immediately apparent. Lasting improvement is the result of patient and persistent following of the new way of living. Happy is the person who knows the art of starting again after each defeat.

Precautions for an all-fruit diet

● **Fruitarians may need to eat
greens if they live in polluted environments.**

*"Although fruit is the food best adapted to human digestion, a diet limited to
fruit would make the city dweller's organism too sensitive to the damaging
effects of air pollution. If you live in the unhealthful environment of polluted
cities, you will continue to need greens. However, once you move to the higher
altitudes of subtropical mountains, or...take residence in a warmer climate away
from polluted areas, you no longer need greens."*[1]

● **Drink freshly squeezed vegetable juice often?**

According to Dr. Norman Walker, raw-fresh vegetable juices are a necessary
supplement to **every diet**, even when no special diet is followed and especially
when individuals eat any and everything they please. **Even if one is a
rawfooder, they still need the fresh juices**. Why? Because a large percentage
of the atoms making up rawfood nourishment is used up as fuel by the digestive
organs in the process of digesting /assimilating the food, which usually requires
as long as 3-5 hours after every meal. This leaves only a small percentage
available for nourishing and regenerating the cells /tissues. **But when we drink
raw vegetable juices, they are digested and assimilated within 10-15 minutes
after drinking them, and are used almost entirely in the nourishment and
regeneration of the cells, tissues, organs.**[2]

● **Be careful of over-consuming acid fruit.**

*"A diet with emphasis on citrus and pineapple can dissolve any fruitarian. One
purchases in the city inorganic fruit in an unripened state which is embalmed
with chemicals. Even when organic, the fruit is generally picked unripe and has
gone through nutritional losses due to the timelapse between the harvest and the
time of eating. These highly acid fruit will inactivate some of the hemoglobin,
produce gum bleeding and dissolve teeth."*[3]

● **A salt-free *vegetarian* diet may not be safe.**

Sodium (and other minerals) are apparently deficient in the cultivated and
genetically altered unnatural vegetables and fruit grown by humans (even if
organically grown). Therefore, *"because fruits and vegetables are near salt-
free, such a raw vegetarian diet will create an anemic condition and other salt-
starvation diseases. This often triggers strong cravings for salted snack foods,
or for rare meat as fresh killed animals –that have retained some urine and
blood– are not there to provide the needed salt. ..A case in point is a well-
known author of several books who advocates vegetarianism but no salt as well.
She was often observed backstage eating rare steaks right after lecturing on the
merits of vegetarian raw foods on the speaker's platform."*[4] Spinach, celery,
beets, lemons, strawberries, and Celtic salt are healthy sources of sodium.

1) Kulvinskas, STC. 2) Walker, FV, 15. 3) Kulvinskas, STC, 104. 4) de Langre, 30, 31.

● Avoiding mold-toxins and rancidity in Nuts and Seeds

Many nuts are contaminated with mold-toxins, including aflatoxin, one of the most potent liver-cancer causing agents known. In experiments, levels of Aflatoxin B1 as low as 1ppb (part per billion) –fed continuously in the diet produced cancer in 100% of the poor rats tested.[1] A large dose (5 milligrams) given just once also caused cancer in rats. Aflatoxins are produced by molds on peanuts, Brazil nuts, pistachio nuts, almonds, walnuts, pecans, filberts (and corn, millet, grain sorghum, figs, cottonseed). Symptoms of aflatoxin ingestion includes loss of appetite, weight loss, jaundice, cirrhosis, and cancer.

Shelled nuts & roasted nuts can be demolded /decontaminated of mold-toxins by using Vitamin C as follows: *First rinse nuts well in water (this removes a lot of mold). Cover with water, add about 1/4 tsp. vitamin C powder for a pint of nuts and mix. Let stand for 5 minutes. The water penetrates the nuts, taking the C with it. Pour off the water and dry nuts in gas oven at low heat.* (See p140)

The safest way to eat nuts is to buy nuts in their shells and do your own cracking. Most nuts keep fresh in shells for as long as a year. Shelled nuts deteriorate gradually, some faster than others. Walnuts, pecans, Brazil nuts and sunflower seeds tend to oxidize more quickly than most other nuts/seeds. Avoid rancid (spoiled) nuts and seeds. Almonds are usually safe. Walnuts and cashews are less durable. Hulled sunflower seeds rapidly deteriorate. Especially bad are nuts which are not whole but sold as pieces, or diced. When you buy a package of sunflower seeds, pick out and discard all the damaged seeds (brown, dark, yellow or different from the normal light-gray color). Taste sesame seeds before you buy them. Rancid or old sesame seeds taste bitter and look muddy gray (avoid them). Fresh sesame seeds are light beige /yellow.

● Avoiding mold-toxins in fruits

Fresh Fruit: Patulin is the major fruit mold-toxin, present in most common fruit if they are bruised. Choose fruit meticulously. Wash and peel everything so you can see and avoid every bruise. Cut out bruises, dark spots. Yes, I know, the highest concentration of nutrients is just under the skin. You'll have to decide about peeling. If the skin looks perfect, it's probably just fine; then just cut out / off the bruises and dark or discolored spots. **Dried Fruit:** Soak them in vitamin C water. Rinse and bake on low heat to dry again; store in refrigerator or freezer. (See page 140 for more information)

● For optimum nutrition, your food should be organically grown.
● If you live up north, being a healthy fruitarian may be impossible.

● Be careful of over-consuming bottled fruit juice, etc.

Consuming concentrated sources of sugars (fructose, glucose, sucrose, honey, etc.), bottled fruit juice and orange juice greatly reduces the ability of the white blood cells to kill bacteria, according to one study [2] (which probably did not use any *freshly pressed juice* –which may not have had this effect). They recommend diluting fruit juices with water before drinking.

1) Winter, PIF, 76.   2) Murray, EN,63, 229.

Stay in the *BLACK* with Health:
Eat the *DARKest* of natural wholefoods

For the highest level of nutrients choose the darkest colored wholefoods: The darker the natural color of a fruit, vegetable, wholefood, the more enzymes, vitamins, minerals, anti-oxidants, bioflavonoids and nutrients it has. Conversely, the lighter it is the poorer it is nutritionally. And if artificially white –it's a big nutritional zero that even steals nutrients from your tissues. The rich color of dark bing cherries has more nutrition than red cherries. Same for red grapes vs. white; dark leafy greens vs. iceberg lettuce; red or sweet potatoes vs. white potatoes. And sun-ripened produce is richer nutritionally than produce picked green and gas-ripened.

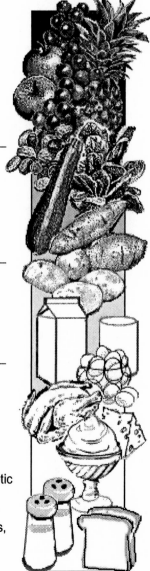

Water-rich, crispy, RAW, DARK, LIVING (↑)	**BEST food for Humans.** Health-producing. Required for optimum health	• Darkest colored fresh fruit • Darkest leafy greens, raw • Non-starchy raw vegetables • Nuts
	Though not optimum, can be handled in moderate amounts if combined properly.	• Starchy Vegetables, yams, potatoes • Sprouted seeds, Seeds • Grains, Cereals • Legumes, Beans
Dried out, hard, limp, COOKED, WHITE, DEAD (↓)	Not well-adapted for human physiology. Strains our organism.	• Dairy, Milk, Cream, Yogurt • Cheese, Butter • Extracted Oils
	WORST foods for Humans. Incompatible with Humans' physiology. Full-fledged health-wreckers. Killer drugfood. UnFood.	• Meat, fleshfood, eggs • Cooked, nuked, dead food • Processed, chemicalized, preserved food • Artificial or Irradiated food • Genetically engineered food • Fractionated nutrients, synthetic vitamins • Salt, Spices, Condiments • White, denatured foods (flours, sugars, grease...) • Snow-White "refined" sugar

A successful fruitarian diet used in a study

The following diet was used successfully in a university study to establish that humans can stay healthy on a fruitarian diet.[1] The guinea-humans were required to follow this diet for six months. Only fresh fruit (not dried, sugared, or canned) and fresh juice (not bottled or canned) were used:

Breakfast	Calories
1 cup of fruit juice	100
4 portions of fruit	300
10:30 a.m.	
2 tablespoons of nuts	100
Lunch	
1 cup of fruit juice	100
6 portions of fruit	450
3:30 p.m.	
1 cup of fruit juice	100
2 tablespoons of nuts	100
Supper	
7 portions of fruit	525
2 tablespoons of nuts	100
9:00 p.m.	
3 portions of fruit	225
Total	2100

Rawfood Recipes

I selected these recipes on the basis of their healthfulness, simplicity, ease of preparation, and minimal or non-inclusion of drugfood ingredients (spices, pepper, vanilla, tamari, extracted oils, tofu, etc.). Rawfood recipes often have drugfood ingredients –or they have too many ingredients. **Less is best!** A mono-meal of just one type of fruit /vegetable (or multiple but compatible combinations) is preferable and healthier. *Experiment and create your own unique combinations...*

Seed-Nut Dressings /Sauces

An enjoyable way of eating live rawfoods is to dice or slice up your favorite vegetables or fruit; then pour on a tasty sauce or dressing. (It can even be a drugfood dressing). Yum. Or use the sauce/dressing as a dip. Yum. Or best yet, just straight out eat the veggie or fruit as is. Yum.

Using **apple cider vinegar** makes a salad dressing acid-forming. Using **lemon juice** (fresh) makes a salad dressing alkaline-forming (alkalizing). **Soaking seeds and nuts** moves these foods in the direction of being neutral to alkaline. By varying the thickness, seed & nut sauces /dressings can also be used as soups, dips, and even whole meals in themselves.

1) Honiballl, 76.

Flaxseeds are the best and safest source of the essential omega-3 fatty acids. They also provides lignands, which boost the immune system. Flaxseeds are not well-absorbed unless they are soaked (overnight) and blended. When flaxseeds are combined with sunflower seeds, which supply the essential omega-6 fatty acids, one gets a supply of all fatty acids. Flaxseeds give a creamy texture to whatever they are blended with. Following are wholesome sauce/dressing recipes.

Apple Double O-3 Dressing
1 Tbs. soaked flaxseed
2 Tbs. raw walnuts
1 cup raw apple juice
2 Tbs. raw apple cider vinegar
Add ingredients and blend until smooth.

Papaya-Carrot Dressing or Creme Sauce
1 Tbs. soaked flaxseed
1 cup carrot juice
1 papaya
1 tsp. fresh grated ginger to taste
Add ingredients and blend until smooth.

Zucchini-Sun Dressing
1 cup chopped zucchini
1/2 cup soaked sunflower seeds
1 Tbs. soaked flaxseeds
1 cup raw apple juice
(optional) 1 clove garlic or 1/2 tsp.
   sun-dried garlic powder
1 1/2 tsp. dill
Blend all ingredients.

Veggie Spice Dressing
1 cup chunked carrots, added to blender
1 cup beets, in chunks
1 cup broccoli, in chunks
1/2 avocado
1 clove garlic or 1/2 tsp.
   sun-dried garlic powder
1 tsp. grated ginger
1 tsp. or more of curry
Blend all ingredients.

Banana Sunseed Sauce
2 bananas
1/2 cup soaked sunflower seeds
1/2 cup water (or raw apple
   juice for sweeter taste)
Blend and serve over fruit, or drink directly. The carbohydrate from the banana and the predigested protein from the seeds makes this a powerful rebuilder and a good snack for hypoglycemia. Also helpful for people with poor absorption.

Tahini Lemon Dressing
1 Tbs. raw tahini
1/4 cup lemon juice
1/2 cup water
2 tsp. dill
Blend.

Sweet Sour Dressing
1 cup water
1/2 cup sunflower seeds
3 Tbs. raw apple cider vinegar
2 dates or 1 Tbs. pure maple
   syrup or Sucanat, or raw honey
1 large tomato
Put all ingredients into blender and liquefy.

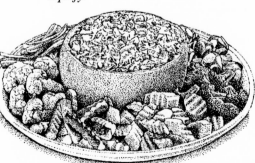

Kreamy Kuke Dressing

2 heaping Tbs. raw tahini
1 large kukumber (cucumber)
2 tsp. dill
1/3 cup water
Blend all ingredients.

Mayonnaise

1/2 cup lemon (lime juice or
　　apple cider vinegar)
3 Tbs. seed or nut butter
1/4 cup unrefined oil
1 tsp. kelp
Blend the lemon and seed or nut butter.
At low speed add oil slowly.
For a thinner or thicker mayonnaise,
add less or more oil. Store in glass jar.

Fruit Salad Dressing

3/4 cup fruit juice (apple, orange, pine-
　　apple, or any combination of fruit juices)
2 Tbs. coconut meal (or any nut butter)
1 tsp. pure maple syrup or raw honey
1 tsp. unrefined oil (optional)
Mix all together by hand or blending.
Serve over any single raw fruit or cut
up fruit. Serves 4 people.

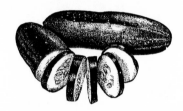

Soups

Spinach Soup

1 bunch fresh spinach
1 avocado
1/2 cup parsley
1/2 to 1 cup water, depending
　　on desired thickness
1 Tbs. lemon juice
Add ingredients and blend. For a warm
soup, add water heated to 118 degrees.

CornAvo

2 cobs corn
1 avocado
1 1/2 cups warm water
1 tsp. kelp
3 sprigs watercress
Cut corn from cob. Blend with water at
low speed to smooth consistency.
Blend in avocado. Season
with kelp. Serve with
watercress sprinkled over
top.

Carrot Creme

2 cups carrot juice
1/4 cup almond butter
1/2 tsp. kelp
Adding juice gradually, blend to a
cream

Beetiful Soup

1/2 cup grated beets
1/2 cup grated carrots
1 avocado
2 cups fresh carrot juice
Blend all ingredients until smooth.
Garnish with sprouts. For chunkier
soup, reserve 1/4 cup grated beets &
carrots; add/mix in to soup last.

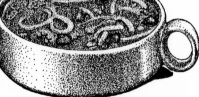

Entrees

Virtual Chicken Salad

2 cups finely sliced cabbage
1 cup celery
2 Tbs. finely chopped onion
1/2 cup green peppers, finely chopped
1 cup cubed nut loaf, cold
2 Tbs. mayonnaise
Mix thoroughly. Serve on crisp lettuce leaves. Decorate with olives.

Tri-Nut Loaf

1 cup cashews coarsely ground
1 cup almonds coarsely ground
1 cup ground coconut
1 cup diced carrots
1/2 cup raisins
6 spinach leaves
12 sprigs of parsley
Put all ingredients through food grinder except avocado. Mash avocado and mix with ingredients, Form into loaf.

Apple Celery Salad

2 cups cubed apples
fresh lemon juice (added to the
    apples to prevent discoloring)
1 cup chopped celery
1/4 cup fine chopped parsley
1 handful raisins
2 Tbs. mayonnaise
Mix thoroughly. Serve on crisp lettuce.

Stuffed Cabbage Rolls

1/2 cup nuts (pecans or
    almonds) coarsely ground
1/2 cup raisins or currants
1/4 cup minced parsley
1 cup diced apples
Mix together. Fill cabbage leaves and fasten with toothpicks.

Virtual Turkey

1 bunch celery
1 cup pecans or almonds
1 green onion
1 avocado
parsley
sage
lettuce
cranberry sauce
Grind celery, onion, & parley through food grinder. Drain off juice; use for soup. Blend the almonds or pecans in nut mill or blender and grind until fine. Mash avocado with a fork until well mashed. Add nuts, avocado and sage to celery mixture. Shape into patties with a spoon and serve on a lettuce leaf with cranberry sauce.

Nut Milks n' Ice Cream

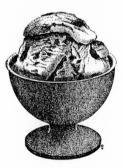

- **Almond Milk**
- **Sesame Seed Milk**
- **Banana Marble Ice Cream**
    See page 112 in Chapter 5 for the Recipes. Yum!

Edible Flowers / Blossoms

For flavoring and garnishing your fruit & vegetable salads or other dishes. All fruit were flowers before becoming fruit!

Apple	Gladiolus	Orange Blossoms	Raspberry Leaves
Broccoli	Grape Leaves	Pansy	Rose Petals
Cauliflower	Lavender	Primrose	Rosehips
Chamomile	Marigold	Quince	Rosemary
Chive	Milkweed		Sage
Chrysanthemum	Mulberry		Sorrel
Crabapple			Spearmint
Dandelion Petals			Squash
Elderberry			Strawberry Leaves
Fuchsia			Sweet Potato
Garlic			Thyme
Geranium			Violet

Recommended Further Reading on Rawfood Recipes

Many delicious fruitarian and raw-food recipes are presented in most of following books, which also give hard-to-find information regarding the rawfood diet.

– *The Essene Gospel of Peace (book one)*	Szekely, E. (translator)
– *The UN Cook Book*	Elizabeth Baker
– *Live Foods: Nature's Perfect*	
System of Human Nutrition	George & Doris Fathman
– *Dick Gregory's Natural Diet for Folks*	
Who Eat: Cookin' with Mother Nature	Dick Gregory
– *Sunfired Foods Cookless Recipes*	Aris LaTham
– *I Live On Fruit*	Essie Honiball & T.C. Fry
– *The Mucusless Diet Healing System*	Arnold Ehret
– *Conscious Eating*	Gabriel Cousens
– *Fresh Vegetable & Fruit Juices*	Norman Walker
– *Survival in the 21st Century*	Viktoras Kulvinskas

Feas(t)able Diet Pyramid for Good Health

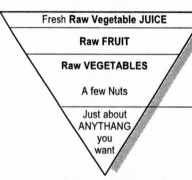

5%-10% of diet. Glass of juice at least thrice weekly. The more drugfood you eat, the more you need this!

Fresh **Raw Vegetable JUICE**

Raw FRUIT

Raw VEGETABLES

A few Nuts

60-80% of diet. Organically grown if possible. Go easy on the nuts. Tips: preceed most of your meals with a fruit or two. Then have your raw vegetables or a salad or drugfood. Fruit is a meal unto itself. Many little meals a day is better than 3 big meals a day.

Just about ANYTHANG you want

5%-20% of your diet. Cooked food, drugfood. Wean off the more harmful foods (white, denatured, refined, chemicalized, unfood, factory-farm-grown, etc.)

Note: The FDA's food pyramid, though improved from before, is still a health hazard. It points up, and has sugar at the very capstone and sugar (in form of starches) at the base, making your body a "sandwich" heading for eventual diabetes, etc.

Breatharianism is even higher than Fruitarianism

Breatharianism, the most perfect state of the Original Human, *the Black HUE-man.*

Humans were Fruitarians eons before becoming Vegetarians, Grainarians, Flesharians, –and just over the last century– becoming omnivorous Drugfoodarians. But Humans were *Breatharians* before becoming Fruitarians. Breatharians? The *Breatharian* is able to take all the energy her body needs directly from sunlight and air without the intermediary called food. Food itself is but condensed sunlight. Breatharianism was the most perfect state of the Human, the *Melanated Original Hue-man.* And such Hue-mans lived on solar radiation. You can bet they were Black... especially at the beginning. For when the Sun kisses you, you darken. The skin is the organ for assimilating light nutrition, just as the lungs are the organs for assimilating air nutrition.

Breatharian? –really a *"Solarian."* Melanin and Chlorophyll are essentially twins.

Black Melanin absorbs and stores light (energy). Melanin is the *chlorophyll* of HUE-mans. *Chlorophyll* transmutes sunlight into a form called *plants,* which we eat as food. Melanin also has the ability to transmute light. HUE-manity has degenerated and is not able to do this as efficiently as we did in the past when we were Breatharians. Eons ago, the Black original Hue-man had the ability to transmute sunlight and air into whatever nutrients s/he needed, not just vitamin D (one of the last vestiges of this ability), but all the vitamins and minerals too. (Are not minerals crystallized light in all the "gemstone" colors of the *rainbow*? –and if you strike a crystal in the dark, it even flashes light.) And protein was made from *nitrogen* in the *air,* which even today is still the most abundant gas (80%) of the atmosphere. The original Human, the *Black Hue-*man, evolved in the Earth's sunlit tropical regions. Sunlight and Melanin = divine marriage. They go together. Thus, the term "Breatharian" is incomplete or even a misnomer; it should be *Solarian* (or *Sunarian).* No wonder the ancient Afrikans called themselves "The Children of the Sun."

You Breatharian, you!

Are you breathing now? Of course. And you breath all day, 24 hours a day. So did Breatharians. You still take into your body *PRANA* from the air, just like the Breatharian you *still* essentially are. *In fact, each day you consume more weight in AIR than in food and water combined!* Humans breathe in *34 pounds* of air daily! –and ingest 2 pounds of food; 4 pounds of liquids. But if you stopped drinking water or eating food you would die. The reason you still need to eat any food at all, whether vegetables, grains, meat or hard-drugfood, is because you are an *addict.* Hooked. The orders of foodarians (Waterians, Juicearians, Fruitarians, Vegetarians, Grainarians, Flesharians, Drugfoodarians) signify increasing degrees of toxicity, addiction, and biological degeneration. One day, despite current alarming appearances to the contrary, Earth and *surviving* Humanity will be healed. The glorious Human body will again be honored as the Temple of the Divine, –a Living, Radiating Jewel of Light!

Recommendations for Better Health

- A *total* **fruitarian diet is _not_ necessarily recommended** since good quality, organically grown fruit, in good variety and supply, is often not consistently available. It seems that the *ideal diet* goes best with the *ideal environment* (a rarity on our polluted planet). Today's fruits are not as nourishing, natural & whole as they should be, since like veggies, fruits are hybrid, gene-altered, have unnatural high levels of sugar, and are picked unripe. Best to eat from a wide variety. **Supplement your diet with raw-fresh veggie juice** (see pg 233).

- **For best results, your change to a healthier way of eating should be** *gradual* (unless you are sick), stress-free, not forced or rushed. Take your *sweet* time, for you are undoing a lifetime of perverted eating habits and drugfood addictions. You need time to adjust on all levels.
  - **If you are a flesh-eater**: *gradually* ease into a *more-vegetarian* diet by eating more raw leafy greens especially, and fruit. Eat flesh less often and in smaller portions. Cut back on starches. Supplement your diet with raw veggie juice.
  - **If you are a vegetarian /starcharian** (heavy eater of starches): gradually include more fruit in your diet. Eat less starches and fake fleshfoods. Supplement your diet with raw-fresh veggie juice.
  - **If you are a rawfooder or fruitarian:** review precautions on page 233. Supplement your diet with raw-fresh veggie juice.

- **Make fruit your first meal of the day** (or have at least one meal a day consisting only of fruit); eat till satisfied. Consider eating raw fruit 10-30 minutes before *all* your regular meals. Fruit should be eaten alone, on an empty stomach, and only when ripened –else it may cause digestive distress. The safest way to eat nuts is to buy them in shells and do your own cracking.

- **Gradually make your diet mostly fruit.** You'll attain a high state of health, mental well-being, and great vigor as a *near-fruitarian*. If you drink fresh veggie juice and occasionally eat salads and a protein food such as bee pollen, nuts or seeds, you're ensuring more than sufficient nourishment.

- **Parents should feed fruit to their children**, raising them on a largely fruitarian diet. Such children escape many diseases and grow up healthy, strong, gentle, lovable, and free from unnatural propensities and vices.

- **Habitually use *kinesiology*** to tell whether a food, anything, is good for you.

- **To remove mold /mold-toxins** from nuts & fruit, see directions on pages 140, 234. **To effectively cleanse produce**, see directions on page 152.

- **The pain of denying yourself a food** you vastly crave can create toxins. So if you're vastly craving a drugfood, go ahead and indulge! (perhaps once a month). *Savor* each bite! (To help neutralize toxic effects, have raw veggies with it) When finished, brush the crumbs off yo smiling face and get back on track, you drugfood-addict you! Don't give up! Restart after each defeat, like a babe learning to walk. The rewards are worth the perserverance.

Food Guide Summary

Recommendations for Better Health

SWEETS (p 73, 79)

Avoid /Limit:	Replacements:
• white sugar • brown sugar • raw or turbinado sugar • date sugar • fructose, dextrose • maltose, "oses" • all refined sugars • "evaporated cane juice" • molasses • blackstrap molasses • syrups, corn syrup • ice cream • all honey • candy, chocolate • pasteurized fruit juices • jelly & jam • sugary cereal • any foods with sugar • all artificial sweeteners	BEST: • ripe bananas • *fresh* fruit juice • dates • raisins (unsulfured) • unsulfured dried fruit Improvement: • Sucanat • 100% pure maple syrup • carob instead of chocolate

OIL /FATS (p 83, 90)

Avoid /Limit:	Replacements:

• all margarines
• shortening
• baking sprays
• most "cold pressed" & "expeller pressed" oils
• extracted oils
• canola oil
• corn oil
• soybean oil
• peanut oil
• coconut oil
• palm or palm kernel oil
• cottenseed oil
• *pasteurized* butter
• lard, all animal fat
• cooked fatty foods:
  – mayonnaise
  – ice cream
  – peanut butter
  – dressings
  – fried foods
	BEST:
	uncooked oily wholefoods such as
	• avocados
	• hemp seed
	• sesame seeds
	• nuts & seeds
	
	Improvement:
	Use sparingly, for oils are fractionated, hence drugfoods:
	• virgin olive oil (unfiltered)
	• sesame oil
	• flax seed oil
	• wheat germ oil
	• evening primrose oil
	• raw butter or cream (is better than margarine)

STARCH /Grains (p 80, 82)

Avoid /Limit:	Replacements:

• white flour
• breads, cereals, pasta, pastry, gravies... made with white flour or any refined grains
• white rice
• white grits
• "wheat bread" or multi-grain bread made with blend of white flour & whole grain flour
• Packaged breads / starches, including health varieties (contaminated with mold-toxins)
	BEST:
	NONE, since ALL grains are harmful to humans
	
	Improvement:
	• red potatoes
	• wholegrains:
	  – kamut
	  – amaranth
	  – quinoa
	  – spelt
	  – millet
	  – wild rice
	  – buckwheat
	• (limit eating wheat, rye, oats, barley, brown rice)

SALT (p 91, 95)

Avoid /Limit:	Replacements:

• all white salt
• "sea salt"
• salty foods:
  – cheese
  – potato chips
  – soy sauce
  – pretzels, crackers
  – bacon, jerky
  – dressings
  – hot dogs
	• Celtic salt (undried gray ocean salt)
	• filtered seawater
	• kelp, dulse
	• seaweed
	• herbal seasoning (salt-free)

WATER (p 96, 102)

Avoid /Limit:	Replacements:
• tap water • drinks, ice, food made with tap water • purchased ice • all bottled water • mineral water • well water • spring water	• reverse osmosis mineral-free water • purified water from water-dispensers • filtered tap water • clean rain water • distilled water mixed with any of the above

continued...

Food Guide Summary

MILK (p 103, 112)

Avoid /Limit:	Replacements:

• pasteurized milk
• homogenized milk
• ice cream
• dairy products from
  pasteurized milk (skim
  milk, butter, cream,
  cheese, yogurt, whey)
• babies' milk formulas
• powdered milk
• nondairy creamers
• yeast powders
	BEST:
	• seed or nut milk
	• coconut milk
	• frozen ripe bananas
	
	Improvement:
	• raw, unpasteurized
	  milk (from goats if
	  possible)
	• raw milk cheese

PROTEIN (p 113, 127)

Avoid /Limit:	Replacements:

• commercially
  grown flesh
• cured meats
• hotdogs, spam
• liver
• all fish /seafood
• all shellfish, tuna
• fish with skin
  instead of scales
• infertile
  commercial eggs
• peanuts
	BEST:
	• nuts & seeds
	• fruit & leafy greens
	• bee pollen
	
	Improvement:
	• beans
	• fake fleshfood *(limit)*
	• organic, fertile eggs
	• fish with scales
	• range-fed, additive/
	  hormone-free meats

BEVERAGES (p 128, 132)

Avoid /Limit:	Replacements:

• carbonated drinks
• soda pop, colas
• carbonated water
• coffee, tea
• all bottled fruit &
  vegetable juices
• all bottled beverages
• powdered beverages
	• pure water
	• fresh organic
	  fruit juices
	• fresh organic
	  vegetable juices
	• steeped herbal teas
	  (not boiled)

OTHER (p 140, 193, 196, 242)

Avoid /Limit:	Replacements:

• microwaved, grilled,
  fried or smoked food
• fermented/soured food
• pickled foods
• yeasted /fungus food
• mushrooms
• foods you're allergic to
	• raw plant food
	• steamed, baked, or
	  lightly cooked food
	• foods you are *not*
	  allergic to

CONDIMENTS (p 141, 143)

Avoid /Limit:	Replacements:

• condiments
• spices, salt
• black, white pepper
• cayenne pepper
• white vinegar
• onions & garlic
• MSG, tartar sauce
• soy sauce
• tamari sauce
• barbecue sauce
• ketchup
• mustard
	• lemon juice
	• kelp (seaweed)
	• non-irritating herbs
	• Celtic salt
	• filtered seawater
	• herbal seasoning
	  (salt-free)
	• apple cider vinegar
	  (organic)

PRODUCE (p 145, 152)

Avoid /Limit:	Replacements:

• commercially grown
  fruits, vegetables,
  nuts, spices, herbs.
• canned fruit &
  vegetables
• commercial frozen
  produce
• commercial dried fruit
  & raisins
• commercial herbs,
  seasonings
	• organically grown,
	  pesticide-free, fruits,
	  leafy greens,
	  vegetables, nuts
	• organic produce you
	  grow yourself
	• non-irradiated herbs
	• non-sulfured,
	  demolded dried fruit
	  & raisins

SUPPLEMENTS (p 155, 177-179)

Avoid /Limit:	Replacements:

• fractionated nutrients
• vitamin supplements
• synthetic vitamins
• so-called
  "natural vitamins"
• mineral supplements
• vast majority of
  nutritional
  "supplements"
• supplements in
  drugstores and
  supermarkets
• protein powders
• most lecithin products
	• fresh JUICE of fruits
	  & vegetables
	• *wholefood* supple-
	  ments like spirulina,
	  bluegreen algae,
	  chlorophyll-powders
	• wolfberries
	• hemp seed
	• organic MSM
	• pollen, royal jelly
	• dehydrated veg juice
	• wholeherb
	  supplements
	• apple cider vinegar
	  (organic)
	• digestive enzymes
	• buffered vitamin C (ok)

30 Health/Survival Books by Afrikans

Afrika, Dr. Llaila	**African Holistic Health**
Afrika, Dr. Llaila	**Nutricide: The Nutritional Destruction of the Black Race**
Afua, Queen	**Heal Thyself – For Health and Longevity**
Ali, Shahrazad	**How Not To Eat Pork (or life without the PIG)**
Ali, Shahrazad	**Things Your Parents Should Have Told You**
Ali, Shahrazad	**Urban Survival for the Year 2000:** ...with Special Instructions for Blacks, Latinos, Asians & Indians
Amen, Ra Un Neter	**A Holistic Guide to Family Disorders**
Awadu, Keidi Obi	**AIDS: Confessed –It's a Hoax**
Awadu, Keidi Obi	**Food – It's About Survival**
Awadu, Keidi Obi	**Vaccines: An Ounce of Prevention or a Pound of Death?**
Awadu, Keidi Obi	**Epidemic: The Rise of New Childhood Diseases in the U.S., a Manmade Disaster**
Browder, Anthony	**Survival Strategies for Africans in America**
Chappell, Drs. Arvel & Bobbie	**The Double-You ("W") Book**
Dixon, Dr. Barbara M.	**Good Health for African Americans**
Doctah B	**Doctah B's Food for Mind Body and Soul**
Goss, Dr. Paul	**Forever Young**
Goss, Dr. Paul	**The Rebirth of the Gods**
Gray, Robert	**The Colon Health Handbook**
Gregory, Dick	**Dick Gregory's Natural Diet for Folks Who Eat: Cookin' with Mother Nature**
Hollis, Norma Thompson	**Teach Your Child to Honor God**
Hollis, Norma Thompson	**The Candida Epidemic**
M. Walker & K. Singleton	**Natural Health for African Americans The Physicians' Guide**
Newton, Dr. Patricia A.	**Post Traumatic Slavery Disorder**
Powell, Alfred "Coach"	**Message 'N A Bottle –The 40oz. Scandal**
Sista Yuki (Dr. Yukiko Kudo)	**Aromatherapy**
Smith, Dr. Meri Morgan	**Parenting By Rhyme and Reason**
Southall, Dr. Willie	**Hyssop – Superior Healing Power**
Suzar	**Drugs Masquerading As Foods**
Suzar	**Unfood By The UnPeople**
Suzar	**Don't Worry, Be Healthy**

Selected Bibliography

Abramowski, O. M. — **Fruitarian Diet and Physical Rejuvenation**
Fremont CA: Custodian Publishing Co.

Afrika, Llaila — **African Holistic Health**
Silver Spring MD: Adesegun, Johnson & Koram Publishers, 1989.

Afrika, Llaila — **Nutricide: The Nutritional Destruction of the Black Race**
Dr. L. Afrika: The Herb Pantry, Box 2475, Beaufort SC 29901
(843) 525-1885. 1994.

Afrika, Llaila — **Understanding Homosexuality & Homosexual Detox** (video)
Dr. L. Afrika: The Herb Pantry, Box 2475, Beaufort SC 29901
(843) 525-1885. 1998.

Afua, Queen — **Heal Thyself - For Health and Longevity**
Brooklyn NY: A & B Publishers, 1993.

Aihara, Herman — **Acid & Alkaline**
Oroville CA: George Ohsawa Macrobiotic Foundation, 1986.

Airola, Paavo — **Are You Confused?**
Phoenix AZ: Health Plus Publishers, 1979.

Airola, Paavo — **How to Keep Slim, Healthy and Young with Juice Fasting**
Sherwood Oregon: Health Plus Publishers, 1971.

Airola, Paavo — **How to Get Well**
Phoenix AZ: Health Plus Publishers, 1974.

Anderson, N./Benoist, A. — **Your Health and Your House**
New Canaan CT: Keats Publishing, Inc., 1994.

Anderson, Rich — **Cleanse & Purify Thyself**
Tucson AZ: Arise & Shine, 1992.

Astor, Stephen — **Hidden Food Allergies**
Garden City Park NY: Avery Publishing Group, Inc., 1988.

Awadu, Keidi Obi — **Epidemic**
Longbeach CA: Conscious Rasta Press, 1997.

Awadu, Keidi Obi — **Food - It's About Survival**
Longbeach CA: Conscious Rasta Press, 1996.

Awadu, Keidi Obi — **Population War...Report from the Frontline**
Longbeach CA: Conscious Rasta Press, 1997.

Ayto, John — **Dictionary of Word Origins**
New York NY: Arcade Publishing, 1990.

Baker, Arthur — **Awakening Our Self Healing Body**
Los Angeles CA: Self Health Care Systems, 1994.

Baker, Elizabeth — **The UN Cook Book**
San Diego CA: ProMotion Publishing, 1995.

Balch, James; Balch, Phyllis — **Prescription for Cooking & Dietary Wellness**
Greenfield IN: PAB Books, Inc.

Balch, James; Balch, Phyllis — **Prescription for Nutritional Healing**
Garden City Park NY: Avery Publishing Group Inc. 1990

Banik, Allen — **The Choice is Clear**
Raytown, Missouri: Acres U.S.A, 1975.

Barnes, Carol — **Melanin: The Chemical Key to Black Greatness**

Houston TX, Carol Barnes, 1988.

Bartnett, Beatrice — **Urine Therapy: It May Save Your Life**
Lifestyle Institute (505) 257-3406,
P.O. Box 4735, Ruidoso, NM 88345, 1993.

Bartnett, B; & Adelman, M.	**The Miracles of Urine Therapy** Lifestyle Institute (505) 257-3406, P.O. Box 4735, Ruidoso, NM 88345, 1987.
Becker, Robert	**Cross Currents** Los Angeles CA: Jeremy P. Tarcher, Inc., 1990.
Bird, Christopher	**The Persecution and Trial of Gaston Naessens** Tiburon CA: H. J. Kramer, Inc., 1991.
Block, Zenas	**It's All On the Label** Boston Mass.: Little, Brown & Company, 1981.
Bragg, Paul	**Apple Cider Vinegar Health System** Santa Barbara CA: Health Science, 1988.
Bragg, Paul /Patricia	**The Miracle of Fasting** Santa Barbara CA: Health Science, 1990.
Boone, J. Allen	**Kinship With All Life** New York, NY: Harper & Row, 1976.
Burroughs, Stanley	**The Master Cleanser** Auburn CA: Burroughs Books, 1993.
Burton Goldberg Group	**Alternative Medicine –The Definitive Guide** Fife, Washington: Future Medicine Publishing, Inc. 1995.
California Sun Newspaper	**(Hydrogenated Oils article)** Volume 21, pages 10-11, March 1997. Ojai CA.
Canning, Peggy	**Exotic Supplements** Vista CA: Margaret Canning, 1995.
Clark, Hulda Regehr	**The Cure For All Diseases** San Diego CA: ProMotion Publishing, 1995.
Clark, Linda	**Secrets of Health & Beauty** New York NY: Jove Publications, Inc., 1981.
Clark, Linda	**A Handbook of Natural Remedies for Common Ailments** Old Greenwich CT: Devin-Adair Company, 1976.
Clark, Linda	**Know Your Nutrition** New Canaan CT: Keats Publishing, Inc., 1981.
Clements, G.R.	**The Law of Life and Human Health** Mokelumne Hill CA: Health Research, 1972.
Colborn, Theo; Dumanoski, D.; Myers, P.	**Our Stolen Future** New York: Penguin Books, 1997.
Colgan, Michael	**The New Nutrition** Vancouver BC Canada: Apple Publishing Company Ltd, 1994.
Cooper, J.C.	**Symbolism, The Universal Language** Wellingborough, Northhamptonshire. Britain: The Aquarian Press, 1982.
Cummings, Robert	**Truffles, Death Caps and the Chanterlelle** Santa Barbara CA: Santa Barbara City College, 1993.
Cohen, Robert	**MILK The Deadly Poison** Englewood Cliffs NJ: Argus Publishing Inc., 1998.
Cousens, Gabriel	**Conscious Eating** Santa Rosa CA: Vision Books International, 1993.
Cousens, Gabriel	**Spiritual Nutrition and the Rainbow Diet** Boulder CO: Cassandra Press, 1986.
David, Marc	**Nourishing Wisdom** New York NY: Bell Tower, 1991.
Davidson, John	**Subtle Energy** England: C. W. Daniel Company Limited, 1987.

de Langre, Jacques   **Seasalt's Hidden Powers**
Magalia CA: Happiness Press, 1994.

DeRohan, Ceanne   **Right Use of Will**
Four Winds Publications, 535 Cordova Road, #112; Santa Fe, NM 87501. 1986.

Dixon, Barbara M.   **Good Health for African Americans**
New York NY: Crown Publishers, Inc., 1994.

EarthWorks Group   **50 Simple Things You Can Do To Save The Earth**
Berkely CA: Earthworks Press, 1989.

Ehret, Arnold   **Mucusless Diet Healing System**
Beaumont CA: Ehret Literature Publishing Co., 1922 /1953.

Ehret, Arnold   **Rational Fasting -For Physical,
Mental and Spiritual Rejuvenation**
• New York NY: Benedict Lust Publications, 1971.
• Beaumont CA: Ehret Literature Publishing Co.

Enright, John   **In Our Face: Impolite Essays on
Humanity's War Against Our Children and the Earth**
Menlo Park CA: Intermedia, 1993.

FASE Reports   Volume 11 No. 1 Spring 1993, S-5
Foundation for Advancements in Science and Education
Park Mile Plaza, 4801 Wilshire Blvd, Los Angeles, CA 90010

Fathman, George & Doris   **Live Foods - Nature's Perfect Sysem of Human Nutrition**
Beaumont CA: Ehret Literature Publishing Co., 1973.

Flanagan, Patrick & Gael   **Elixir of the Ageless**
Flagstaff AZ: Vortex Press, 1986.

Fry, T.C.   **The Great AIDS Hoax**
Manchaca TX: Health Excellence Systems, 1989.

Gagne, Steve   **Energetics of Food**
Sante Fe NM: Spiral Sciences, 1990.

Goss, Paul   **The Rebirth of the Gods**
Los Angeles CA: Paul Goss, 1995.

Gray, Robert   **The Colon Health Handbook**
Reno NV: Emerald Publishing, 1990.

Gregory, Dick   **Dick Gregory's Natural Diet for Folks Who Eat:
Cookin' with Mother Nature**
Perennial Library / Harper & Row, Publishers, Inc., NY, 1973.

Havender, William R.   **Does Nature Know Best? Natural Carcinogens
and Anticarcinogens in America's Food**
5th Edition Report written for ACHS (American Council on Science and Health). Published on the Internet, revised 1996.

Healthiatry   **Healthiatry Course II**
Oroville CA: American College of Healthiatry, 1992.

Hills, Christopher   **Rejuvenating the Body Through
Fasting with Spirulina Plankton**
Boulder Creek CA: University of the Trees Press, 1979.

Ho, Mae-Wan   **Genetic Engineering - Dream or Nightmare?**
Bath, UK: Gateway Books, 1998.

Honiball, Essie; Fry, T.C.   **I Live On Fruit**
Health Excellence Systems
1108 Regal Row, Manchaca, TX 78652. 1990.

Hotema, Hilton   **Man's Higher Consciousness**
Mokelumne Hill CA: Health Research, 1962.

Inglass, Leslie   **Diet for a Gentle World**
Garden City Park NY: Avery Publishing Group, Inc., 1993.

Igram, Cass   **Self Test Nutrition Guide**
Buffalo Grove Ill., Knowledge House, 1994.

Jubal, J. Asar	**The Black Truth** Longbeach CA: Black Truth Enterprises, 1991.
Kent, Ray	**Independently Healthy -The Ultimate Freedom** Canton TX: Our Place, 1993.
Kirban, Salem	**Health Guide for Survival** Huntingdon Valley PA: Salem Kirban, Inc., 1976.
Kroeger, Hanna	**Parasites - The Enemy Within** Boulder, CO: Hanna Kroeger Publications, 1991.
Kulvinskas, Viktoras	**Life in the 21st Century** Fairfield IA: 21st Century Publications, 1981.
Kulvinskas, Viktoras	**Love Your Body** Wethersfield CT: Omangod Press, 1972.
Kulvinskas, Viktoras	**Survival Into the 21st Century** Wethersfield CT: Omangod Press, 1975.
Law, Donald	**A Guide to Alternative Medicine** Garden City NY: Dolphin Books, 1976.
Lifestyle News	**Zap Your Food Sparingly** (article) Lifestyle News, January 1995, volume 4, Issue 1 P.O. Box 4735, Ruidoso, NM 88345.
Loomis, E; Paulson, J.	**Healing for Everyone** Marina del Ray CA: DeVorss & Company, 1975.
Lynes, Barry	**The Cancer Cure That Worked** Queensville, Ontario Canada: Marcus Books, 1992.
Mander, Jerry	**Four Arguments for the *Elimination* of Television** New York NY: Quill, 1978.
Michael, Russ	**Miracle Cures: Catalyst Altered Water** Olympia WA: Russ Michael Books, 1984.
Murray, M.; Pizzorno, J.	**An Encyclopedia of Natural Medicine** Rocklin, CA: Prima Publishing, 1991.
Nelson, Dennis	**Food Combining Simplified** Tampa FL: Natural Hygiene Press, 1988.
Nelson, Dennis	**Maximizing Your Nutrition** Tampa FL: Natural Hygiene Press, 1988.
Ott, John	**Health and Light** Atlanta GA: Ariel Press, 1976.
Ott, John	**Light, Radiation, and You** Greenwich Connecticut: Devin-Adair, 1985.
Rector-Page, Linda	**Detoxification and Body Cleansing** Sonora CA: Healthy Healing Publications, Inc., 1993.
Pappas, Theoni	**The Magic of Mathematics** San Carlos CA: Wide World Publishing /Tetra, 1994
Preston, Robert	**Healthology: Your Master key to Perfect Health** Salt Lake City UT: Hawkes Publishing, Inc., 1977.
Professional Research Institute	**Your Vitamins...Supplements** **Are Being POISONED!!!** (Report) Amherst VA: Professional Research Institute, 1998.
Quillin, Patrick	**Healing Secrets From the Bible** N. Canton OH: The Leader Company, Inc., 1995.
Rappoport, Jon	**AIDS, INC. —Scandal of the Century** Foster City CA, Human Energy Press, 1988.
Robbins, Anthony	**Unlimited Power** New York NY: Ballantine Books, 1986.
Robbins, John	**Diet for a New America** Walpole NH: Stillpoint Publishers, 1987.

Secret Country, The	(see: *Talking Drum*)
Saulson, Donald & Elisabeth	**A Pocket Guide to Food Additives** Huntington Beach CA: VPS Publishing, 1991.
Schroeder, Henry	**The Poisons Around Us** New Canaan CT: Keats Publishing, Inc., 1994.
Schul & Pettit	**Pyramid Power A New Reality** Walpole NH: Stillpoint, 1979.
Silver, Helene	**The Body-Smart System** Sonora CA: Healthy Healing Publications, 1994.
Southall, Willie	**Hyssop Superior Healing Power** Hollywood CA: Southall Research, 1993. Hyssop Enterprises: superior hyssop products (323) 465-3221.
Steadman, Alice	**Who's The Matter With Me?** Marina del Ray CA: DeVorss & Company, 1997.
Steinman, D., & Wisner, M.	**Living Healthy In A Toxic World** New York NY: Perigee & The Berkeley Publishing Group, 1996.
Suzar	**Don't Worry, Be Healthy** Pasadena CA: A-Kar Productions, 2000.
Szekely, E, translator	**The Essene Gospel of Peace** (Book One) Matsqui BC Canada: International Biogenic Society, 1981.
Talking Drum	**How Homosexuality Originated in the Black Community: Afrika vs. Manago** (video) Los Angeles CA: Talking Drum, 1998: (323) 296-0768)
Talking Drum	**The Secret Country** (a documentary film detailing white-settler intrusion in Australia) Inquire through *The Talking Drum*: (323) 296-0768.
Tien, Juliet	**Breaking the Yeast Curse** Las Vegas NV: Infinite Success International Publishing House, 1997.
Valerian, Valdamar	**Matrix III: The Psycho-Social, Chemical, Biological and Electronic Manipulation of Human Consciousness** Valdamar Valerian, 1992.
Walker, Norman	**Fresh Vegetable and Fruit Juices** Phoenix AZ: O'Sullivan Woodside & Company, 1978.
Weinberger, Stanley	**Healing Within: The Complete Colon Health Guide** Larkspur CA: Colon Health Center, 1988.
Welsing, Frances Cress	**The Isis Papers** Chicago IL: Third World Press, 1991.
West, Samuel	**The Golden Seven Plus One** Orem UT: Samuel Publishing Co., 1983.
Whittlesay, Marietta	**Killer Salt** New York NY: Avon Books, 1978.
Whole Life Times	April 1991, page 17; January 1990, page 14 Malibu, CA
Wiles, June	**RBTI Diet and Guidebook** Tampa FL: Nutritional Counselors of America, Inc., 1979.
Williams, David G.	**Secrets of Life Extension** Ingram TX: Mountain Home Publishing, 1995.
Williams, David G.	**The Doctor's Worldwide Encyclopedia of Natural Healing** Ingram TX: Mountain Home Publishing, 1995.
Winter, Ruth	**A Consumer's Dictionary of Food Additives** New York NY: Crown Trade Paperbacks, 1994.
Winter, Ruth	**Poisons In Your Food** New York NY: Crown Publishers, 1991.

Index

A

AANS, Acquired Anti-Nappy Syndrome 65
acerola 163, 179
Acesulfame-K 29
acetaldehyde 54
acetic acid 228
acetone 52, 54, 129, 130
acetylcholine 170
acid 159, 206, 228
    fruit 233
    organic 228
    rain 28
    which give metabolic problems 228
acid-forming dressings 236
acidity 92
acidosis 92, 143, 176
acorns 225
Acquired Anti-Nappy Syndrome (AANS) 65
active ingredients 156, 172, 212
ADD, Attention Deficit Disorder 49
addicting substances 181
addiction 8, 158, 181, 242
    to drugfood 2
    to fractionated nutrients 158, 175
    to supplements 158
Addicts, Drugfood 181
additives 64
Adenosine Triphosphate (ATP) 87, 141
ADH 95
adrenal glands 94, 114, 131
adrenaline 113, 131
adverse reactions from prescription drugs 66
aflatoxin 25, 90, 130, 136, 137, 139,
    140, 212, 234
Afrika 46, 208
    Nile Valley 167
Afrika, Dr. 124
Afrikans
    addicted to Euro culture 11
    advanced mental ability 16
    advanced physical ability 16
    athletics 16
    babies 16, 40
    Genocide through Pesticides 22
    highest rates of hypertension 94
    mortality rates 10
    overmedicated by hospitals 48
    salt sensitivity 94
    seek to be like their colonizers 11
    Slave Trade 73
agar-agar 82
Agaricus bisporus (mushroom) 212
agaritine 212
agent orange 22
agglutination, blood 195, 196
aging 16, 31, 142, 161, 184, 201
agriculture 45
AIDS 50, 53, 129
air 70, 173
    humans breathe in 34 pounds daily 241
    nutrition 241
    sunlit, has prana 179
Akhenaten 174
Alanine 167, 169
albinism 12
Albinos (whites)
    campaign for fractionated nutrition 158
    Disconnected from Nature 158
    heartless treatment of farm animals 159
    make supplements from horrible stuff 159
    started isolated nutrition 158
ALCOA 99
alcohol 25, 47, 48, 65, 67, 87,
    133, 137, 138, 141, 142, 161,
    166, 181, 186, 215, 217
    kills brain cells 137
alcoholic beverages 140, 204
    in Black neighborhoods 44
alcoholics 186
alcoholism 53
Aldehyde C-17 27
ale 27, 133
alfalfa 167, 177, 178, 208
    seeds 207, 209
    sprouts 207
Algae, Bluegreen 179
Alginic acid 27
alkaline 228
    mineral reserves 125
    saliva 220

alkaline-forming dressings 236
alkalis 228
alkaloids 210, 213
alkalosis 228
alkamines 202
Alkenylbenzenes 142
allergies 110, 138, 194, 196, 216, 217
allergy mechanism 195
allyl isothiocyanate 205
Almond Milk 112
almonds 178, 206, 209, 225, 234
Aloe Vera 178, 179
aloin 212
alpha-linolenic acid 84
alternative medicine 6, 7
aluminosilicate 28
aluminum 28, 43, 52, 65, 81, 94,
    99, 101, 130, 160
    cans 130
    neuro-toxin 99
    sulfate 29
Alvenia Fulton 192
alveoli 174
Alzheimer's disease 52, 61, 65, 99, 101,
    108, 170, 176
AMA 4, 5, 6, 8, 50, 53
Amalgam fillings 66
amaranth 27, 82
Amendment to the Constitution 6
America 57
    first flag, of hemp fiber 169
    sickest nation 4
    trillion dollar-a-year healthcare 4
American
    Dental Association 66
    food 146
    Medical Association 4, 5, 7
    Medical News 5
    supermarket diet 32
Americans
    minerally deficient 146
    number of animals consumed in lifetimes
    117
amines 183
amino acids 115, 117, 167, 169, 170,
    177, 183, 225, 226
    chains 164
    isolated 156
    raw plantfood sources 179
ammonia 28, 35, 114, 125, 129,
    139, 204, 209
amphetamines 47, 48
amygdalin 209
amylase 137
analgesics 48
ananda, bliss 169
anandamide 169
anaphylactic shock 53
anemia 87, 151, 168, 196, 211, 227
anemic condition 233
Anger-provoking agents in beer 44
animal
    crackers 127
    fat 118, 127
    feed 35
animals 107, 199, 203, 208,
    215, 220, 222
    castrated, neutered, sterile 124
    commercial 121
    cruelty 121
    Earth's biggest are plant eaters 226
    Factory-Farms 122
    farm, albinos 126
    killed 233
    mass-brutality to 121
Anionic minerals in water 97
Ankhs 174
anthers of flowers 170
Anthropological findings 220
anti-cancer compounds 45
    in Nuts 225
anti-carcinogens 214
anti-freeze 52, 65, 77
anti-oxidants 16, 214, 235
anti-psychotic drugs 48
antiacid tablets 77
antibiotics 37, 52, 76, 116, 160
    plant 214
antigenic elements 216
antigens 195
Antimony 93
anxiety attacks 135
apathy 31
apes 220

appetite 31, 234
apple cider vinegar
    98, 140, 172, 177, 178, 236
apples 149, 151, 178, 209, 226
    peels 178, 179
apricots 149, 178, 179
    pits 209, 225
Arachidic Acid 169
arachidonic 84, 227
arbon dioxide 174
Arginine 167, 169
Argon 93
Aris LaTham 192
Arnold Ehret 231, 232
Arrowroot 82
arsenic 93, 207
arsenicals 35
arterial degeneration 110
arteries 89, 117, 223
    clogged 104
    disorders 131
    hardened 100, 175
arteriosclerosis 81, 201
arthritis 3, 4, 78, 81, 97, 100, 106,
    131, 144, 161, 175, 185,
    194, 200, 215, 217
artificial
    environment 164
    lifestyle 164
    light 59
        harmful effects 59
    sweeteners 77
arugula 205
Asara Tsehai 192
asbestos 28, 137, 139
ascorbate form of vitamin C 177
ascorbic acid 145, 162, 176, 177
Asia 46
Asian Americans 48
Asparagine 169
asparagus 203, 207
aspartame 77
    deadly effects 77
aspartate 141
aspartic acid 77, 167, 169
aspirin 47, 48, 51, 77
assimilation of food 138
asthma 10, 28, 78, 105, 110,
    168, 194, 196, 217
ataxia 208
atheroma 201
atherosclerosis 78, 89, 104, 106,
    110, 125, 176
athlete's foot 135
atmosphere 199
    Earth's 128
atomic bombs 3
ATP 87, 141, 143
Attention Deficit Disorder 49
attorneys 49
aura 179, 189
Australia 192, 213
auto-intoxication i 201
autolyzed yeast protein 136, 141
automaticity of heart 14
Aversion therapy 54
avocados 149, 178, 179, 198
    oil 84
Awadu, Keidi Obi 52
AZT 50

B

B1 167, 169
B12 167
B2 167, 169
B6 125, 167, 169
Baby(s)
    4000 Colored, die daily from milk formula
    105
    Afrikan 40
    baby oil 65
    blue baby 45
    Bottle Baby Disease 105
    electro-activity of infant's brain 151
    human 103, 226
    making babies right 41
    milk formulas 112
    milk-substitutes 109
    mortality rate 103
    Natural Blender Formulas 109
    on raw milk 185
back pains 135
bacon 38, 95, 118

bacteria 135, 186, 187, 195, 234
  colon 114
bacterial
  life of soil 20
  mutagen 128
bad breath 114
Baked Goods 140
baker's yeast 136
baking
  powders 81, 161
  soda 81
  sprays 90
Balance 222
  body 228
  osmotic 117
bamboo sprouts 208
Banana Marble Ice Cream 112
bananas 79, 112, 149, 178,
  179, 224, 228
Barium 93, 169
barley 82, 134, 200, 215
  juice 179
barley-green 167, 177
Barnes, Carol 48
battery, Melanin 16
Bayer 67
beans 127, 140, 182, 194, 198,
  205, 210, 216, 235
  sprouts 208
beasts 188
bee pollen 127, 170, 177,
  178, 179, 242
  lifeforce containing 179
beechnuts 225
beef 23, 121, 127, 183, 194
  fat 120
beepers 55
beer 27, 133, 134, 136,
  137, 138, 139
  ANGER-provoking agents in 44
  industry 160
bees 76
beets 95, 178, 198, 204,
  206, 207, 210, 233
  greens 206
behavior modifiers 64
behavioral disorders 78
Behenic Acid 169
bell peppers 149, 202, 218
bemomyl 151
Benjamin Rush 6
benzaldehyde 76, 128
benzalkonium 160
benzene 25, 27, 54, 116, 128,
  129, 130, 160
  rings 88
benzethonium chloride 52
benzo(a)pyrene 128, 131, 183
benzofurans 128
benzoic acid 228
benzopyrene 182
benzoyl peroxide 110
Beryllium 93
beta-carotene 157, 171, 177
beta-glucuronidase 209
Beverages
  avoid /replacements summary 244
beverages (bottled), harmful effects 130
BGH hormones 103, 124
BHA 28, 51
BHT 28, 51
Bibb Lettuce 204
Bible 170
  hemp in the 169
binder 161
bio-accessible 209
bio-availability 162, 206
bio-available nutrients 166
bio-electric field 179, 189
bio-energy field 24
bio-fuel 169
biodegradable 135
bioflavonoids 45, 151, 157, 223, 235
Biological Transmutations 173
biomagnetic field 55
Biotech companies 19, 146
Biotin 167
birds 220
birth defects 31, 41, 137, 151
birthrate 31
bishydroxyanisole 28
bishydroxytoluene 28
Bismuth 93
bitter
  almonds 208

lettuce 204
nuts 209
Bittersweet 178
Black
  currants 178, 179
  Melanin 16
  men, malt liquor consumption 137
  neighborhoods 137
  pepper 142, 210
  slave women 121
  sour bread 133
  walnuts 179
black-eyed peas 205
Black-on-Black crimes 44
Blacked Out Through Whitewash 68
blackstrap molasses 79, 160
bladder 141, 143, 205
  disorders 100
  inflammation 196
bleached-white stuff 23
blindness 78, 87, 211
bloating 135
blood 14, 190, 206, 233
  agglutination 196
  chemistry 61
  colloids 93
  crystallization 204
  fats 78
  sugar levels 73, 131, 144, 196
  sugar problems 89
  type 195, 217
  vessel fragility 51
blood-proteins 68
Blossoms, Edible 240
blue
  baby syndrome 45
  cheese 135
  mold 135
  water, bleach 76
Blueberries 178
Bluegreen Algae 167, 177, 178, 179
Body 14, 228, 241
  Balance 228
  detoxifying 230
  odor 136
  polluted 31
  Purified 228
  purified by rawfood 224
  repair, twarted by supplements 161
  toxic 228
body & vibratory rates 15
body-parts market 15
bodycare products 43
Boiling 140
bologna 38, 115
Bombesin 111
bombs 28, 38
  nuclear 70
bones 15, 156, 159, 171, 220, 228
  diseases 100
  marrow 15
  meal 160
Bookbinder's paste 80
bordeaux 27
Boron 93, 169
Botha, P.W. 44, 137
Bottle Baby Disease 105
bottled
  beverages 140
    harmful effects 130
  drinks 132
  fruit juice 234
  juices 132
botulism 38
bourbon whiskey 138
Bovine Somatotropin 107
Bovine Spongiform Encephalopathy 108
Bowel disease 216
boys 215
brain 14, 16, 57, 125, 139, 169, 223
  cannabinoid-receptors 169
  cells 137, 139
  composed of fat 84
  damage 53, 151
    from lead 42
    from neuroleptics 48
    from pesticides 43
  development 103
  intake of oxygen 179
  ossification 100
  toxin 139
  tumors 59, 61
brain-dissolving Prions 111
Bran 160, 176, 200, 217
brandy 138

Brassica oleracea 214
Brazil nuts 178, 179, 209, 234
breads 133, 136, 140, 218
Breakfast 236
breast 22
  cancer 110, 118
  enlargement in men 207
  milk 109
    toxic 43
Breatharian is a Solarian 241
Breatharianism 241
breathe in 34 pounds of air, humans 241
Breathing 14, 174
  exercises 190
brewer's yeast 133, 134, 136, 160
Britain 213
broccoli 149, 178, 179, 205,
  210, 214, 218
broilers 121
bromate 27, 130
bromated vegetable oil 27
bromelain 179, 185
brominated vegetable oil 130
bromine gas 145
brown rice 136, 215
Brown sugar 76
brussel sprouts 149, 210
BSE 108
BST 107
bubble bath 64
buckwheat 82
buffered vitamin C 177
Bulgarians 133
bunions 100
buns 82
Burdock 178
burgers 153
Burroughs, Stanley 174, 179
butter 43, 84, 86, 104, 112, 118,
  120, 133, 134, 136, 138, 235
butter beans 208
butterfat 134
butterfly 188
buttermilk 133, 134, 138
butters, nut 127
butyl benzyl phthalate 46
Butyraldehyde 27
BVO 27, 130
by products 115

C

cabbage 179, 198, 205, 207, 208,
  210, 214, 218, 239
cadmium 54, 93, 131, 223
caffeine 48, 125, 128, 130, 131,
  142, 144, 165, 205
cakes 9, 82, 136
calciferous degeneration 201
calcium 93, 98, 103, 110, 125, 131,
  160, 164, 167, 169, 170, 176,
  216, 217, 227, 228
  aluminosilicate 28
  caseinate 112
  citrate 162
  deficiency 110
  gluconate 162
  inorganic 81
  metabolism 95
  organic, raw plantfood sources 178
  oxalate 206
  phosphate 161
  sulfate 28
calcium-phosphorous relationship 78
calf 103, 122
Calories, fruit 236
Canada 213
Canada oil 87
Canavanine 207
cancer 3, 51, 53, 78, 83, 85,
  110, 122, 125, 151, 184
  100 million cancer cells form daily in body 86
  58 anti-cancer compounds in citrus 223
  anti-cancer compounds 45
  anti-cancer indoles 210
  anti-cancer Laetrile 209
  Breast 118
  caused by nitrates in fleshfood & produce 118
  Cervical 118
  Colon 118
  Leukemia 118
  Ovarian 118
  Prostate 118

252   Drugs Masquerading As Foods...

H

haemoglobin 45
Hafnium 93
hair 142, 191, 224
  of the gods 65
  sprays 27
hairdryers 55
hallucinatory effects 202
hallucinogen 139, 215
hallucinogenic toxin 210
ham 38, 127
hamburgers, killing forests 123
hands 221
hangover deficiency disease 230
hard drugfoods 202
hardened arteries 81, 100
hardening of the arteries 156, 161
harmony 231
Harvard Medical School 31
hashish 169
hay fever 196
hay, plastic 35
hazelnuts 225
HDL 84
headaches 4, 47, 135, 194, 196, 216, 217
headsets 55
heal FAST 192
Healer, Water 99
Health Freedom News 53
heart 14, 31, 151, 156, 207
heart attacks 4, 10, 83, 101, 110,
  125, 131, 176
heart disease 3, 4, 78, 83, 85, 89,
  122, 125, 184, 194
heart palpitations 194
heart problems 81, 185, 217
heartbeat 194
heartburn 89, 114
Heaven 222
heavy metals 157, 160, 175, 223
heebie-geebies 159
Helium 93
hemaglutins 205
hemoglobin 233
hemolytic anemia 196
hemorrhage 203
hemorrhoids 4, 78, 81, 185, 215, 217
Hemp 109, 225
  a complete food 168
  active ingredient 169
  Bible references 169
  can save Earth 169
  cleanses the lungs 169
  edestin globulin 168
  habit forming 168
  healer of many diseases 168
  healing medicine 169
  holy herb 168
  medicinal value 169
  not addictive 168
  Oil 90
    fatty acids 169
    green tinged 168
  oxygenates the blood 168, 179
  ozone layer healer 170
  products 169
  protein globulin 109
  purifies the air 169
  Rich Spectrum of Nutrients 169
  Seed 90, 168, 177, 178, 179
    sterilized 168
  Sickle Cell Anemia fighter 168
  smoking to get high 169
  versatile 169
  waterpipe 169
  why made illegal 169
hens 116
hepatitis B 52
hepatitis-A vaccine 52
heptachlor 22, 43
Heptadecanoic Acid 169
Heptylparaben 29
herbal seasoning 95, 140
herbal supplements 172
herbal teas 132, 173, 213
herbiage 220
herbicides 21, 22, 43, 111
  bind minerals 145
herbivores 220
herbs 6, 161, 166, 172, 179, 181, 212
  lose effectiveness when taken often, too
    long 173
  tips 177
  whole 177

heroin 181
heterocyclic amines 183
Hexane 131
Hibiscus 179
high blood pressure 3, 117
  medications 51
higher vibratory food 230
Hilton Hotema 204
histamines 104, 105, 139
Histidine 167, 169
Hitler 64
hives 196
Hoechst 67
hogs 117, 160, 187
holistic schools 6
Holmium 93
Holstein Frisian cow 109
holy people 232
homeopathic cell salts 177
Homeostasis 173, 228
homeostatic neutralization 177
homogenized milk 104, 110, 112
homosexuality 124, 125
  and hormones in meat 124
honey 76, 79, 136, 140, 170, 234
  reference to hemp 169
honeycomb 169
hooves 127, 159
Hops 137
hormone 171
  disrupters 45, 161
  imbalances 170
  impostors 41, 45
hormoned drugmeat 124
hormones 35, 109, 170
  cow 111
  synthetic 107
  vitamin D 179
hormony meat 124
horseradish 141, 205
horses 220
Hospitals 32
hot dogs 38, 95, 115, 118, 125, 127, 153
hot peppers 142
hot sauce 141
Hotema 204
Huckleberries 179
Hue-mans 222, 241
Hulda Clark 129, 135, 140, 161
Human 220
  Baby 226
  Body 199, 241
    can make protein, nutrients from
      sunlight & air 173
    not made to handle fractioned nutrients
      175
  genes, added to livestock 34, 117, 126
  milk 226
Human-Pig animal 19
Humanity 220, 241
Humans 70, 198, 241
  BEST food for 235
  breathe in 34 pounds of air, daily 241
  WORST foods for 235
humectant 65
Hunza people 32, 98
HVP 28
hybred 198
hybrid fruit 242
hybrid produce 19
hydraulic fluid 65
Hydrazines 212
hydrocarbons 42, 183
hydrochloric acid 152, 220
hydrocyanic acid 208
hydrocyanic gas 76
hydrogen 93, 117, 174
hydrogen cyanide 54
hydrogen peroxide 23, 110, 152
hydrogen sulfide gas 114
hydrogenated fats
  deadly effects 89
hydrogenated oils 83, 86, 144
hydrogenated vegetable oils 83
hydrolyzed vegetable protein 136, 141
hydrophile 185
hydrophobe 185
hydroquinone 128
hydrous magnesium silicate 28
hydroxide 65
hyperactive children 49
hyperactivity 78, 196
hypertension 78, 89, 94
hypoglycemia
  3, 77, 78, 89, 135, 141, 156, 237

hypoglycemic 205
Hyssop 179
Hyssop Enterprises 179
Hyssop Extract 179

I

ice 69
  chemicalized 36
ice cream 9, 27, 104, 112
  Banana Marble (substitute) 112
iceberg lettuce 204, 235
iced tea 132
ICI 67
ideal diet 242
ideal environment 242
IGF hormones 106
  in milk 106
IGF-1 106
imitation fleshfoods 153
immune function, disrupted by mold-toxins 136
immune system 46, 50, 61, 85, 86, 87, 89,
  105, 129, 136, 151, 195, 237
immunity, low 135
immunization 52
  compulsory 53
impotence 125, 171
impotency 31
IMS America 49
Incense 168
incubators 174
incurable diseases 122
India 32, 98
indigestion 89, 131, 194
Indigotine 29
indoles 114, 210
industrial farming companies 4
Industrial waste as healthfood 160
industries 160
infertility 22, 78, 79
inflammation 85
Inflammatory Bowel disease 216
inner peace 225
inoculations 52, 53
inorganic minerals 97, 185, 190
Inositol 167
insanity 108, 117
insect life 128
Insect Wax-Moth Potato 19
insecticides 35, 116, 151
insects 21, 199
insoluble 162
insomnia 130, 168
insulin-like
  action of wolfberries 171
  Growth Factor 106
insulin-sugar intake 196
intermedine 213
internal drowning 93
intestinal bacteria 195
intestinal gas 135
intestines
  134, 138, 142, 205, 216, 220, 223, 227
intoxication of digestive system 183
Iodine 93, 169, 176
ionic state, minerals 192
ionic substances 192
ions 169
Iridium 179
Irish Moss 178, 179
iron 93, 98, 132, 167, 169, 170,
  173, 176, 216, 217, 227
  organic, raw plantfood sources 178
  sulfate 81
irradiated food 25, 37, 235
irradiated grains 151
irradiation 24, 161
  harmful effects 25
irritability 31, 130, 159, 211
isobutenol (natural gas) 44, 139
isoeugenol 210
isolated nutrients 155, 156
isolated nutrition 158
Isoleucine 167, 169
isothio-cyanates 87, 141, 143
isothiocyanate 205
isotopes 62
ivory 27

J

jackals 220
JAMA (Journal of the American Medical
  Association) 5

S

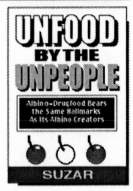
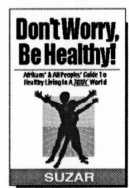

Blacked Out Through Whitewash

by Suzar
Paperback : Vol. 1 of 7, Unabridged
450 pages, Illustrated, Indexed
Black Resources Guide included
$49.00

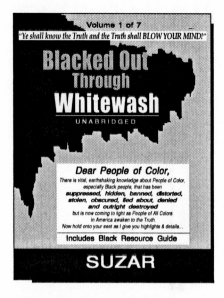

"Ye shall know the Truth and the Truth shall BLOW YOUR MIND!" Blacked Out Through Whitewash may be **the greatest Exposé of the last two millenniums.** It exposes the **Quantum Deception** composing the Foundation of Western Culture, Religion & His-Story. It exposes the greatest Coverups in **"His-Story"**, along with the massive **Mind-Control** and **Deception** perpetrated in the name of **"the Lord."** Among other things, **irrefutably exposes and proves that the entire Bible is disguisedly a** "Book of StarScience," composed of **disguised zodiacs** and **Egyptian astrological allegories.** The abundant evidence for this is from the Bible itself! For example, Suzar has discovered that the **true etymology** or meaning of the **names** of all the many **groups of 12** in the Bible, **aligns with a major trait of the astrological sign** which that name /individual represents. Thus, the name **Thomas Didymus** (a disciple of Christ) literally means twin-twin, and stands for **Gemini.** The name **Gad** (a son of Jacob) means goat, hence is **Capricorn.** This is 100% consistent throughout the Bible. Turn to **Genesis, chapter 49** where astrology is especially evident. Here, in each "blessing" which dying Jacob (representing the setting, hence, dying Sun) gives to each of his "sons" is a major astrological trait identifying that son with the zodiac sign he stands for: Joseph= Sagittarius and is linked with archers; Judah= Leo and is linked with lions; Zebulon= Pisces and is linked with the sea; Simeon & Levi "are brethren" —distinguished from their other "brethren" because they represent Gemini, and so on. **Turn to chapter 3 of Nehemiah.** "In his account of the reconstruction of the walls of Jerusalem, Nehemiah appropriately begins at the **Sheep Gate,** which of course is Aries. As to be expected, there are 12 gates. Unlike the names of personages, half of these gate names are stark clear about which zodiacal sign they represent. Nehemiah's 'wall' symbolizes the Zodiac...." **It is critical for Afrikan people and ALL Peoples to awaken to these quantum truths which have been hidden from Humanity for 2000 years.** Recovering these suppressed Truths is vital for the full Awakening, Upliftment, Liberation, Healing, Kinship, Empowerment, and thus the *SURVIVAL,* of *all* Humanity. **Other topics:**

- What **Cosmic Principle** causes **hair** (antennae) to be **Nappy?** (page 7)
- In what ancient symbols is **Jesus's sex life** disguised in the Bible? (pgs 138, 193, 195)
- How did **Afrikans spark the European Renaissance?** (page 43)
- Who were the **world's 25 crucified risen saviors?** (page 121)
- Where is **Santa Claus in the Bible** & what is his true identity? (page 355)
- Why did Napoleon's soldiers blow off the **nose of the Sphinx?** (page 23)
- Why are the **world's top religions all Anti-Female,** fear-based and militaristic ?

If you have the courage to finish reading this book, you won't be the same by the time you finish.

Creation's Great Blak Mother & The Blak Woman

by Suzar (Tentatively available by spring of year 2000)

This is volume 2 of the 7 volumes of *Blacked Out Through Whitewash*. This book resurrects awareness of **The Great BLAK Mother of Creation** and restores the **Blak Feminine** part of the equation which has been blacked out the most, even more than Blak history. You thought the Blak Male was the endangered species. No, it's the Blak Woman and her precious Womb. The ongoing Great War on *The Great Mother* and the Female Principle is why women of all races on all continents are being oppressed, repressed, suppressed, depressed, demeaned and subjugated. In reality, **the Blak Afrikan Woman is the Original Most Powerful Being on Earth**. She is in a *Spell*, along with the entire Blak Race –the Parents of Humanity and usurped Guardians of Planet Earth. The Blak Afrikan Woman –Mother of Humanity– unknowingly holds the key to Humanity's salvation.

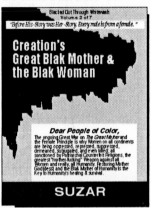

- The Blak Feminine Origin and Foundation of Civilization and "Culture."
- Female Biological Superiority –fact or fiction?
- The Sexual Foundation of Religion.
- Why "Pussy" is a name for the Cat & Vagina.
- Afrikan extraterrestrial legacy and Blak People from outta space –founders of legendary super-civilizations?
- The Great Mother's Gift of Blak Melanin.
- How the Controllers stay fat off Her Power.
- Disguised *StarScience* is still the *Global* Cosmology.

Resurrecting BAB-EL, the Book of Books of Books

by Suzar (Tentatively available by spring of year 2000) Volume 3 of the 7 volumes of *Blacked Out Through Whitewash* resurrects BAB-EL, the Book of Books of Books, a Cosmic Power-Generator and Core of the (True) Bible —personified as the Bab-El of the Great Pyramid, Tree, Melanin Molecule, Eternal Ankh, Ark of the Covenant, "777", but especially the Bab-El of your Temple-Body. Exposes the diabolical *Reversed Bab-Els* empowering "white supremacy" and *UnHeaven USA* –the Counterfeit-Godhead of the Planet (False Egypt).

The Double-You (W) Book

by Drs. Arvel & Bobbie Chappell
Edited by Dr. S. Epps
Paperback, 146 pages. Color Illustrated **$29.95**

Dare discover who YOU truly are. Dare risk knowing the true WHY of your life. Dare to stop giving away your power ... through undermining your own Will, the magnetic Mother-Principle of God within you. Get ready for significant change in your life, sparked by "little you" discovering "BIG YOU." Get ready for Personal Empowerment that does not require taking power from anyone, or giving away your power to anyone. Discover the Unseen Role of **Self-Denial** in your life. Everybody on the planet –especially Women– are taught and trained to systematic-ally deny themselves (give away their power) right from babyhood. In little things and big thangs. NO is usually the first word children learn. You often deny yourself in favor of others: Staying in conversations longer than you prefer in order to be "polite." Going out with someone when you'd rather stay home. Wearing beautiful tight shoes that are "killing" your feet. Daily going to a job you can't stand. "Self sacrifice." Staying in a relationship that is not working. Not speaking up for yourself. Self-Denial is WRONG Use of Will. Self-Denial (Will-Denial) leads to steady loss of Personal Power by degrees. Because Will and Power are one and the same. As you diminish your Will through Self-Denial, you also diminish your Personal Power. **WILL, the magnetic Mother-Principle within you** holds your essence together. When we deny our Will, we lose some of it...and thereby lose some of our Personal Power. As a result, we periodically "fragment", losing some of our "essence." We literally are not all there. Where there is Self-Denial, full consciousness is not present, hence full Personal Power is not present. Reveals new revelations /channeled insights which helps resolve these problems –and empower the individual. Reveals a **simple powerful technique for balancing your whole being.** If practiced daily and before endeavors (making an important decision, appointments, etc.), it helps ensure a favorable and "balanced outcome." Aligns, integrates, and balances your Four Aspects: Spirit, Heart, Will, and Body.

Exposing the Top
Reversed Bab-Els Secretly Empowering "White Supremacy"

Washington DC, the Vatican, Bible, U.S. Dollar Bill, etc., all harness and draw Power by secretly being layed out and structured according to the Cosmic Geometry of the "Zodiac" and Great Pyramid. But because of their deliberate reversal of certain key elements, they are not true Bab-Els but "UnBabs" (Reversed Bab-Els). Hence, they are not true *power generators* but anti-life *power suckers* which fuel global Albino Domination. (Vol. 3, #36: Parts I & II) **$9.95 ea.**

How the Bible & Dollar-Bill are a Great 555, 666 and 777

For starters, the Bible begins on 5 as the Pentateuch, has exactly 66 books, and 7 of its books are double-books. Why are 5, 6 and 7 singled out from the other numbers? What do trippple digits signify? How the Bible, Dollar Bill & Masonic Logo have the exact same hidden numeric /geometric traits built into them, and why. (Vol. 3, #36c) **$9.95**

How the Great Pyramid & "Zodiac" are Built into the Bible & Dollar Bill

The Bible, U.S. Dollar Bill, and Mason Logo all possess the key traits & geometry of the Great Pyramid. The whole Zodiac –all 12 signs– are hidden in the U.S. Dollar Bill. (Vol. 3, #36d) **$9.95**

America, the Counterfeit Godhead of Earth

The Throne of Kamit (ancient Blak Egypt) was the Godhead of planet Earth and Seat of the greatest Power. The capstone, apex, top *Bab-El.* As such, Egypt represented Heaven on Earth. Whites apparently usurped & supplanted Blak Egypt, replicating her key elements into their structures to secure power. America is presently the latest & greatest Counterfeit Egypt, thus the False Godhead of Earth and "Counterfeit Heaven." No wonder most people around the world wanna come to America...just like they wanna "go to heaven." (Vol. 3, #37)

The Hidden Sweet Truth About "666"

Like we've been given huge Lies for history, we've been given huge Lies, plus slander and reversals about "666"...and "13." Now the precious Truth is available, ruining the Lies, restoring denied Power, and exposing the true identity of "the Beast," "the Man," and "the Mark of the Beast." (Vol. 6, #46) **$9.95**

You "Come To Power" Only When You "Come To A Point"

Power is at the Point. Exudes, shoots, radiates from the Point, as shown by Kirlian photographs of pyramids. Only when the spellbound-but-Awakening Blak Race, the Parent Race of Humanity, "Comes-To-A-Point," will it "Come-To-Power." Regain its hijacked power. The Point is the Intersection of Life's two Polarities. This Intersection is where "Creation Happens." The CenterPoint is supposed to be BLAK, like the Pupil of the Eye. When the Pupil or Center is white it is DEAD, a "dead center." Cannot generate Power, thus is a Vampire. Like no other people, Blaks (especially Blak women), have been /are being vampirised for their abundant power, which they have been trained to give away. Revelations, insights and solutions. (Vol. 4, #38: Parts I & II) **$9.95 each**

Blak Survival Guide Now

Effective, practical strategies and tools for our Personal Empowerment and Survival. Effective ways to protect and heal ourselves, awaken and "Come-To-A-Point" thus "Come-To-Power." Work these strategies in increments. Make this serious business FUN. (Vol. 7, #51) **$9.95**

The Hidden "Zodiacs" Composing the Bible

Irrefutable evidence that the entire Bible is a "Great Book of StarScience," disguisedly composed of numerous hidden "zodiacs." The abundant evidence is from the Bible itself! Though the Bible has been "tampered with," in reality its original hidden astrological blueprint has been completely preserved. This book is mainly an overview of chapters 12 & 13 in volume 1 of BOTW **$9.95**

Printed in the United States
27194LVS00005B/85-93